Your *Clinics* subscriptio[...]er!

You can now access the FULL TEXT of this publication online at no additional cost! Activate your online subscription today and receive...

- Full text of all issues from 2002 to the present
- Photographs, tables, illustrations, and references
- Comprehensive search capabilities
- Links to MEDLINE and Elsevier journals

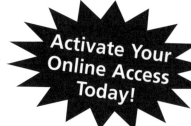

Plus, you can also sign up for E-alerts of upcoming issues or articles that interest you, and take advantage of exclusive access to bonus features!

To activate your individual online subscription:

1. Visit our website at **www.TheClinics.com**.

2. Click on "Register" at the top of the page, and follow the instructions.

3. To activate your account, you will need your subscriber account number, which you can find on your mailing label (note: the number of digits in your subscriber account number varies from six to ten digits). See the sample below where the subscriber account number has been circled.

This is your subscriber account number

```
****************************************3-DIGIT 001
FEB00   J0167   C7   ( 123456-89 )  10/00   Q: 1

J.H. DOE, MD
531 MAIN ST
CENTER CITY, NY  10001-001
```

4. That's it! Your online access to the most trusted source for clinical reviews is now available.

theclinics.com

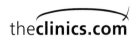

RADIOLOGIC CLINICS
of North America

PET Imaging II

ABASS ALAVI, MD
Guest Editor

January 2005 • Volume 43 • Number 1

SAUNDERS

An Imprint of Elsevier, Inc.
PHILADELPHIA   LONDON   TORONTO   MONTREAL   SYDNEY   TOKYO

W.B. SAUNDERS COMPANY
A Division of Elsevier Inc.

The Curtis Center • Independence Square West • Philadelphia, Pennsylvania 19106

http://www.theclinics.com

THE RADIOLOGIC CLINICS OF NORTH AMERICA **Volume 43, Number 1**
January 2005 **ISSN 0033-8389**
Editor: Barton Dudlick

Reprints: For copies of 100 or more, of articles in this publication, please contact the Commercial Reprints Department, Elsevier Inc., 360 Park Avenue South, New York, New York 10010-1710. Tel. (212) 633-3813; Fax: (212) 633-3820; email: reprints@elsevier.com.

The Radiologic Clinics of North America (ISSN 0033-8389) is published bimonthly by W.B. Saunders Company. Corporate and editorial offices: 170 S Independence Mall W 300 E, Philadelphia, PA 19106-3399. Accounting and circulation offices: 6277 Sea Harbor Drive, Orlando, FL 32887-4800. Periodicals postage paid at Orlando, FL 32862, and additional mailing offices. Subscription prices are USD 220 per year for US individuals, USD 331 per year for US institutions, USD 110 per year for US students and residents, USD 255 per year for Canadian individuals, USD 405 per year for Canadian institutions, USD 299 per year for international individuals, USD 405 per year for international institutions and USD 150 per year for Canadian and foreign students/residents. To receive student and resident rate, orders must be accompanied by name of affiliated institution, date of term, and the *signature* of program/residency coordinator on institution letterhead. Orders will be billed at individual rate until proof of status is received. Foreign air speed delivery is included in all *Clinics* subscription prices. All prices are subject to change without notice. POSTMASTER: Send address changes to *The Radiologic Clinics of North America,* W.B. Saunders Company, Periodicals Fulfillment, Orlando, FL 32887-4800. **Customer Service: 1-800-654-2452 (US). From outside of the US, call 1-407-345-4000.**

The Radiologic Clinics of North America also is published in Greek by Paschalidis Medical Publications, Athens, Greece.

The Radiologic Clinics of North America is covered in *Index Medicus, EMBASE/Excerpta Medica, Current Contents/Life Sciences, Current Contents/Clinical Medicine, RSNA Index to Imaging Literature, BIOSIS, Science Citation Index,* and *ISI/BIOMED.*

Printed in the United States of America.

GOAL STATEMENT

The goal of the *Radiologic Clinics of North America* is to keep practicing radiologists and radiology residents up to date with current clinical practice in radiology by providing timely articles reviewing the state of the art in patient care.

ACCREDITATION

The *Radiologic Clinics of North America* is planned and implemented in accordance with the Essential Areas and Policies of the Accreditation Council for Continuing Medical Education (ACCME) through the joint sponsorship of the University of Virginia School of Medicine and W. B. Saunders, an Imprint of Elsevier Science, Inc. The University of Virginia School of Medicine is accredited by the ACCME to provide continuing medical education for physicians.

The University of Virginia School of Medicine designates this educational activity for a maximum of 90 category 1 credits per year, 15 category 1 credits per issue, toward the AMA Physician's Recognition Award. Each physician should claim only those credits that he/she actually spent in the activity.

The American Medical Association has determined that physicians not licensed in the US who participate in this CME activity are eligible for AMA PRA category 1 credit.

Category 1 credit can be earned by reading the text material, taking the CME examination online at *http://www.theclinics.com/home/cme*, and completing the evaluation. Each test question must be answered correctly; you will have the opportunity to retake any questions answered incorrectly. Following successful completion of the test and the evaluation, you may print your certificate.

FACULTY DISCLOSURE

As a provider accredited by the Accreditation Council for Continuing Medical Education (ACCME), the Office of Continuing Medical Education of the University of Virginia School of Medicine must ensure balance, independence, objectivity, and scientific rigor in all its individually sponsored or jointly sponsored educational activities. All authors/editors participating in a sponsored activity are expected to disclose to the readers any significant financial interest or other relationship (1) with the manufacturer(s) of any commercial product(s) and/or provider(s) of commercial services discussed in an educational presentation and (2) with any commercial supporters of the activity (significant financial interest or other relationship can include such things as grants or research support, employee, consultant, stock holder, member of speakers bureau, etc.) The intent of this disclosure is not to prevent authors/editors with a significant financial or other relationship from writing an article, but rather to provide readers with information on which they can make their own judgments. It remains for the readers to determine whether the author's/editor's interest or relationships may influence the article with regard to exposition or conclusion.

The authors/editors listed below have identified no professional or financial affiliations related to their presentation:
Abass Alavi, MD; Norbert E. Avril, MD; James E. Baumgardner, MD, PhD; Michael Bono, BS; Britton Chance, PhD, ScD; Edward J. Delikatny, PhD; Barton Dudlick, Acquisitions Editor; Kiarash Emami, MS; Martin C. Fisher, PhD; Alan J. Fischman, MD, PhD; Warren B. Gefter, MD; Roland Hustinx, MD, PhD; Xavier Intes, PhD; Masaru Ishii, MD, PhD; Maxim Itkin, MD; Hossein Jadvar, MD, PhD; Stephen J. Kadlecek, PhD; Kenneth A. Krohn, PhD; David A. Lipson, MD; David A. Mankoff, MD, PhD; Ayse Mavi, MD; Andrew B. Newberg, MD; Harish Poptani, PhD; Michael Pourdehnad, BS; Joseph G. Rajendran, MD; Rahim R. Rizi, PhD; Anthony F. Shields, MD, PhD; Joseph B. Shrager, MD; Barry L. Shulkin, MD, MBA; and, Wolfgang A. Weber, MD.

Disclosure of discussion of non-FDA approved uses for pharmaceutical products and/or medical devices: The University of Virginia School of Medicine, as an ACCME provider, requires that all authors/editors identify and disclose any "off label" uses for pharmaceutical products and/or for medical devices. The University of Virginia School of Medicine recommends that each reader fully review all the available data on new products or procedures prior to instituting them with patients.

All authors/editors who provided disclosures will not be discussing any off-label uses except:
Norbert E. Avril, MD and **Wolfgang A. Weber, MD** will discuss the use of [18F] fluorodeoxyglucose for the treatment monitoring in malignant tumors.
Alan J. Fischman, MD, PhD will discuss the use of fluorodeoxyglucose (FDG) for imaging movement disorders.
Xavier Intes, PhD will discuss the use of indocyanine green for optical mammography.
Hossein Jadvar, MD, PhD will discuss the use of fluorine-18–fluorodeoxyglucose (FDG).
David A. Lipson, MD will discuss the use of hyperpolarized helium-3 gas that is experimental in humans.
David A. Mankoff, MD, PhD will discuss PET radiopharmaceuticals other than FDG.

The authors/editors listed below have not provided disclosure or off-label information:
Luis Araujo, MD; Gonca Bural, MD; Naresh C. Gupta, MD; Bruno Kaschten, MD; Rakesh Kumar, MD; Paras Lakhani, BA; Daniel H.S. Silverman, MD; Zebulon Z. Spector, BS; Amol Takalkar, MD; Jian Q. Yu, MD; Jiansheng Yu, MS; Jianliang Zhu, MD; and, Hongming Zhuang, MD, PhD.

TO ENROLL
To enroll in the Radiologic Clinics of North America Continuing Medical Education program, call customer service at 1-800-654-2452 or sign up online at *http://www.theclinics.com/home/cme*. The CME program is available to subscribers for an additional annual fee of USD 195.

FORTHCOMING ISSUES

RECENT ISSUES

THE CLINICS ARE NOW AVAILABLE ONLINE!

Access your subscription at:
http://www.theclinics.com

GUEST EDITOR

ABASS ALAVI, MD, Professor, Radiology and Neurology; and Chief, Division of Nuclear Medicine, Department of Radiology, Hospital of the University of Pennsylvania, Philadelphia, Pennsylvania

CONTRIBUTORS

ABASS ALAVI, MD, Professor, Radiology and Neurology; and Chief, Division of Nuclear Medicine, Department of Radiology, Hospital of the University of Pennsylvania, Philadelphia, Pennsylvania

LUIS ARAUJO, MD, Associate Professor, Radiology, Division of Nuclear Medicine, Department of Radiology, Hospital of the University of Pennsylvania, Philadelphia, Pennsylvania

NORBERT E. AVRIL, MD, Division of Nuclear Medicine, Department of Radiology, University of Pittsburgh Medical Center, Pittsburgh, Pennsylvania

JAMES E. BAUMGARDNER, MD, PhD, Department of Anesthesiology, University of Pennsylvania Health System, Philadelphia, Pennsylvania

MICHAEL BONO, BS, AMICI, Spring City, Pennsylvania

GONCA BURAL, MD, Visiting Scholar, Division of Nuclear Medicine, Department of Radiology, Hospital of the University of Pennsylvania, Philadelphia, Pennsylvania

BRITTON CHANCE, PhD, ScD, Eldridge Reeves Johnson University Professor Emeritus, Department of Biophysics, Physical Chemistry, and Radiologic Physics, University of Pennsylvania, Philadelphia, Pennsylvania

EDWARD J. DELIKATNY, PhD, Assistant Director, Molecular Imaging Laboratory; and Assistant Professor, Department of Radiology, University of Pennsylvania School of Medicine, Philadelphia, Pennsylvania

KIARASH EMAMI, MS, Department of Radiology, University of Pennsylvania Health System, Philadelphia, Pennsylvania

MARTIN C. FISCHER, PhD, Department of Radiology, University of Pennsylvania Health System, Philadelphia, Pennsylvania

ALAN J. FISCHMAN, MD, PhD, Director, Division of Nuclear Medicine, Department of Radiology, Massachusetts General Hospital; and Professor, Department of Radiology, Harvard Medical School, Boston, Massachusetts

WARREN B. GEFTER, MD, Department of Radiology, University of Pennsylvania Health System, Philadelphia, Pennsylvania

NARESH C. GUPTA, MD, Staff Physician, Frederick Imaging Centers, Frederick, Maryland

ROLAND HUSTINX, MD, PhD, Head, Division of Nuclear Medicine, University Hospital of Liège, Liège, Belgium

XAVIER INTES, PhD, Senior Staff Scientist, Biomedical Optical Imaging, Advanced Research Technologies (ART), Saint-Laurent, Quebec, Canada

MASARU ISHII, MD, PhD, Department of Otolaryngology–Head and Neck Surgery, Johns Hopkins University, Baltimore, Maryland

MAXIM ITKIN, MD, Department of Radiology, University of Pennsylvania Health System, Philadelphia, Pennsylvania

HOSSEIN JADVAR, MD, PhD, Assistant Professor, Division of Nuclear Medicine, Departments of Radiology and Biomedical Engineering, Keck School of Medicine, University of Southern California, Los Angeles; and Visiting Associate, Bioengineering Program, California Institute of Technology, Pasadena, California

STEPHEN J. KADLECEK, PhD, Department of Radiology, University of Pennsylvania Health System, Philadelphia, Pennsylvania

BRUNO KASCHTEN, MD, Chef de Clinique, Department of Neurosurgery, University Hospital of Liège, Sart Tilman, Belgium

KENNETH A. KROHN, PhD, Professor, Division of Nuclear Medicine, Department of Radiology; Department of Radiation Oncology; and Adjunct Professor, Chemistry, University of Washington, Seattle, Washington

RAKESH KUMAR, MD, Research Fellow, Division of Nuclear Medicine, Department of Radiology, Hospital of the University of Pennsylvania, Philadelphia, Pennsylvania

PARAS LAKHANI, BA, Medical Student, Division of Nuclear Medicine, Department of Radiology, Hospital of the University of Pennsylvania, Philadelphia, Pennsylvania

DAVID A. LIPSON, MD, Department of Pulmonary Medicine, University of Pennsylvania Health System, Philadelphia, Pennsylvania

DAVID A. MANKOFF, MD, PhD, Associate Professor, Radiology and Medicine, Division of Nuclear Medicine, Department of Radiology, University of Washington, Seattle, Washington

AYSE MAVI, MD, Visiting Scholar, Division of Nuclear Medicine, Department of Radiology, Hospital of the University of Pennsylvania, Philadelphia, Pennsylvania

ANDREW B. NEWBERG, MD, Assistant Professor, Pathology and Psychiatry, Division of Nuclear Medicine, Department of Radiology, Hospital of the University of Pennsylvania, Philadelphia, Pennsylvania

HARISH POPTANI, PhD, Assistant Professor, Molecular Imaging Laboratory, Department of Radiology, University of Pennsylvania School of Medicine, Philadelphia, Pennsylvania

MICHAEL POURDEHNAD, BS, Medical Student, Finch University of Health Science–Chicago Medical School, North Chicago, Illinois

JOSEPH G. RAJENDRAN, MD, Assistant Professor, Division of Nuclear Medicine, Department of Radiology; and Department of Radiation Oncology, University of Washington, Seattle, Washington

RAHIM R. RIZI, PhD, Department of Radiology, University of Pennsylvania Health System, Philadelphia, Pennsylvania

ANTHONY F. SHIELDS, MD, PhD, Professor, Medicine and Oncology, Wayne Sate University; and Associate Center Director for Clinical Research, Karmanos Cancer Institute, Detroit, Michigan

JOSEPH B. SHRAGER, MD, Section of General Thoracic Surgery, University of Pennsylvania Health System, Philadelphia, Pennsylvania

BARRY L. SHULKIN, MD, MBA, Professor, Department of Radiology, University of Michigan, Ann Arbor, Michigan

DANIEL H.S. SILVERMAN, MD, PhD, Head, Neuroimaging Section; Associate Director, University of California at Los Angeles Alzheimer's Disease Center Imaging Core; and Associate Professor, Ahmanson Biological Imaging Division, Department of Molecular and Medical Pharmacology, David Geffen School of Medicine, University of California at Los Angeles Medical Center, Los Angeles, California

ZEBULON Z. SPECTOR, BS, Department of Radiology, University of Pennsylvania Health System, Philadelphia, Pennsylvania

AMOL TAKALKAR, MD, Nuclear Medicine Resident, Division of Nuclear Medicine, Department of Radiology, Hospital of the University of Pennsylvania, Philadelphia, Pennsylvania

WOLFGANG A. WEBER, MD, Department of Medical and Molecular Pharmacology, University of California at Los Angeles, Los Angeles, California

JIAN Q. YU, MD, Clinical Fellow, Division of Nuclear Medicine, Department of Radiology, Hospital of the University of Pennsylvania, Philadelphia, Pennsylvania

JIANGSHENG YU, MS, Department of Radiology, University of Pennsylvania Health System, Philadelphia, Pennsylvania

JIANLIANG ZHU, MD, Section of General Thoracic Surgery, University of Pennsylvania Health System, Philadelphia, Pennsylvania

HONGMING ZHUANG, MD, PhD, Assistant Professor, Division of Nuclear Medicine, Department of Radiology, Hospital of the University of Pennsylvania, Philadelphia, Pennsylvania

CONTENTS

in recent years, all protocols can lead to various degrees of radiation injuries. Radiation necrosis is the most worrisome of these injuries and occurs several months or years after completing the treatment. It is essential to differentiate radiation necrosis from tumor recurrence, which requires specific treatment. Fluorodeoxyglucose-PET (FDG-PET) has been used for this indication for 2 decades and is generally recognized as a useful clinical tool, providing clinicians with both diagnostic and prognostic information.

and automated synthesis modules, FD-PET will soon become an important component of the clinical armamentarium.

PET in Cardiology 107

Amol Takalkar, Ayse Mavi, Abass Alavi, and Luis Araujo

Myocardial perfusion imaging with single-photon emission CT (SPECT) is a key investigation in the work-up of patients with coronary artery disease. PET, however, with inherently better spatial and temporal resolution, offers several advantages over SPECT. The last decade has witnessed extensive application of PET techniques to assess myocardial viability and has provided valuable information important in analyzing the risk: benefit ratio for several therapeutic measures. Recent advances in PET instrumentation and radiopharmaceuticals have generated considerable interest to use PET for evaluating an array of cardiovascular disease.

Applications of Fluorodeoxyglucose-PET Imaging in the Detection of Infection and Inflammation and Other Benign Disorders 121

Hongming Zhuang, Jian Q. Yu, and Abass Alavi

Fluorodeoxyglucose-PET (FDG-PET) has become an important imaging modality in daily practice in oncology. FDG, however, is not tumor-specific and can accumulate in a variety of nonmalignant lesions. A limited but gradually increasing number of publications has shown the potentials of FDG-PET in the detection of infection and inflammation.

PET in Pediatric Diseases 135

Hossein Jadvar, Abass Alavi, Ayse Mavi, and Barry L. Shulkin

Positron emission tomography (PET) is emerging as an important diagnostic tool in the imaging evaluation of pediatric disorders. The recent advent of the dual-modality PET–computed tomography (PET-CT) imaging systems has provided unprecedented diagnostic capability by providing precise anatomic localization of metabolic information. This article reviews the clinical applications of PET and PET-CT in pediatrics with an emphasis on the more common applications in epilepsy and oncology. General considerations in patient preparation and radiation dosimetry are also discussed.

PET Imaging of Cellular Proliferation 153

David A. Mankoff, Anthony F. Shields, and Kenneth A. Krohn

Increased cellular proliferation is a hallmark of the cancer phenotype. Cellular proliferation imaging has a number of potential advantages over in vitro assay and glucose metabolic imaging using fluorodeoxyglucose PET, which is the mainstay of current clinical PET imaging. This article reviews the biology underlying proliferation imaging, radiopharmaceuticals used for proliferation imaging, preclinical studies of proliferation imaging, and clinical results through 2003.

Imaging Hypoxia and Angiogenesis in Tumors 169

Joseph G. Rajendran and Kenneth A. Krohn

There is a clear need in cancer treatment for a noninvasive imaging assay that evaluates the oxygenation status and heterogeneity of hypoxia and angiogenesis in individual patients. Such an assay could be used to select alternative treatments and to monitor the effects of treatment. Of the several methods available, each imaging procedure has at least one disadvantage. Rather than develop new and improved hypoxia agents, or even quibbling about the pros and cons of alternative agents, the nuclear medicine community needs to convince the oncology community that imaging hypoxia is an important procedure that can lead to improved treatment outcome.

ELSEVIER
SAUNDERS

RADIOLOGIC
CLINICS
of North America

Radiol Clin N Am 43 (2005) xiii – xv

Preface

PET Imaging II

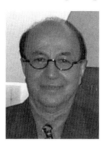

Abass Alavi, MD
Guest Editor

In 1973, Godfrey Hounsfield introduced radiographic CT, which truly revolutionized the field of radiology. Later that year, the concept of $[^{18}F]$-fluorodeoxyglucose PET (FDG-PET) was born when three investigators from the University of Pennsylvania (Penn)—Martin Reivich, David Kuhl, and myself—discussed the feasibility of labeling deoxyglucose (DG) with a gamma-emitting radionuclide for in vivo imaging of regional brain function in humans. Up until that time, researchers at the National Institutes of Health (NIH) and Penn had tested the beta-emitting ^{14}C-DG in rats as a novel radiotracer to image regional cerebral glucose metabolism and, therefore, function in a variety of physiologic and pathologic states. Because ^{14}C is a beta-emitter and the electrons emitted are stopped internally, a technique called autoradiography was used to map its distribution in the brain and elsewhere in the body. In animal experiments, 40 to 45 minutes following the administration of this radiotracer, slices of the tissue such as the brain are placed on a radiographic film that is exposed to the beta particles emitted by ^{14}C. The film is then processed to capture the biodistribution of this compound, which reflects regional glucose metabolism with exquisite detail. By the early 1970s, the potential of this preparation as a probe to map regional metabolism and function in humans had become increasingly evident to the scientific community. Therefore, it was quite logical to plan on furthering the power of this methodology by imaging its kinetics externally with an appropriate instrument.

Soon after this initiative, we discussed the concept of labeling DG with a radionuclide with Alfred Wolf of the Brookhaven National Laboratory (BNL), who suggested 18F as the best option for this purpose and expressed a great desire to collaborate with us in undertaking the required tasks to synthesize this compound. During the ensuing years, a great deal of effort was spent by the chemistry group at the BNL to label DG with ^{18}F, and by 1975, the synthesis schemes had been perfected, and we were in a position to start planning for human studies in the succeeding year. The 2-hour half-life of ^{18}F allowed shipment of a dose of FDG to Penn in August 1976 when the first brain and whole body images of a human being were acquired. The first brain images were acquired by using only one of the two 511-keV gamma rays emitted following a positron decay and using a single photon emission CT instrument (the Mark IV, which was designed and built at Penn) that was equipped with high-energy collimators for this purpose. Whole body images were acquired by employing an Ohio Nuclear dual head scanner that also was capable of imaging high-energy gamma rays

0033-8389/05/$ – see front matter © 2004 Elsevier Inc. All rights reserved.
doi:10.1016/j.rcl.2004.10.001

(510 keV from strontium 85). This was a memorable day for investigators from both institutions who had worked tirelessly toward achieving this goal. Simultaneous with our attempts to synthesize FDG, investigators at Washington University (Drs. Terpogossian, Phelps, and Hoffman) and Searle Radiographics (Dr. Muehelenner) had initiated and successfully built instruments that would allow for optimal in vivo imaging of positron-emitting radionuclides in humans. Because of these successes, the NIH within a few years decided to establish several research centers to explore the potential of this powerful modality in mapping body metabolism and function as quantitative images.

The initial focus of the research in these centers was brain imaging by using FDG and several neuroreceptor compounds to determine alterations that occur in the central nervous system in a variety of neuropsychiatric disorders. In fact, during most of the 1980s, the majority of the work reported in the literature dealt with the applications of this methodology in assessing derangements in the central nervous system physiology and metabolism in a multitude of diseases.

However, based on the observation made by Warburg in the 1930s that Malignant cells prefer glucose over other substrates as a source of energy, some attempts were made in the late 1970s and the early 1980s to use FDG in assessing disease activity in cancer. Pioneering work in animals by Som and collaborators at the BNL and by Di Chiro and colleagues at the NIH, in addition to the work done in human brain tumors by our group at Penn, clearly demonstrated the importance of FDG-PET imaging in the evaluation of cancer. In the meantime, performance of whole body imaging with PET was optimized during the 1980s. By the early 1990s, investigators from the University of California–Los Angeles, and later from the Universities of Michigan, Duke, Nebraska, and Heidelberg, demonstrated the importance of FDG-PET imaging in the management of several common malignancies. These efforts were applicable to diagnosis, staging, monitoring response following treatment, and detecting recurrence of cancer. By the late 1990s, a large body of literature on FDG-PET imaging had clearly shown that FDG-PET imaging was essential for optimal assessment of patients with a number of malignancies, and its routine use was well justified. Among these clinical applications, certain entities appeared most impressive, including differentiating benign from malignant lung nodules, staging lung cancer, detection of recurrent colon cancer, and assessing lymphomas at various stages of the disease.

The use of FDG-PET as an effective method for determining myocardial viability is well established and is considered the gold standard for this purpose. Increasingly, FDG-PET imaging is being employed for the detection of orthopedic infections, fever of unknown origins, and inflammatory disorders. In addition, FDG-PET may prove to be an important method for detecting atherosclerosis, blood clots, and muscle dysfunction.

The introduction of PET/CT in the late 1990s added a major dimension to the utility of this powerful methodology, particularly in certain clinical settings. By combining the structure and function in the same image and therefore precise localization of the diseased sites will play an important role in optimal use of this technology. This is particularly true for preoperative and prebiopsy interventions in patients who have cancer and possibly other disorders. An area in which PET/CT imaging will become the standard of care is in radiation oncology, which, in my view, may prove to be the most important application of this powerful modality. In head and neck pathologies, because of the complexity of the structures visualized using radiologic and functional imaging techniques, precise coregistration of PET and CT images is essential for accurate interpretation. In certain anatomic sites, such the brain and the lower extremities, the impact of PET/CT may not be as dramatic as in other sites in the body. We expect that over the next 5 to 10 years the majority of nuclear medicine procedures will be generated employing PET. Therefore, it is essential that the imaging community makes every effort to define the necessary indications for which combined modalities (PET/CT as a unit) are required for optimal results. This is a challenge that should be addressed soon so that the cost and the space requirements will not interfere with the widespread use of PET in the day-to-day practice of medicine.

Several new tracers will be approved and routinely used in the coming years. Agents that measure regional hypoxia in malignant tumors and possibly in some benign disorders will be frequently employed. Hypoxia is considered the main factor in lack of response following radiation and or chemotherapy. Therefore, in patients who have hypoxia, radiation or chemotherapy may be postponed until optimal oxygen levels have been restored in the tumor. In certain cancers radiolabeled fluorothymidine may prove to be of value in monitoring response to therapy instead of FDG. This tracer, however, does not appear optimal for diagnostic purposes because it is insensitive for detecting slow-growing tumors. ^{18}F-labeled DOPA is expected to be used for the diagnosis of

Parkinson's disease and will be widely adopted for this purpose. There are several amyloid imaging agents that may become the test of choice in the early diagnosis of Alzheimer's disease.

The introduction of FDG and a multitude of novel radiotracers has clearly demonstrated the enormous potential of nuclear medicine as an emerging discipline in the field of molecular imaging. Molecular imaging in its broad definition represents methodologies and probes that allow visualizing vents at the molecular and cellular levels. The intended targets for this purpose include cell surface receptors, transporters, intracellular enzymes, or messenger RNA. The source of the signal detected by these techniques could originate directly from the molecule or its surrogates.

The NIH Road Map Initiative has placed molecular imaging as a main focus for this major undertaking, which further demonstrates the importance of this approach in the scientific community. It is not farfetched to speculate that in the future molecular imaging will be the "centerpiece" of medical practice where early and accurate diagnoses will be made by appropriate imaging probes. Treatment for most diseases and disorders will be individualized by using labeled pharmacologic agents that would be predictive of a favorable outcome. Molecular and cellular imaging techniques will be successfully employed for monitoring response and detecting early evidence for failure or recurrence of disease activity.

In addition to nuclear medicine techniques, many different methodologies have been studied for the purposes of molecular imaging, including optical imaging, magnetic resonance spectroscopy, and functional magnetic resonance imaging. The merits and current applications of these techniques are also described elsewhere in this issue of the *Radiologic Clinics of North America*.

The challenges faced by the imaging community include the shortage of properly trained personnel to perform various tasks that are associated with this complex technology. This is applicable to running cyclotron facilities, synthesizing routine and new novel compounds, and operating the imaging instruments. Obviously, there is a great demand for physicians who are adequately trained to provide this type of service with high standards. Efforts are underway to include training in PET as an additional component for conventional education in nuclear medicine.

I should conclude by stating that FDG-PET, as a single modality, has made an everlasting impact on the specialty of nuclear medicine. In fact, it has rejuvenated the field and has changed its image in the medical community. It is not an exaggeration to speculate that in the coming years, the number of FDG-PET images performed in most facilities will exceed that of all other procedures performed with radiolabeled compounds. It is therefore quite appropriate to applaud our distinguished colleague Henry Wagner, who called FDG the "molecule of the century" because of its unparalleled impact on the evolution of the specialty of nuclear medicine.

Abass Alavi, MD
Professor
Radiology and Neurology
Chief
Division of Nuclear Medicine
Department of Radiology
Hospital of the University of Pennsylvania
3400 Spruce Street
110 Donner Building
Philadelphia, PA 19104, USA
E-mail address: abass.alavi@uphs.upenn.edu

ELSEVIER
SAUNDERS

Radiol Clin N Am 43 (2005) 1 – 21

RADIOLOGIC
CLINICS
of North America

Fluorodeoxyglucose-PET in characterizing solitary pulmonary nodules, assessing pleural diseases, and the initial staging, restaging, therapy planning, and monitoring response of lung cancer

Ayse Mavi, MD[a], Paras Lakhani, BA[a], Hongming Zhuang, MD, PhD[a], Naresh C. Gupta, MD[b], Abass Alavi, MD[a],*

[a]Division of Nuclear Medicine, Department of Radiology, Hospital of the University of Pennsylvania,
3400 Spruce Street, Philadelphia, PA 19104, USA
[b]Frederick Imaging Centers, 46 B Thomas Johnson Drive, Frederick, MD 21702, USA

Radiologic imaging modalities play a critical role in the diagnosis and the overall management of many pulmonary disorders, including solitary pulmonary nodules, lung cancer, and pleural diseases. In these conditions, a correct and timely diagnosis is essential and can result in decreased morbidity and mortality for the patient. Traditionally, chest radiography and CT have been used to assess the nature of the disease in these clinical settings. Although both modalities serve as primary diagnostic tools in these patients, functional imaging with fluorodeoxyglucose-PET (FDG-PET) complements the observations made with structural techniques and improves the outcome in many circumstances. Such information usually leads to alterations in the management and treatment of patients. As a result, the use of FDG-PET has gained a major role in the evaluation of patients with thoracic disorders. In this review the authors discuss the role of FDG-PET in characterizing pulmonary nodules, in assessing pleural diseases, and in the initial diagnosis, staging and re-staging, monitoring response following treatment, and detecting recurrence of lung cancer.

Solitary pulmonary nodules

A solitary pulmonary nodule (SPN) is usually defined as a lung lesion that is well defined, round or oval, smaller than 3.0 cm in diameter, and entirely surrounded by normal pulmonary parenchyma. Lesions that are larger than 3 cm are typically designated as masses and are usually malignant [1]. Solitary pulmonary nodules are a relatively common clinical finding and are seen in approximately 1 in 500 chest radiographs and computed tomograms [2]. Of the nearly 130,000 new SPNs found each year in the United States, about 50% to 60% are benign. If the true nature of these lesions could be determined noninvasively, patients with benign lesions could be spared surgical resection [3]. In two thirds of these nodules, however, chest radiography and CT imaging may not be able to differentiate malignant from benign lesions by the pattern of calcification or even by CT densitometry [4]. The two most common underlying pathologies of SPNs are primary lung carcinomas and benign granulomas, which constitute more than 80% of pulmonary nodules with equal distribution of about 40% in each category [5]. The goal of modern imaging studies, therefore, is to improve the accuracy of distinguishing benign from malignant lesions.

---

* Corresponding author.
   E-mail address: abass.alavi@uphs.upenn.edu (A. Alavi).

0033-8389/05/$ – see front matter © 2004 Elsevier Inc. All rights reserved.
doi:10.1016/j.rcl.2004.09.001

Conventional diagnostic approach in lung nodules

Although various diagnostic procedures have been used to evaluate patients with SPNs, plain radiography and CT are the most commonly used modalities [4]. In SPNs, estimating the probability of malignancy depends on both the imaging findings and on the clinical history of the patient. Clinical factors that are associated with a high probability for malignancy include advanced age, a history of smoking, and evidence of a prior malignancy [6]. Radiologic findings that are suggestive of a malignant process include the thickness of the cavity wall, presence of a speculated or nodular edge, and a diameter greater than 3 cm [6]. On the other hand, SPNs with central, laminated, or diffuse calcifications are more likely to be benign. In general, stability of a nodule over an extended period of time is considered an indicator of a benign lesion. It has been shown, however, that absence of measurable growth over a 2-year period has a predictive value of only 65% for a benign lesion [7]. Thus, the notion that a stable lesion is predictive of a favorable prognosis should be interpreted with caution in most clinical settings.

Most noncalcified SPNs may remain indeterminate on the basis of findings on CT and plain-film radiographs [5]. In addition, it is often difficult to distinguish between diffuse benign and malignant parenchymal abnormalities that cannot be classified as SPNs on radiographic studies [5].

The optimal work-up of a patient with a solitary pulmonary nodule depends on the level of suspicion for cancer based on the established criteria for this purpose and on the availability of previous imaging studies. If no previous radiographs are available, or if such images were acquired close in time to the detection of the SPN, subsequent serial follow-up radiographs may be adequate to determine the nature of the incidentally detected lesion if the patient is younger than 30 years of age. Also, if the SPN has a benign radiographic appearance, and there is no history of extrathoracic malignancies, the patient can be observed and no further work-up for cancer may be necessary. Otherwise, aggressive investigation is warranted to determine the underlying pathology in these nodules.

The least invasive nonimaging method for the evaluation of an SPN is sputum cytology. Although this method has a high specificity, it has a relatively low sensitivity, particularly for peripheral malignancies and for patients with cough, hemoptysis, or airway involvement. Bronchoscopic biopsy, transbronchoscopic biopsy, transthoracic needle aspiration (TTNA), and transthoracic fine-needle biopsy (TTFB) are semi-invasive methods that can be employed for further pathologic characterization of indeterminate SPNs. Bronchoscopic biopsy is preferred for centrally located lesions and achieves a sensitivity of only 65% in the diagnosis of malignant nodules [8]. With transbronchoscopic biopsy the sensitivity increases to 79% in this population [8]. With both methods, the false-positive rates are sufficiently low, and the diagnosis of malignancy can be made with confidence with a positive result. The sensitivity is not optimal for excluding malignancy with confidence in a segment of this population, however. In addition, transbronchoscopic biopsy carries a small risk of intrabronchial bleeding. For peripherally located SPNs, TTNA is preferred over other techniques and has a sensitivity of 85% to 90% [9]. The sensitivity of TTNA is 70% to 75% for small or centrally located lesions. Additionally, there is a relatively high risk of pneumothorax (24.5%) and bleeding with central biopsies, and chest tube placement may be required in 6.8% of patients who undergo this procedure [9]. Furthermore, TTNA cannot assess the status of nodes unless the TTNA is specially directed toward central lymph nodes. TTNA should, therefore, be reserved for assessing cases in which the sputum cytology and subsequent bronchoscopy are negative and the patient is not a surgical candidate or refuses surgery. TTNA may then allow initiation of cytotoxic chemotherapy and or radiotherapy, and it may also be helpful in cases where the likelihood of cancer is intermediate [10]. TTFB is more accurate than TTNA, and achieves a sensitivity of 94% to 98% and a specificity of 91% to 96%. Complications are frequently noted following this procedure, however; pneumothoraces occur in 19% to 26% of patients, and 10% to 15% of patients require pleural drainage after TTFB [8]. The most invasive procedures that can be employed in the work-up of an SPN are video-assisted thorascopic surgery and thoracotomy. These surgical interventions are reserved for lesions that are suspected to be malignant based on various clinical and imaging criteria and when less-invasive attempts for establishing the diagnosis have failed.

Overall, the use of FDG-PET imaging along with minimally invasive techniques may prove to be a cost-effective approach. It has been shown that the use of CT-guided needle biopsy combined with FDG-PET scanning for the evaluation of SPNs discovered on screening chest radiographs is quite cost-effective and frequently provides accurate results [11].

The role of fluorodeoxyglucose-PET imaging in lung nodules

Application of fluorodeoxyglucose-PET in the evaluation of lung nodules

Many studies have demonstrated the accuracy of FDG-PET in evaluating SPNs. The sensitivities and specificities for this technique, as reported in the literature, have ranged from 83% to 97% and from 69% to 100%, respectively, pointing to its important role in the evaluation of SPNs [12]. In a recent meta-analysis, FDG-PET imaging was found to have cumulative sensitivity of 96.8% and specificity of 77.8% for identifying malignant lung nodules and masses [13]. Moreover, FDG-PET may provide a reliable means for noninvasive diagnosis of malignancy in patients with SPNs that are less than 3 cm size. It has been shown that a negative FDG-PET study represents less than a 5% probability for cancer in an SPN [14,15]. Investigators have applied the Bayesian analysis for the evaluation of SPNs [16]. The likelihood ratio for malignancy in an SPN with increased FDG uptake is 7.11, suggesting a high probability for malignancy, and is 0.06 when the PET scan is normal, indicating a high likelihood for a benign process [15]. For radiologically indeterminate nodules, FDG-PET has been shown to have a sensitivity of 92%, specificity of 90%, positive predictive value of 92%, negative predictive value of 90%, and an overall diagnostic accuracy of 91%, when a standardized uptake value (SUV) of 2.5 is used as the cutoff threshold for malignancy [17]. Because of its high negative predictive value, a pulmonary lung nodule or mass without increased FDG activity is unlikely to be malignant (Fig. 1) [18].

Data in the literature to date suggest that PET imaging for the diagnosis of pulmonary lesions is more useful in patients with an intermediate probability for lung cancer as estimated by considering symptoms, risk factors, and radiographic appear-ances. An FDG-PET scan is also warranted when there is discordance between the pretest probability of cancer and the appearance of the nodule on CT [19]. On the other hand, in lesions that are suspected to represent bronchoalveolar carcinomas or typical carcinoid tumors, the usefulness of PET may be limited. FDG-PET imaging has a relatively high false-negative rate in this population [20]. Moreover, in patients with lesions smaller than 1 cm, FDG-PET imaging has been shown to provide a relatively high false-negative rate for cancer [1,15]. A recent study, however, showed that FDG-PET is useful in evaluating indeterminate lesions found on CT that are less than 1 cm [21]. In this series, the prevalence of malignancy was found to be 39%. These investigators reported a sensitivity of 93%, specificity of 77%, positive predictive value of 72%, and negative predictive value of 94% [21]. Thus, FDG-PET may have a role in evaluating small lesions (< 1 cm) that are indeterminate on CT. These promising results can be partly attributed to the improved resolution of instruments used for PET imaging in recent years.

Benign causes of fluorodeoxyglucose uptake

Increased FDG activity has been observed in a variety of benign conditions that can result in false-positive (for cancer) interpretation of PET studies evaluating solitary pulmonary nodules. The benign conditions in the chest with increased FDG accumulation include

1. Infectious processes [22–27]
2. Noninfectious inflammatory diseases [28–31]
3. Iatrogenic disorders or artifacts [32–37]

Certain active infectious processes tend to reveal higher FDG uptake than others. For example, some active granulomatous infections such as histoplasmosis may show intense FDG concentration. FDG is

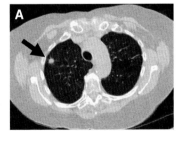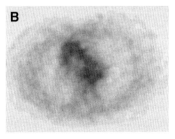

Fig. 1. An 83-year-old woman underwent an FDG-PET examination for the assessment of a 1.0 × 1.2–cm right upper lung nodule with spiculated margins. (*A*) The CT scan appearance was suggestive of a malignant process (*arrow*). (*B*) No increased metabolic activity was noted at the corresponding site on PET images.

incorporated into acute inflammatory lesions that may include both acute (polymorphonuclear) and chronic cells such as macrophages or lymphocytes [38]. Recognizing specific patterns for certain inflammatory conditions may improve the ability to distinguish between benign and malignant causes of positive FDG scans. There is a considerable degree of variability in the FDG uptake among these non-malignant causes. In vitro studies have shown that the levels of FDG uptake correlate well the number of macrophages that are noted by histologic analysis [39]. In the authors' experience, several acute inflammatory or infectious conditions such as pneumonia or other bacterial or viral infections are associated with a relatively mild degree of FDG uptake. Granulomatous diseases or chronic infections usually demonstrate significant levels of FDG uptake, overlapping with the levels noted in malignant diseases [14]. This overlap in uptake levels can pose a difficulty in distinguishing low-grade lung malignancies such as bronchoalveolar carcinoma from granulomatous infections.

Although increased FDG uptake in benign conditions may decrease the specificity of FDG-PET scanning when a malignant disease is suspected, familiarity with the metabolic patterns of benign conditions may decrease the rate of false-positive results. For example, a pattern of bilateral, symmetrical hilar/mediastinal uptake without lung parenchymal abnormality usually represents inflammatory or nonmalignant lymphadenopathy [40].

Dual time point or delayed imaging for differentiating benign and malignant nodules

Because tumor cells avidly take up FDG for many hours after injection compared with normal tissues, delayed imaging should improve the contrast ratio between the tumor and background tissue and therefore allow enhanced visualization of cancer. In a preliminary study the authors' group performed PET imaging in patients with non–small cell lung cancer (NSCLC) at 1 hour, 2 hours, 4 hours, and 6 hours after injection with FDG. In these patients, the investigators noticed a significant change in tumor-to-lung FDG uptake over time (Fig. 2; 136.90%, 167.78%, and 157.97% at 2 hours, 4 hours, and 6 hours, respectively). Furthermore, they demonstrated that the tumor-to-lung ratio peaks at 4 hours after injection and remains flat after that time point. This information is valuable because it may allow optimal use of FDG-PET imaging in detecting cancer. These findings confirm that delayed imaging should allow improved and more accurate staging in patients with NSCLC and increase the sensitivity of PET in

detecting lesions missed on scans at earlier time points. More research should be performed to confirm these findings [41]. It is advisable that patients with lung cancer be imaged at least 2 or possibly 3 hours after the administration of FDG to improve the sensitivity of the technique and allow optimal staging in these patients. Delayed imaging is particularly important in the initial staging of the cancer when accurate determination of the extent of the disease is of great importance in planning optimal treatment strategies. In addition, delayed imaging may improve the specificity of the technique in assessing lymph nodes in the mediastinum and allow an accurate diagnosis of inflammatory lesions.

Dual time point FDG-PET scanning can be useful for differentiating benign from malignant lung nodules. This technique was first described by the authors' group for assessing head and neck malignancies. Hustinx et al [42] performed dual time point scanning in 21 patients with 18 head and neck malignant tumors and 9 inflammatory/infectious lesions. These authors noted that malignant tumors had an average increase of SUVs between the first and second scan of 12%, whereas inflammatory lesions and structures with physiologic uptake of FDG (tongue, larynx) showed essentially stable uptake over time or a slight decline. In later, comprehensive in vitro, animal, and human studies, the authors further demonstrated that lesions with increasing SUVs over time are likely to be malignant and that dual time point FDG-PET imaging may become a promising method for distinguishing malignant from benign lesions [43]. Other investigators using dynamic imaging also observed increased FDG uptake over time in malignant lesions [44]. In a study using a turpentine-induced inflammation in a rat model, Yamada et al [45] found that FDG uptake in inflammatory tissue increased gradually until 60 minutes after injection and then decreased gradually. In a study of 40 patients, Nakamoto et al [46] determined the difference between the SUVs obtained at 60 and 120 minutes after FDG injection in a sample of benign and malignant lesions. They showed that the SUVs in 23 of 31 malignant lesions increased over time, whereas the SUVs in 12 of 13 benign lesions decreased over time. They also found that FDG uptake in 20 of 27 tumor lesions increased between the first hour and the second hour. In another study the authors [47] reported that dual time point imaging with FDG-PET considerably improved both the sensitivity and the specificity of detecting malignant pulmonary nodules. In this study the nodules were scanned by PET at approximately 60 and 90 minutes after the injection of FDG. The tumor SUVs

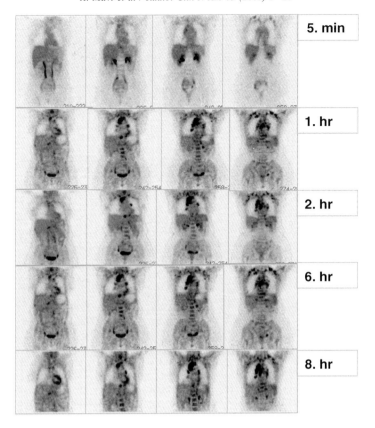

Fig. 2. This patient with diagnosis of non-small cell lung cancer underwent FDG-PET examinations after the intravenous injection of FDG and was imaged at 5 minutes, 1 hour, 2 hours, 6 hours, and 8 hours. The number of lesions and the intensity of uptake increased over time. The authors believe that delayed imaging up to 2 to 3 hours will be increasingly employed for optimal staging of patients with lung cancer and possibly for other malignancies such as head and neck and colon tumors.

increased from 3.66 to 4.43 between the first and second scans, representing an increase of 20.5% ($P < 0.01$). This technique achieved a sensitivity of 100% and specificity of 89% for detecting malignant pulmonary nodules, using a threshold value of a 10% increase between scan 1 and scan 2 (Fig. 3) [47].

Partial volume correction for accurate measurement of standardized uptake value

The spatial resolution of PET systems varies substantially among models and is typically between 5 to 10 mm for most machines in clinical use. There is a significant difference between the resolving powers of modern CT and MR imaging scanners and those of PET and single photon emission computed tomography (SPECT) instruments, and this difference poses a challenge when structural abnormalities are compared with metabolic findings for the assessment of the nature of the disease process. This shortcoming of the functional imaging techniques

may result in low sensitivities when instruments with limited resolutions are used for the diagnosis of small malignant lesions [48]. Under these circumstances, the measured SUV underestimates the true metabolic activity of lesions when their size is less than twice the spatial resolution of the camera.

One method to correct for the resolution effect is to consider the use the lesion size, as determined on CT scan, as the basis to calculate the SUV. Hickeson et al [49] reported that accuracy increased from 58% to 89% with the use of this technique for lung nodules that measured less than 2 cm in 42 patients when a SUV threshold of 2.5 was used to differentiate benign from malignant lesions.

Measuring the SUV by using the CT size to correct for resolution effect may improve the role of FDG-PET in distinguishing malignant from benign nodules in this population. Partial volume correction along with dual time point imaging may further improve the accuracy of this technique in assessing lung nodules and possibly many other malignancies.

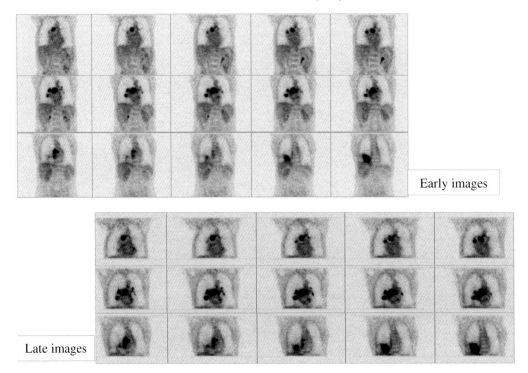

Early images

Late images

Fig. 3. In this patient with a primary lung cancer in the right lung base, the early PET images were acquired 60 minutes following the intravenous administration of FDG. The late set was generated at the completion of the first whole-body scan. Although most lesions are seen on both sets, the intensity of FDG uptake increased in the late set at the primary site and metastatic nodes in both hila, in the mediastinum, and in the right paratracheal region. The maximum SUVs of a metastatic left hilar node were calculated and revealed a 28.9% increase on the late image (3.8 and 4.9, respectively). In addition, additional sites were visualized in the late set that were not clearly defined on the early images.

Role of somatostatin scintigraphy in lung nodules

Somatostatin is a peptide that naturally exists in two forms: one with 14 amino acids and the other with 28 amino acids. Human somatostatin receptors (SSTRs) are expressed on many cells of neuroendocrine origin and also on lymphocytes. In addition, many tumors, including bronchogenic carcinomas, express high densities of SSTRs. Therefore, radiolabeled somatostatin analogues are another class of radiopharmaceuticals used for the evaluation of SPN.

One such radiopharmaceutical is indium-111 (^{111}In)-octreotide, which contains eight amino acids. It has variable binding affinities to SSTRs. Five subtypes of SSTRs have been identified so far [50,51]. ^{111}In-octreotide has the highest binding affinity to SSTR2, followed by SSTR3 and SSTR5 [52]. Because of the relatively long half-life of this radionuclide, images are acquired 24 to 48 hours after administration, but if indicated a repeat image at 72 hours after injection can be acquired to enhance the sensitivity of the technique. Kwekkeboom

et al [53] and other investigators have reported encouraging results in the imaging of lung cancers with ^{111}In-octreotide.

Technitium-99m (^{99m}Tc)-depreotide is another synthetic somatostatin analogue with a low molecular weight of 1358 [51]. This agent also has been used for imaging pulmonary nodules in an effort to differentiate malignancies from infectious processes [54]. Imaging with ^{99m}Tc-depreotide results in high-quality scans, lowers radiation burden to the patient, and decreases the costs of the study. In addition, SPECT images with ^{99m}Tc-depreotide seem to be of higher quality than those acquired with ^{111}In-octreotide. ^{99m}Tc-depreotide imaging provides a rapid, effective, and noninvasive method for the evaluation of SPNs. In patients with SPNs the reported sensitivity of this technique ranges from 93% to 100%, and specificity ranges from 43% to 88%, [55,56]. The somewhat low specificity of somatostatin scintigraphy in the evaluation of lung nodules may result from increased somatostatin binding sites in activated lymphocytes [57].

Previous reports have failed to demonstrate clinical advantages for using ^{99m}Tc-depreotide imaging over FDG-PET in the assessment of lung nodules [54,58]. Thus, FDG-PET is considered the standard modality for this purpose and has been established as the noninvasive test of choice in the differential diagnosis of SPNs.

Lung cancer

Lung cancer is the leading cause of cancer worldwide and results in more than 1 million deaths each year [59]. This malignancy is the leading cause of cancer-related death in the United States, with a 5-year survival of only 15% [60]. Nearly 80% of patients with lung cancer are inoperable at the time of diagnosis. A major role of imaging studies is to diagnose the disease in early stages when the potential for cure is relatively high. In the past decade, significant advances in PET imaging seem to have substantially changed the traditional role of conventional radiological techniques in the work-up of patients with suspected or proven lung cancer.

Primary diagnostic methods

At the initial presentation, most patients with lung cancer are symptomatic. Patients may present with a wide variety of nonspecific symptoms, which can include cough, dyspnea, hemoptysis, chest pain, wheezing, hoarseness, and weight loss. In approximately 10% of patients the diagnosis of cancer is made incidentally by findings on chest radiography or CT performed for unrelated reasons [61]. Traditionally, when lung cancer is suspected, the diagnostic work-up may include chest radiography, CT of the chest and upper abdomen, sputum cytology, and bronchoscopy [62]. Once the diagnosis of lung cancer has been established, it is essential that every effort be made to stage the extent of the disease to allow appropriate treatment planning.

The optimal management of lung cancer depends largely on the type of tumor and the stage of the disease. It has been estimated that only 20% to 35% of lung cancer patients are considered candidates for surgical resection at the time of presentation. Therefore, accurate staging is essential for appropriate therapeutic interventions, which include surgery or radiation and chemotherapy [63–66]. Noninvasive methods such as imaging play a critical role in the staging of lung tumors.

The American Thoracic Society and the European Respiratory Society currently recommend the use of CT scanning for initial staging in NSCLC [67]. CT imaging assists in the staging of NSCLC by permitting an accurate measurement of tumor size and by aiding in the detection of enlarged lymph nodes. CT scanning, however, does not reliably detect tumor invasion into the chest wall [68]. In addition, the CT evaluation of metastasis to the mediastinal lymph nodes has some limitations. In one meta-analysis of 42 studies, CT had a sensitivity of 79% and a specificity of 78% in detecting mediastinal lymph node involvement [69]. CT scanning can also be used to search for distant metastasis in extrathoracic organs such as the adrenal glands and the liver. The presence of radiographic lesions in these organs does not always indicate malignant spread, however, because incidental benign lesions can mimic malignant disease at those sites. Also, some metastases may go unnoticed with these techniques [70].

The role of fluorodeoxyglucose-PET in lung cancer staging

Hilar and mediastinal lymph node staging

FDG-PET is an effective, noninvasive method for staging hilar and mediastinal lymph nodes in patients with lung cancer and is superior to CT scanning in differentiating patients with N1/N2 disease from those with unresectable N3 stage [71]. A recent meta-analysis has established the superiority of PET over CT scanning for staging lymph node metastasis, with median sensitivities of 85% and 90%, respectively, and specificities of 61% and 79%, respectively [72].

One of the main criteria for determining the presence or lack of nodal metastasis by conventional imaging is the size of the lymph node. Because lymph node size correlates poorly with tumor involvement, morphologic imaging techniques such as CT have been shown to have insufficient sensitivity for detecting lymph node metastases [73,74]. Therefore, CT is insensitive for detecting metastasis in lymph nodes that are smaller than 1 cm [75,76]. Furthermore, it has been determined that approximately 30% to 40% of enlarged lymph nodes (2–4 cm in diameter) exhibit no tumor cells by histopathologic examination [73]. Thus, morphologic criteria for determining nodal disease are not as accurate as functional methods based on FDG-PET. This conclusion has remained unchanged in the last decade following the introduction of spiral CT. Meta-analysis demonstrated that spiral CT is inferior to FDG-PET for this purpose (sensitivity of 64% and specificity of 62% for spiral CT versus sensitivity of 85% to 95% and specificity of 81% to 100% for FDG-PET) [72]. It has been reported that FDG-PET has a high negative predictive value in the exclusion of N2 or N3 disease so that mediastinoscopy can be omitted in most patients with a negative PET scan for mediastinal involvement [77].

Distant metastases

In addition to detecting involved mediastinal nodes, PET may be used to detect distant extrathoracic metastases. By detecting distant metastases in 10% to 25% of patients, whole-body PET plays a critical role in accurate preoperative staging of

patients with lung cancer [78]. Extrathoracic sites of metastases (Figs. 4 and 5) from bronchogenic cancer include the brain, adrenal glands, liver, bone marrow, soft tissues, and kidneys. With the exception of the kidneys and the brain, most sites could be successfully detected on a whole-body PET scan. A whole-body PET scan can accurately characterize indeterminate adrenal masses found on CT scan and detect metastatic disease in normal-appearing adrenal glands [70]. Incidentally detected enlarged adrenals, which occur in up to 20% of this population at initial presentation, pose a difficult challenge in the work-up

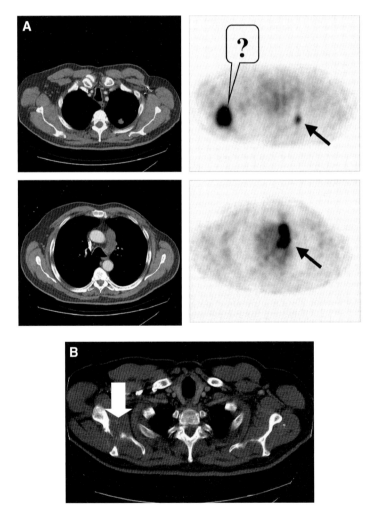

Fig. 4. (*A*) A 67-year-old woman with history of breast cancer years ago presented with a left upper lung nodule and mediastinal adenopathy on a thoracic CT scan. (*B*) An FDG-PET scan was performed for further characterization of these lesions. In addition to the foci of metabolic activity in the left upper lung and mediastinum, which correspond to the lesions detected by CT (*A, arrows*), a large region of hypermetabolism was detected in the region of right scapula which was missed on the initial interpretation of the structural examination. Bone metastasis in the right scapula was clearly identifiable in retrospect when the CT scan was re-reviewed and would have gone unnoticed without the benefit of the PET scan (*B, large arrow*).

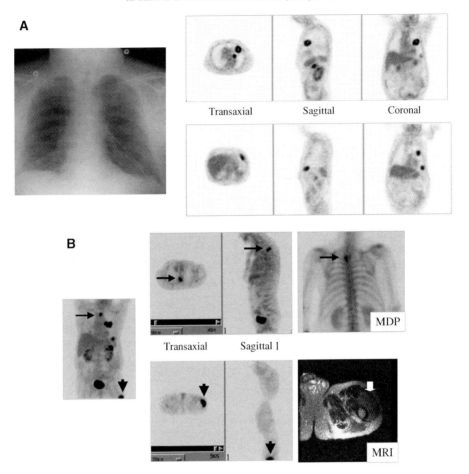

Fig. 5. This 77-year-old man was examined with FDG-PET to characterize a pulmonary nodule detected on chest radiograph. (*A*) The PET images demonstrated multiple regions of intense activity in the chest, which were interpreted as suggesting metastatic lung cancer. (*B*) In addition to sites of disease activity in the lung and the lymph nodes, a bone metastasis (*long thin arrow*) was detected in the upper thoracic spine and a large soft tissue lesion was noted (*short thick arrow*) in the left upper thigh. The bone metastasis was confirmed by bone scintigraphy, and the malignancy in the left upper thigh was clearly demonstrated by MR imaging and subsequent biopsy.

of patients with lung cancer [79]. FDG-PET has been shown to detect adrenal metastases with a sensitivity of 100% and a specificity of 80% to 94% [70,80]. Therefore, the combination of an enlarged adrenal gland found on CT and a negative PET scan may obviate the need for further examination of this site for metastasis. FDG-PET has a higher specificity (98% versus 61%) [81] and a slightly lower sensitivity [82] than conventional bone scanning for detecting bone metastasis. Bone scintigraphy may seem to be more sensitive than PET because any abnormality is attributed to metastatic disease. The authors believe that a single PET scan may accurately detect metastatic sites in the soft tissues and the skeletal structures. In contrast to bone scintigraphy,

which usually remains positive for years following fracture [83], FDG uptake is increased only transiently at fracture sites and therefore is less likely to cause false-positive results [84]. This observation can partially explain the high specificity of FDG-PET in detecting bone metastasis.

PET may have a limited role in the evaluation of certain types of distant metastases. For example, PET is less sensitive than MR imaging or CT in detecting brain metastases because of the limited spatial resolution of PET instruments and the intense uptake of FDG in normal cortical structures [85].

The PET and CT images acquired by a single combined unit may allow greater accuracy than the use of either instrument alone (Fig. 6) [86–88].

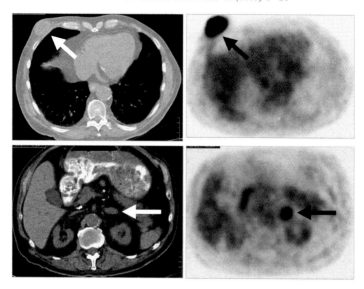

Fig. 6. In this patient with lung cancer and multiple metastases, the complementary roles of FDG-PET and CT are clearly demonstrated. Whereas CT is of great value in demonstrating the exact anatomic location of these lesions, PET has greater sensitivity in defining the extent of the disease and can distinguish active disease from inactive structural abnormalities. PET images in this patient clearly demonstrate metastases to the left adrenal gland and the soft tissues of the right chest wall.

Role of fluorodeoxyglucose-PET in clinical management, treatment planning, and monitoring

Impact on surgical planning

Recently published findings from the American College of Surgeons Oncology Group trial indicate that PET can prevent nontherapeutic thoracotomy in a significant number of patients with suspected and proven lung cancer [77]. Because of PET's superior ability, compared with conventional imaging modalities, to detect locoregional and distant metastasis, the use of FDG-PET can alter the stage in many patients. In one prospective study, the use of FDG-PET compared with conventional staging techniques upstaged 30% of patients with NSCLC [89]. In another prospective study, compared with conventional staging, FDG-PET uncovered new sites of metastases and upstaged 20% of patients enrolled in the study [90]. In another prospective study FDG-PET upstaged 26% of the patients and appropriately downstaged 10 of 16 patients who were scheduled for palliative therapy [91]. Finally, in the largest prospective study with NSCLC (400 patients), FDG-PET accurately upstaged 7% of patients with unsuspected metastasis and accurately downstaged 6% of patients [92]. Accurate preoperative staging is required to reduce the number of futile surgeries and other interventions [93]. In surgically managed lung cancer patients, the degree of SUV on the initial FDG-PET images proved to be highly predictive of overall survival after resection [94]. In patients whose maximum SUV was greater than 9, the 2-year survival was only 68%. In contrast, in patients with a maximum SUV less than 9, the 2-year survival equaled 96%. Therefore, the maximum SUV of lung cancer lesions may be an accurate predictor of prognosis and outcome.

Applications in radiation oncology

In patients with locoregional advanced disease, or when surgery is contraindicated, radical radiotherapy may offer a chance for prolonged survival. Improvements in radiotherapy delivery using conformal techniques and intensity-modulated radiotherapy offer the hope of improving local tumor control and survival by delivering higher doses to tumor while sparing normal adjacent tissues. FDG-PET has been shown to be helpful in delineating the extent of malignant tissues and therefore further enhancing the role of the CT examination by accurately identifying affected sites in the lungs and in the mediastinal lymph nodes.

Accurate determination of gross tumor volumes is important in radiotherapy planning. Studies comparing gross tumor volumes as assessed by both CT and PET showed that FDG-PET significantly changed the measurement of gross tumor volume in to up 56% of patients when the information gained from metabolic imaging was used in the planning process [95–97].

In using FDG-PET to assess tumor volume, several issues are still under investigation. First, an accurate standardized SUV threshold that can be used to differentiate active tumor sites from nonmalignant masses for the purposes of radiation treatment planning has not yet been adequately established. Second, respiratory gating to optimize the validity of the fused PET/CT data is a source of controversy. When lesions are close to the diaphragm or in the lower mediastinum, respiratory motion results in misplacement of the true sites of the malignant tumor and therefore may adversely affect radiotherapy planning. Gating would sharpen the outline of the lesions, which in turn should allow precise radiation treatment planning [95,96].

FDG-PET will increasingly play a role in radiotherapy planning and may be a better predictor of survival than conventional staging technique, because it can stage nodal and extrathoracic metastases more accurately [90].

Assessment of response to chemo-/radiotherapy

Structural imaging has several limitations in assessing treatment response in NSCLC following chemo- or radiation therapy. On CT images, for example, the tumor site and size may not be clearly definable because of atelectasis, fibrosis, or inflammation. Similarly, large lymph nodes seen on conventional imaging may not truly represent evidence for metastasis, and, conversely, those that are generally considered nonmalignant (ie, < 1 cm in size) may actually harbor tumor. Moreover, reductions in metabolic activity on FDG-PET following treatment precede changes in tumor volume detected by structural imaging techniques. Therefore, a decrease in metabolic activity detected by FDG-PET may be a reliable indicator of early response following various therapeutic interventions.

These advantages favoring PET over CT have been reasonably well validated by the studies reported in the literature. In one study of 57 patients with stage IIIB or IV NSCLC, a reduction of FDG activity after one cycle of chemotherapy was closely correlated with the final outcome of therapy [98]. The authors concluded that using metabolic response as an end point may decrease the morbidity and costs of therapy in nonresponding patients. PET may be well justified after chemotherapy (especially induction chemotherapy) for restaging the disease and assessing the treatment response. PET may accurately detect residual viable tumor following chemotherapy [99]. Surgery after induction chemotherapy for N2 disease is most effective when there is pathologic evidence of response [100]. Survival rates of up to 54% can be achieved in patients treated with induction chemotherapy who have no residual mediastinal disease [101,102]. Persistent FDG uptake in the primary tumor site following chemo- or radiation therapy indicates residual viable tumor in most patients with lung cancer [103].

The main argument against using FDG-PET in managing patients with cancer is its relatively high cost. This objection may be valid for the initial diagnosis of lung cancer, for which CT scanning or bronchoscopy may be more cost-effective. For patients who are scheduled to undergo extensive treatment protocols with questionable results, the cost of PET scanning is rather small compared with the savings realized by avoiding unnecessary treatments, and the significant morbidity and side effects suffered by these patients as a result of such interventions are avoided. In addition, based on the excellent diagnostic accuracy of PET, the routine use of bone and whole-body CT scanning for monitoring these patients following treatment may not be justifiable in the future. Eliminating such posttreatment imaging can further reduce the costs of managing these patients.

Role of PET in the detection of recurrence

Approximately 50% of patients with resected NSCLC present with a recurrent tumor during the course of the disease. FDG-PET can detect local recurrences of previously treated lung carcinomas with a sensitivity of 98% and a specificity of 87%, substantially superior to those of the other imaging methodologies [104,105].

New radiotracers and implications for the future

Many inflammatory processes show FDG activity and therefore are potential sources of false-positive results on PET scan when this technique used to detect suspected malignancy. Therefore, the search for new tracers continues. It is expected that PET examination with new molecular tracers will provide information complementary to that gained by FDG and will allow selection of appropriate treatment modalities and detection of early response during and following chemotherapy or radiotherapy.

The thymidine analogue 3-deoxy-3[^{18}F]-fluorothymidine (FLT) is a new PET tracer that specifically targets proliferative cells in malignant lesions [106]. FLT-PET seems to have lower sensitivity, higher specificity, and more accuracy in assessing lung malignancies compared to FDG-PET [106]. Therefore, the number of false-positive results may be reduced with FLT-PET imaging. FLT uptake correlates well with proliferative activity of malignant cells and therefore may prove to be a selective biomarker for tumor proliferation [106]. In a study involving 30 patients with FLT-PET scans for evaluating SPN, the authors conclude that FLT uptake is more specific for malignant lesions and may be used for the differential diagnosis of SPNs, assessment of the degree of cell proliferation, and estimating prognosis [107].

Hypoxia is considered a major factor in lack of response following chemo- and radiation therapy. In recent years attempts have been made to synthesize compounds that allow visualization of tumor hypoxia before such therapies are initiated [106,108–110]. In a study using 60-diacetyl-bis(N(4)-methylthiosemicarbazone) (^{60}Cu-ATSM), tumor hypoxia was imaged in 19 patients with NSCLC. The SUV of 60Cu-ATSM in the lung malignancies proved to be a reliable predictor of tumor response following radiation [111].

In a study by Hustinx et al [112], 2-^{18}F-fluoro-L-tyrosine (^{18}F-TYR) was found to be inferior to ^{18}F-FDG PET for staging patients with NSCLC and lymphomas.

Higashi et al [113] evaluated 23 patients with ^{11}C-acetate with lung cancer and noted that this compound was inferior to FDG in visualizing tumor sites. The authors suggest that ^{11}C-acetate may play a complementary role to that of FDG in the identification of low-grade malignancies that are missed with the latter PET tracer, however.

In pursuit of new tracers, [^{18}F]-fluoro-L-proline has been synthesized and has been shown to demonstrate encouraging results in the diagnosis of active pulmonary fibrosis [114].

Pleural diseases

The pleura is a serous membrane composed of a single layer of mesothelial cells and consists of a visceral component, which covers the surface of the lung parenchyma, and a parietal layer, which overlies the inner surface of the thoracic cavity. The potential space between these two membranes is named the pleural space.

The pleura and pleural space can be affected by a multitude of pulmonary and extrapulmonary disorders, which can range from simple pleural effusions to fatal malignancies. These pleural changes can be detected by noninvasive anatomic imaging techniques, such as chest radiography, ultrasound, or CT. New evidence suggests that functional and metabolic imaging with FDG-PET may be useful in evaluating many types of pleural diseases, including malignant

disorders like mesothelioma or metastasis. In addition, FDG-PET may be useful in characterizing and monitoring patients with benign inflammatory diseases of the pleura. This section describes the significance of FDG-PET findings in the assessment of pleural disorders and forecasts the utility of this modality in various clinical settings.

Conventional diagnostic approach

Noninvasive imaging modalities

Several anatomic imaging modalities have been used to evaluate pleural disorders, including chest radiography, ultrasound, CT, and MR imaging. Chest radiography was the first imaging modality used to visualize the pleura and the pleural space. Although chest radiography is a good technique for detecting pleural disease and fluid, it is unable to differentiate benign from malignant disease and has a limited resolution for this purpose. The introduction of CT has provided a superior method for assessing pleural disorders and is considered the best overall modality for this purpose. CT of the chest accurately detects changes caused by exposure to asbestos, including malignant pleural mesothelioma, early in the course of the disease [115]. MR imaging is superior to CT in delineating soft tissue structures in various anatomic sites and has been shown to be of value in staging malignant pleural mesothelioma, with an overall accuracy of 50% to 75% for this challenging problem [116,117]. Ultrasonography is another noninvasive imaging method that can be used for evaluating pleural disorders. It provides a simple and inexpensive approach that can distinguish pleural effusion from pleural thickening and could be used to improve the results from diagnostic thoracentesis.

Although structural imaging techniques are critical for evaluating pleural diseases, they suffer from certain limitations in some clinical settings. For example, many infectious disorders such as tuberculosis or empyema cannot be differentiated from pleural malignancies with this approach alone. Benign and malignant pleural diseases have similar appearances on conventional imaging techniques such as CT, ultrasound, and chest radiography. In particular, it has been shown that CT is unable to differentiate pleural fibrosis following therapy from active benign or malignant diseases [118]. MR imaging has limited value in evaluating pleural diseases because of cardiac and respiratory motion artifacts but has the potential to differentiate between benign fibrous mesothelioma (low signal intensity on T2-weighted images) and malignant mesothelioma (high signal intensity) [119].

Semi-invasive procedures

Based on current practice, all patients who are diagnosed or suspected of having a pleural effusion should undergo a thoracentesis. Although there are no absolute contraindications to thoracentesis, relative contraindications include increased risk for bleeding (eg, patients receiving anticoagulation therapy or with a bleeding tendency), very small pleural effusions, and mechanical ventilation [120,121]. The most common complication of thoracentesis is pneumothorax, which occurs in up 30% of patients when the procedure is performed by trainees, but the overall rate is less than 12% [122,123]. Although diagnostic thoracentesis can determine the type of effusion in 75% of cases, an exact diagnosis can be made in only 25% of patients [123]. The combination of pleural fluid cytology and needle biopsy yields a sensitivity of less than 40% for a definitive diagnosis. Moreover, needle biopsy is also associated with a significant risk of pneumothorax, tumor seeding, and bleeding. Although slightly more invasive than needle biopsy, thoracoscopy is the procedure of choice for the diagnosis and management of neoplastic diseases of the pleura, because it can provide direct visualization of the pleural space. Therefore, tissue sampling and pleurodesis can be performed directly with this procedure. There are, however, many potential complications with this method, such as persistent air leaks, hemorrhage, subcutaneous emphysema, wound infections, and the seeding of tumor along the chest wall. Open biopsy allows optimal visualization of the pleural space, but it results in more complications in a substantial number of patients, and thus thoracoscopy is widely used for this purpose [124].

Role of PET in the evaluation of benign and malignant diseases of the pleura

FDG-PET imaging is a unique, noninvasive modality that has been successfully used to evaluate several pleural diseases. The FDG-PET technique has been shown to be highly sensitive in detecting both malignant and inflammatory processes and should be considered as an effective method for the assessment of several pleural diseases. Some of these applications are described in detail here.

Benign causes of pleural fluorodeoxyglucose uptake

Causes of detectable FDG uptake in nonmalignant pleural disorders include inflammatory asbestos reaction, pleuritis of various causes, recent surgery, and radiotherapy. Benign inflammatory processes (eg, bacterial infection, tuberculosis, parapneumonic

effusion, sarcoidosis, fungal infection) can cause increased metabolic activity in the pleura with an SUV that at times may exceed 2.5 [125]. Benign pleural plaques and pleural effusions may have radiologic appearances similar to those of malignant processes, but the degree of FDG uptake in these disorders varies depending on the underlying disorder. No FDG uptake is seen in transudates, but malignant pleural diseases appear metabolically active on PET imaging. Dual time point imaging may be of value in the distinguishing intense uptake of FDG in benign inflammatory disease from that noted in malignant disorders.

Mesothelioma

Exposure to asbestos can lead to thickening and fibrosis of the pleura and can result in an increased risk for mesothelioma. One subtype of mesothelioma is benign fibrous mesothelioma, a rare, nonmalignant, localized tumor of the pleura that is not related to asbestos exposure and can be cured by excisional surgery. Malignant pleural mesothelioma as a consequence of asbestos exposure is a relatively rare disease (incidence of 2000–3000 cases per year) and carries a poor prognosis [126].

Patients with malignant pleural mesothelioma usually present with a unilateral pleural mass or effusion, which is usually detected first by chest radiograph. More than 50% of these patients have pleural effusion at the time of diagnosis, but cytologic examination of pleural fluid is positive only in about 25% of these cases. Distant metastases occur later in the course of the disease, and the median survival after diagnosis is between 12 and 18 months. Currently, early diagnosis and aggressive surgical extirpation are considered important for optimal long-term survival. Imaging plays an essential role in the evaluation of malignant pleural mesothelioma. With MR imaging the degree of tumor extension, especially to the chest wall and diaphragm, can be delineated. [127]. Definitive diagnosis is currently made by thoracoscopic biopsy, which carries the risk of seeding tumor through the operative tract. CT is not specific in the diagnosis of malignant pleural mesothelioma and has limited sensitivity in detecting mediastinal lymph node involvement. The combination of CT with thoracoscopy improves the diagnostic accuracy of the technique and is currently used for staging and restaging of the disease [128]. MR imaging does not provide additional information beyond that which can be noted on the CT scan in patients who suffer from unresectable disease. The sensitivity of either MR imaging and or CT for detecting mediastinal nodal involvement is only 50%, although MR imaging is superior to CT for detecting subdiaphragmatic invasion [117]. Patients with local extension of the tumor into the mediastinum, chest wall, or diaphragm, and those with hematogenous dissemination are considered inoperable and are treated with aggressive combined-modality therapeutic intervention. Thus, accurate detection of local spread and systemic dissemination of the tumor is important in selecting the appropriate treatment modalities, which vary depending upon the stage of the disease.

PET imaging has been used to depict malignant pleural mesothelioma, which appears as a linear area of intense FDG uptake surrounding the lungs (Fig. 7) [129,130]. In one study, FDG-PET achieved a sensitivity of 91% and specificity of 100% for differentiating benign from malignant disease, using an SUV of 2.0 as a cutoff threshold [130]. In this study, the cause of false-negative findings on FDG-PET included a slow-growing epithelioid subtype with a low mitosis rate and a relatively better survival than the other types [131]. In addition, several studies have noted the superiority of PET over CT in differentiating benign from malignant disease in malignant pleural mesothelioma and in detecting extrathoracic and mediastinal nodal metastasis [130,132]. In one study, FDG-PET correctly identified the presence or absence of metastatic sites in 89% of patients [132]. Another prospective study demonstrated the utility of FDG-PET in detecting extrathoracic metastases, which prevented inappropriate thoracotomy in 6 of 60 patients (10%). The study, however, noted mixed results in the ability of FDG-PET to detect mediastinal spread [133]. Other studies have directly compared FDG-PET with CT, mediastinoscopy, thoracoscopy, and pathologic examination and have found that PET is useful in determining the true nature of doubtful CT findings, especially when lymph node involvement and distant metastases are of concern on structural scans [134]. In addition, FDG-PET images provide excellent information about the active tumor sites, especially in patients who are surgical candidates [135]. The degree of

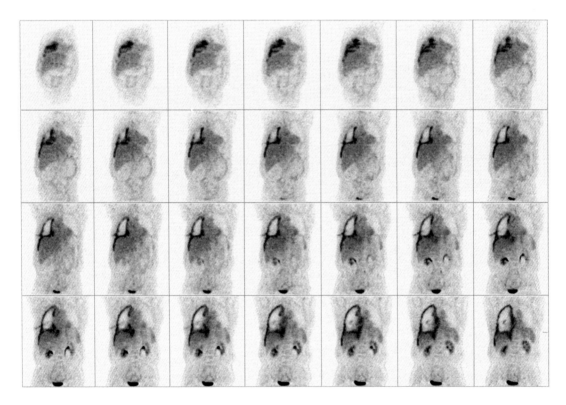

Fig. 7. This patient with a history of mesothelioma underwent FDG-PET imaging to assess the degree of disease activity in the right pleural structures. The images demonstrate abnormally increased radiotracer uptake around the right lung, involving all pleural surfaces as well as the minor fissure suggestive of malignant mesothelioma. No definite evidence of locoregional or distant metastasis was observed on these images.

tumor uptake of FDG is predictive of patient survival, and patients with high uptake in pleural lesions seem to have shorter survival times than those with low metabolic activity [136]. There have been a few reports of false-positive FDG-PET findings, which have resulted from infectious pleuritis, benign causes such as asbestos plaques, and recent abdominal surgery [130,132,137]. Overall, these results suggest that FDG-PET should have a growing role in the evaluation of mesotheliomas, because it is the only noninvasive imaging technique that can reliably differentiate benign from malignant pleural thickenings and more accurately stage malignant pleural mesothelioma. In addition, by quantifying FDG uptake, SUVs may allow monitoring response to therapy or the detection of disease recurrence. Although more research is needed in this area, new developments such as dual time point imaging may improve the accuracy of the technique when existing techniques cannot distinguish between inflammation and malignancy.

Distinguishing metabolic patterns for benign and malignant disorders

Pleural effusion is caused by a variety of benign and malignant disorders. Every year in the United States 200,000 individuals are diagnosed with malignant pleural effusions. Most of these effusions are secondary to metastasis from lung, breast, gastric, and ovarian cancers and lymphomas. Approximately 50% of patients with metastasis to the pleura develop effusion. The prognosis is poor when there is malignant pleural effusion. Pleural effusions are common in patients with NSCLC and are found in one third of patients at the time of presentation. Many of these effusions are benign and may represent reactive fluid collections. Lung cancer is considered unresectable when there is malignant pleural effusion. Therefore, it is important to differentiate between benign and malignant pleural effusions [67,138].

Several recent reports indicate that the degree of the FDG uptake in the pleura and qualitative assessment of pleural thickening can accurately differentiate benign pleural plaques or inflammatory conditions from malignant pleural involvement [137,139–141]. A recently published study including 92 patients with newly diagnosed NSCLC and pleural abnormalities showed that CT findings were indeterminate in 71% of patients and were truly negative in 29% of patients [142]. In this study, the sensitivity of FDG-PET in characterizing pleural malignancies was 100%, specificity was 71%, positive predictive value was 63%, negative predictive value was 100%, and

accuracy was 80%. For CT and FDG-PET combined the sensitivity was 100%, specificity was 76%, positive predictive value was 67%, negative predictive value was100%, and accuracy was 84%. These findings suggest that a negative FDG-PET scan and an indeterminate pleural abnormality on CT usually indicate a benign process, whereas a positive PET scan suggests a malignant disease as the underlying cause for the pleural effusion [142]. In another study of 98 patients presenting with either pleural thickening or an exudative pleural effusion, the sensitivity and specificity of PET in identifying malignancy were 96.8% and 88.5%, respectively, with a positive and negative predictive value of 93.8% and 93.9%, respectively [143].

The authors' group evaluated 106 patients with cancer in whom the degree of FDG uptake was examined in the pleura. Based on the history, findings on the PET scan, the SUV of the pleural FDG uptake, clinical follow-up, and biopsies, the patients were eventually classified as having benign/inflammatory (n = 25) or malignant (n = 81) pleural disease. The average SUV of the malignant pleural lesions was 4.18. CT showed evidence of pleural disease in only 60% of patients with malignant pleural disease and in 64% of patients with benign pleural disease. When an SUV threshold of 2.0 was chosen to separate malignant and benign disease, the sensitivity and specificity of FDG-PET for malignant pleural disease, at 90% and 72%, respectively, was much higher than that of CT . In nine patients, direct extension of FDG activity into the pleura from the primary lung lesion was noted on PET, but such evidence was seen on the CT scan in only three patients (33%) [144].

These reports indicate that FDG-PET is accurate imaging technique for differentiating benign from malignant pleural diseases. FDG-PET can identify other occult foci of metastasis or even a primary site (in the lung or elsewhere in the body) in patients with malignant effusions and an unknown primary tumor. FDG-PET may provide a useful alternative to invasive diagnostic tests diagnostic in patients with a suspected malignant pleural effusion, especially in those with equivocal findings on CT or negative results from pleural cytology after thoracentesis. Incorporating FDG-PET into the diagnostic algorithm may reduce the number of open pleural biopsies and thoracotomies performed for benign pleural disease. Dual time point imaging may also have a role in the evaluation of pleural diseases by FDG-PET [43]. PET-CT co-registered images may substantially enhance the role of FDG-PET imaging in some types of pleural lesions [145]. The authors also believe that early involvement of the pleura with malignant cells that could precede structural changes may allow early detection of this serious complication. Thus, the use of FDG-PET may allow appropriate therapeutic interventions to be initiated early in the course of the disease.

References

[1] Ost D, Fein AM, Feinsilver SH. Clinical practice. The solitary pulmonary nodule. N Engl J Med 2003;348: 2535–42.

[2] Fletcher JW. PET scanning and the solitary pulmonary nodule. Semin Thorac Cardiovasc Surg 2002; 14:268–74.

[3] Valanis BG. Epidemiology of lung cancer: a worldwide epidemic. Semin Oncol Nurs 1996;12:251–9.

[4] Cummings SR, Lillington GA, Richard RJ. Estimating the probability of malignancy in solitary pulmonary nodules. A Bayesian approach. Am Rev Respir Dis 1986;134:449–52.

[5] Khouri NF, Meziane MA, Zerhouni EA, Fishman EK, Siegelman SS. The solitary pulmonary nodule. Assessment, diagnosis, and management. Chest 1987;91: 128–33.

[6] Webb WR. Radiologic evaluation of the solitary pulmonary nodule. AJR Am J Roentgenol 1990;154: 701–8.

[7] Yankelevitz DF, Henschke CI. Does 2-year stability imply that pulmonary nodules are benign? AJR Am J Roentgenol 1997;168:325–8.

[8] Gambhir SS, Shepherd JE, Shah BD, Hart E, Hoh CK, Valk PE, et al. Analytical decision model for the cost-effective management of solitary pulmonary nodules. J Clin Oncol 1998;16:2113–25.

[9] Klein JS, Zarka MA. Transthoracic needle biopsy: an overview. J Thorac Imaging 1997;12:232–49.

[10] Yung RC. Tissue diagnosis of suspected lung cancer: selecting between bronchoscopy, transthoracic needle aspiration, and resectional biopsy. Respir Care Clin N Am 2003;9:51–76.

[11] Tsushima Y, Endo K. Analysis models to assess cost effectiveness of the four strategies for the work-up of solitary pulmonary nodules. Med Sci Monit 2004; 10:MT65–72.

[12] Gupta NC, Frank AR, Dewan NA, Redepenning LS, Rothberg ML, Mailliard JA, et al. Solitary pulmonary nodules: detection of malignancy with PET with 2-[F-18]-fluoro-2-deoxy-D-glucose. Radiology 1992; 184:441–4.

[13] Gould MK, Maclean CC, Kuschner WG, Rydzak CE, Owens DK. Accuracy of positron emission tomography for diagnosis of pulmonary nodules and mass lesions—a meta-analysis. JAMA 2001;285:914–24.

[14] Lowe VJ, Hoffman JM, DeLong DM, Patz EF, Coleman RE. Semiquantitative and visual analysis of FDG-PET images in pulmonary abnormalities. J Nucl Med 1994;35:1771–6.

[15] Gupta NC, Maloof J, Gunel E. Probability of malignancy in solitary pulmonary nodules using fluorine-18-FDG and PET. J Nucl Med 1996;37:943–8.

[16] Dewan NA, Shehan CJ, Reeb SD, Gobar LS, Scott WJ, Ryschon K. Likelihood of malignancy in a solitary pulmonary nodule: comparison of Bayesian analysis and results of FDG-PET scan. Chest 1997; 112:416–22.

[17] Ruiz-Hernandez G, de Juan R, Samanes A, Verea H, Penas JM, Veres A, et al. [Positron emission tomography using 18-FDG-PET in radiologically indeterminate pulmonary lesions]. Med Interna 2004;21: 12–6.

[18] Ghesani NV, Sun XH, Zhuang H, Sam JW, Alavi A. Fluorodeoxyglucose positron emission tomography excludes pericardial metastasis by recurrent lung cancer. Clin Nucl Med 2003;28:666–7.

[19] Ost D, Fein A. Management strategies for the solitary pulmonary nodule. Curr Opin Pulm Med 2004;10: 272–8.

[20] Detterbeck FC, Falen S, Rivera MP, Halle JS, Socinski MA. Seeking a home for a PET, part 1: defining the appropriate place for positron emission tomography imaging in the diagnosis of pulmonary nodules or masses. Chest 2004;125:2294–9.

[21] Herder GJ, Golding RP, Hoekstra OS, Comans EF, Teule GJ, Postmus PE, et al. The performance of (18)F-fluorodeoxyglucose positron emission tomography in small solitary pulmonary nodules. Eur J Nucl Med Mol Imaging 2004;31(9):1231–6.

[22] Bakheet SMB, Powe J, Ezzat A, Rostom A. F-18-FDG uptake in tuberculosis. Clin Nucl Med 1998; 23:739–42.

[23] Bakheet SM, Saleem M, Powe J, Al Amro A, Larsson SG, Mahassin Z. F-18 fluorodeoxyglucose chest uptake in lung inflammation and infection. Clin Nucl Med 2000;25:273–8.

[24] Jones HA, Clark RJ, Rhodes CG, Schofield JB, Krausz T, Haslett C. In vivo measurement of neutrophil activity in experimental lung inflammation. Am J Respir Crit Care Med 1994;149:1635–9.

[25] Zhuang H, Pourdehnad M, Yamamoto AJ, Rossman MD, Alavi A. Intense F-18 fluorodeoxyglucose uptake caused by Mycobacterium avium intracellulare infection. Clin Nucl Med 2001;26:458.

[26] Mackie G. F-18 fluorodeoxyglucose positron emission tomographic imaging of cytomegalovirus pneumonia. Clin Nucl Med 2004;29:569–71.

[27] Zhuang H, Duarte PS, Rebenstock A, Feng Q, Alavi A. Pulmonary Clostridium perfringens infection detected by FDG positron emission tomography. Clin Nucl Med 2003;28:517–8.

[28] Lewis PJ, Salama A. Uptake of fluorine-18-fluorodeoxyglucose in sarcoidosis. J Nucl Med 1994;35: 1647–9.

[29] Yu JQ, Zhuang H, Xiu Y, Talati E, Alavi A. Demonstration of increased FDG activity in Rosai-Dorfman disease on positron emission tomography. Clin Nucl Med 2004;29:209–10.

[30] Yun MJ, Yeh D, Araujo LI, Jang SY, Newberg A, Alavi A. F-18FDG uptake in the large arteries—a new observation. Clin Nucl Med 2001;26:314–9.

[31] Kung J, Zhuang HM, Yu JQ, Duarte PS, Alavi A. Intense fluorodeoxyglucose activity in pulmonary amyloid lesions on positron emission tomography. Clin Nucl Med 2003;28:975–6.

[32] Chiang S, Rebenstock A, Guan L, Burns J, Alavi A, Zhuang H. Potential false-positive FDG PET imaging caused by subcutaneous radiotracer infiltration. Clin Nucl Med 2003;28:786–8.

[33] Lin P, Delaney G, Chu J, Kiat H, Pocock N. Fluorine-18 FDG dual-head gamma camera coincidence imaging of radiation pneumonitis. Clin Nucl Med 2000;25:866–9.

[34] Zhuang H, Cunnane ME, Ghesani NV, Mozley PD, Alavi A. Chest tube insertion as a potential source of false-positive FDG-positron emission tomographic results. Clin Nucl Med 2002;27:285–6.

[35] Yu J, Kumar R, Xiu Y, Alavi A, Zhuang H. Diffuse FDG uptake in the lungs in aspiration pneumonia on positron emission tomographic imaging. Clin Nucl Med 2004;29:567–8.

[36] Bhargava P, Zhuang H, Kumar R, Charron M, Alavi A. Iatrogenic artifacts on whole-body F-18 FDG PET imaging. Clin Nucl Med 2004;29:429–39.

[37] Bhargava P, Zhuang HM, Kumar R, Yu JQ, Alavi A. Ring-shaped FDG uptake in the right lower lung: is it always a tumor? Clin Nucl Med 2004;29:324–5.

[38] Deichen JT, Prante O, Gack M, Schmiedehausen K, Kuwert T. Uptake of F-18 fluorodeoxyglucose in human monocyte-macrophages in vitro. Eur J Nucl Med Mol Imaging 2003;30:267–73.

[39] Valk PE, Pounds TR, Hopkins DM, Haseman MK, Hofer GA, Greiss HB, et al. Staging non-small cell lung cancer by whole-body positron emission tomographic imaging. Ann Thorac Surg 1995;60: 1573–81.

[40] Gupta NC, Tamim WJ, Graeber GG, Bishop HA, Hobbs GR. Mediastinal lymph node sampling following positron emission tomography with fluorodeoxyglucose imaging in lung cancer staging. Chest 2001; 120:521–7.

[41] Kung J, Yu J, Evans T, Zhuang H, Alavi A. FDG uptake at extended time periods in non-small cell lung cancer-implications for improved cancer management [abstract]. J Nucl Med 2004;45(Suppl):378.

[42] Hustinx R, Smith RJ, Benard F, Rosenthal DI, Machtay M, Farber LA, et al. Dual time point fluorine-18 fluorodeoxyglucose positron emission tomography: a potential method to differentiate malignancy from inflammation and normal tissue in the head and neck. Eur J Nucl Med 1999;26:1345–8.

[43] Zhuang H, Pourdehnad M, Lambright ES, Yamamoto AJ, Lanuti M, Li PY, et al. Dual time point F-18-FDG PET imaging for differentiating malignant from inflammatory processes. J Nucl Med 2001;42: 1412–7.

[44] Kubota K, Itoh M, Ozaki K, Ono S, Tashiro M, Yamaguchi K, et al. Advantage of delayed whole-body FDG-PET imaging for tumour detection. Eur J Nucl Med 2001;28:696–703.

[45] Yamada S, Kubota K, Kubota R, Ido T, Tamahashi N. High accumulation of fluorine-18-fluorodeoxy-glucose in turpentine-induced inflammatory tissue. J Nucl Med 1995;36:1301–6.

[46] Nakamoto Y, Higashi T, Sakahara H, Tamaki N, Kogire M, Doi R, et al. Delayed (18)F-fluoro-2-deoxy-D-glucose positron emission tomography scan for differentiation between malignant and benign lesions in the pancreas. Cancer 2000;89:2547–54.

[47] Matthies A, Hickeson M, Cuchiara A, Alavi A. Dual time point F-18-FDG PET for the evaluation of pulmonary nodules. J Nucl Med 2002;43:871–5.

[48] Weber W, Young C, Abdel-Dayem HM, Sfakianakis G, Weir GJ, Swaney CM, et al. Assessment of pulmonary lesions with F-18-fluorodeoxyglucose positron imaging using coincidence mode gamma cameras. J Nucl Med 1999;40:574–8.

[49] Hickeson M, Yun MJ, Matthies A, Zhuang H, Adam LE, Lacorte L, et al. Use of a corrected standardized uptake value based on the lesion size on CT permits accurate characterization of lung nodules on FDG-PET. Eur J Nucl Med Mol Imaging 2002;29: 1639–47.

[50] Patel YC, Greenwood MT, Panetta R, Demchyshyn H, Niznik H, Srikant CB. The somatostatin receptor family. Life Sci 1995;57:1249–65.

[51] Menda Y, Kahn D. Somatostatin receptor imaging of non-small cell lung cancer with 99mTc depreotide. Semin Nucl Med 2002;32:92–6.

[52] Shih WJ, Samayoa L. Tc-99m depreotide detecting malignant pulmonary nodules: histopathologic correlation with semiquantitative tumor-to-normal lung ratio. Clin Nucl Med 2004;29:171–6.

[53] Kwekkeboom DJ, Kho GS, Lamberts SW, Reubi JC, Laissue JA, Krenning EP. The value of octreotide scintigraphy in patients with lung cancer. Eur J Nucl Med 1994;21:1106–13.

[54] Kahn D, Menda Y, Kernstine K, Bushnell D, McLaughlin K, Miller S, et al. The utility of 99mTc depreotide compared with F-18 fluorodeoxyglucose positron emission tomography and surgical staging in patients with suspected non-small cell lung cancer. Chest 2004;125:494–501.

[55] Grewal RK, Dadparvar S, Yu JQ, Babaria CJ, Cavanaugh T, Sherman M, et al. Efficacy of Tc-99m depreotide scintigraphy in the evaluation of solitary pulmonary nodules. Cancer J 2002;8:400–4.

[56] Blum JE, Handmaker H, Rinne NA. The utility of a somatostatin-type receptor binding peptide radiopharmaceutical (P829) in the evaluation of solitary pulmonary nodules. Chest 1999;115:224–32.

[57] Krenning EP, Kwekkeboom DJ, de Jong M, Visser TJ, Reubi JC, Bakker WH, et al. Essentials of peptide receptor scintigraphy with emphasis on the somatostatin analog octreotide. Semin Oncol 1994;21:6–14.

[58] Nguyen DT, Morakinyo T. Discordant Tc-99m

depreotide and F-18FDG imaging in a patient with poorly differentiated small-cell neuroendocrine carcinoma. Clin Nucl Med 2002;27:373–5.

[59] Parkin DM, Bray F, Ferlay J, Pisani P. Estimating the world cancer burden: Globocan 2000. Int J Cancer 2001;94:153–6.

[60] Jemal A, Tiwari RC, Murray T, Ghafoor A, Samuels A, Ward E, et al. Cancer statistics, 2004. CA Cancer J Clin 2004;54:8–29.

[61] Midthun D, Jett J. Clinical presentation of lung cancer. In: Pass HI, Mitchell JB, Johnson DH, Turrisi AT, editors. Lung cancer: principles and practice. Philadelphia: Lippincott-Raven; 1996. p. 421–35.

[62] Prager D, Cameron R, Ford J, Figlin R. Bronchogenic carcinoma. In: Murray JF, Nadel JA, editors. Textbook of respiratory medicine. 3rd edition. Philadelphia: W.B. Saunders; 2000. p. 1415–51.

[63] Lince L, Lulu DJ. Carcinoma of the lung. A comparative series of 687 cases. Arch Surg 1971;102: 103–7.

[64] Hyde L, Wolf J, McCracken S, Yesner R. Natural course of inoperable lung cancer. Chest 1973;64: 309–12.

[65] Overholt RH, Neptune WB, Ashraf MM. Primary cancer of the lung. A 42-year experience. Ann Thorac Surg 1975;20:511–9.

[66] Benfield JR, Julliard GJ, Pilch YH, Rigler LG, Selecky P. Current and future concepts of lung cancer. Ann Intern Med 1975;83:93–106.

[67] The American Thoracic Society and The European Respiratory Society. Pretreatment evaluation of non-small-cell lung cancer. Am J Respir Crit Care Med 1997;156:320–32.

[68] Webb WR, Gatsonis C, Zerhouni EA, Heelan RT, Glazer GM, Francis IR, et al. CT and MR imaging in staging non-small cell bronchogenic carcinoma—report of the Radiologic Diagnostic Oncology Group. Radiology 1991;178:705–13.

[69] Dales R, Stark R, Raman S. Computed tomography to stage lung cancer. Approaching a controversy using meta-analysis. Am Rev Respir Dis 1990;141: 1096–101.

[70] Erasmus JJ, Patz EF, McAdams HP, Murray JG, Herndon J, Coleman RE, et al. Evaluation of adrenal masses in patients with bronchogenic carcinoma using F-18-fluorodeoxy-glucose positron emission tomography. AJR Am J Roentgenol 1997;168: 1357–60.

[71] Halter G, Buck AK, Schirrmeister H, Aksoy E, Liewald F, Glatting G, et al. Lymph node staging in lung cancer using [18F]FDG-PET. Thorac Cardiovasc Surg 2004;52:96–101.

[72] Gould MK, Kuschner WG, Rydzak CE, Maclean CC, Demas AN, Shigemitsu H, et al. Test performance of positron emission tomography and computed tomography for mediastinal staging in patients with non-small cell lung cancer—a meta-analysis. Ann Intern Med 2003;139:879–92.

[73] Arita T, Matsumoto T, Kuramitsu T, Kawamura M,

Matsunaga N, Sugi K, et al. Is it possible to differentiate malignant mediastinal nodes from benign nodes by size? Reevaluation by CT, transesophageal echocardiography, and nodal specimen. Chest 1996; 110:1004–8.

[74] Arita T, Kuramitsu T, Kawamura M, Matsumoto T, Matsunaga N, Sugi K, et al. Bronchogenic carcinoma: incidence of metastases to normal sized lymph nodes. Thorax 1995;50:1267–9.

[75] McLoud TC, Bourgouin PM, Greenberg RW, Kosiuk JP, Templeton PA, Shepard JA, et al. Bronchogenic carcinoma: analysis of staging in the mediastinum with CT by correlative lymph node mapping and sampling. Radiology 1992;182:319–23.

[76] Cascade PN, Gross BH, Kazerooni EA, Quint LE, Francis IR, Strawderman M, et al. Variability in the detection of enlarged mediastinal lymph nodes in staging lung cancer: a comparison of contrast-enhanced and unenhanced CT. AJR Am J Roentgenol 1998;170:927–31.

[77] Reed CE, Harpole DH, Posther KE, Woolson SL, Downey RJ, Meyers BF, et al. Results of the American College of Surgeons Oncology Group Z0050 Trial: the utility of positron emission tomography in staging potentially operable non-small cell lung cancer. J Thorac Cardiovasc Surg 2003;126:1943–51.

[78] Verhagen AFT, Bootsma GP, Tjan-Heijnen VCG, van der Wilt GJ, Cox AL, Brouwer MHJ, et al. FDG-PET in staging lung cancer—how does it change the algorithm? Lung Cancer 2004;44:175–81.

[79] Boland GW, Goldberg MA, Lee MJ, Mayo-Smith WW, Dixon J, McNicholas MM, et al. Indeterminate adrenal mass in patients with cancer: evaluation at PET with 2-[F-18]-fluoro-2-deoxy-D-glucose. Radiology 1995;194:131–4.

[80] Yun M, Kim W, Alnafisi N, Lacorte L, Jang S, Alavi A. 18F-FDG PET in characterizing adrenal lesions detected on CT or MRI. J Nucl Med 2001;42: 1795–9.

[81] Bury T, Barreto A, Daenen F, Barthelemy N, Ghaye B, Rigo P. Fluorine-18 deoxyglucose positron emission tomography for the detection of bone metastases in patients with non-small cell lung cancer. Eur J Nucl Med 1998;25:1244–7.

[82] Kao CH, Hsieh JF, Tsai SC, Ho YJ, Yen RF. Comparison and discrepancy of 18F–2-deoxyglucose positron emission tomography and Tc-99m MDP bone scan to detect bone metastases. Anticancer Res 2000;20:2189–92.

[83] Matin P. Appearance of bone scans following fractures, including immediate and long-term studies. J Nucl Med 1979;20:1227–31.

[84] Zhuang H, Sam JW, Chacko TK, Duarte PS, Hickeson M, Feng Q, et al. Rapid normalization of osseous FDG uptake following traumatic or surgical fractures. Eur J Nucl Med Mol Imaging 2003;30: 1096–103.

[85] Coleman RE. PET in lung cancer staging. Q J Nucl Med 2001;45:231–4.

[86] Metser U, Lerman H, Blank A, Lievshitz G, Bokstein F, Even-Sapir E. Malignant involvement of the spine: assessment by F-18-FDG PET/CT. J Nucl Med 2004; 45:279–84.

[87] Goerres GW, von Schulthess GK, Steinert HC. Why most PET of lung and head-and-neck be cancer will PET/CT. J Nucl Med 2004;45:66S–71S.

[88] Lardinois D, Weder W, Hany TF, Kamel EM, Korom S, Seifert B, et al. Staging of non-small-cell lung cancer with integrated positron-emission tomography and computed tomography. N Engl J Med 2003;348: 2500–7.

[89] Hoekstra CJ, Stroobants SG, Hoekstra OS, Vansteenkiste J, Biesma B, Schramel FJ, et al. The value of [18F]fluoro-2-deoxy-D-glucose positron emission tomography in the selection of patients with stage IIIA-N2 non-small cell lung cancer for combined modality treatment. Lung Cancer 2003;39: 151–7.

[90] Mac Manus MP, Hicks RJ, Ball DL, Kalff V, Matthews JP, Salminen E, et al. F-18 fluorodeoxyglucose positron emission tomography staging in radical radiotherapy candidates with nonsmall cell lung carcinoma—powerful correlation with survival and high impact on treatment. Cancer 2001;92:886–95.

[91] Kalff V, Hicks RJ, MacManus MP, Binns DS, McKenzie AF, Ware RE, et al. Clinical impact of F-18 fluorodeoxyglucose positron emission tomography in patients with non-small-cell lung cancer: a prospective study. J Clin Oncol 2001;19:111–8.

[92] Cerfolio RJ, Ojha B, Bryant AS, Bass CS, Bartalucci AA, Mountz JM. The role of FDG-PET scan in staging patients with nonsmall cell carcinoma. Ann Thorac Surg 2003;76:861–6.

[93] Verboom P, van Tinteren H, Hoekstra OS, Smit EF, van den Bergh J, Schreurs AJM, et al. Cost-effectiveness of FDG-PET in staging non-small cell lung cancer: the PLUS study. Eur J Nucl Med Mol Imaging 2003;30:1444–9.

[94] Downey RJ, Akhurst T, Gonen M, Vincent A, Bains MS, Larson S, et al. Preoperative F-18 fluorodeoxyglucose-positron emission tomography maximal standardized uptake value predicts survival after lung cancer resection. J Clin Oncol 2004;22:3255–60.

[95] Ciernik IF, Dizendorf E, Baumert BG, Reiner B, Burger C, Davis JB, et al. Radiation treatment planning with an integrated positron emission and computer tomography (PET/CT): a feasibility study. Int J Radiat Oncol Biol Phys 2003;57:853–63.

[96] Munley MT, Marks LB, Scarfone C, Sibley GS, Patz Jr EF, Turkington TG, et al. Multimodality nuclear medicine imaging in three-dimensional radiation treatment planning for lung cancer: challenges and prospects. Lung Cancer 1999;23:105–14.

[97] Bradley J, Thorstad WL, Mutic S, Miller TR, Dehdashti F, Siegel BA, et al. Impact of FDG-PET on radiation therapy volume delineation in non-small-cell lung cancer. Int J Radiat Oncol Biol Phys 2004; 59:78–86.

[98] Weber WA, Petersen V, Schmidt B, Tyndale-Hines L, Link T, Peschel C, et al. Positron emission tomography in non-small-cell lung cancer: prediction of response to chemotherapy by quantitative assessment of glucose use. J Clin Oncol 2003;21:2651–7.

[99] Eschmann SM, Friedel G, Paulsen F, Budach W, Harer-Mouline C, Dohmen BM, et al. FDG PET for staging of advanced non-small cell lung cancer prior to neoadjuvant radio-chemotherapy. Eur J Nucl Med Mol Imaging 2002;29:804–8.

[100] Schilder RJ, Goldberg M, Millenson MM, Movsas B, Rogatko A, Rogers B, et al. Phase II trial of induction high-dose chemotherapy followed by surgical resection and radiation therapy for patients with marginally resectable non-small cell carcinoma of the lung. Lung Cancer 2000;27:37–45.

[101] Elias AD, Skarin AT, Leong T, Mentzer S, Strauss G, Lynch T, et al. Neoadjuvant therapy for surgically staged IIIA N2 non-small cell lung cancer (NSCLC). Lung Cancer 1997;17:147–61.

[102] Martini N, Kris MG, Flehinger BJ, Gralla RJ, Bains MS, Burt ME, et al. Preoperative chemotherapy for stage IIIa (N2) lung cancer: the Sloan-Kettering experience with 136 patients. Ann Thorac Surg 1993; 55:1365–73.

[103] Akhurst T, Downey RJ, Ginsberg MS, Gonen M, Bains M, Korst R, et al. An initial experience with FDG-PET in the imaging of residual disease after induction therapy for lung cancer. Ann Thorac Surg 2002;73:259–64.

[104] Baum RP, Hellwig D, Mezzetti M. Position of nuclear medicine modalities in the diagnostic workup of cancer patients: lung cancer. Q J Nucl Med 2004; 48:119–42.

[105] Higashi K, Ueda Y, Arisaka Y, Sakuma T, Nambu Y, Oguchi M, et al. 18F-FDG uptake as a biologic prognostic factor for recurrence in patients with surgically resected non-small cell lung cancer. J Nucl Med 2002;43:39–45.

[106] Buck AK, Halter G, Schirrmeister H, Kotzerke J, Wurziger I, Glatting G, et al. Imaging proliferation in lung tumors with PET: F-18-FLT versus F-18-FDG. J Nucl Med 2003;44:1426–31.

[107] Buck AK, Schirrmeister H, Hetzel M, von der Heide M, Halter G, Glatting G, et al. 3-deoxy-3- F-18 fluorothymidine-positron emission tomography for noninvasive assessment of proliferation in pulmonary nodules. Cancer Res 2002;62:3331–4.

[108] Rajendran JG, Mankoff DA, O'Sullivan F, Peterson LM, Schwartz DL, Conrad EU, et al. Hypoxia and glucose metabolism in malignant tumors: evaluation by F-18 fluoromisonidazole and F-18 fluorodeoxyglucose positron emission tomography imaging. Clin Cancer Res 2004;10:2245–52.

[109] Rajendran JG, Wilson DC, Conrad EU, Peterson LM, Bruckner JD, Rasey JS, et al. F-18 FMISO and F-18 FDG PET imaging in soft tissue sarcomas: correlation of hypoxia, metabolism and VEGF expression. Eur J Nucl Med Mol Imaging 2003;30:695–704.

[110] Ziemer LS, Evans SM, Kachur AV, Shuman AL, Cardi CA, Jenkins WT, et al. Noninvasive imaging of tumor hypoxia in rats using the 2-nitroimidazole 18F–EF5. Eur J Nucl Med Mol Imaging 2003;30: 259–66.

[111] Dehdashti F, Mintun MA, Lewis JS, Bradley J, Govindan R, Laforest R, et al. In vivo assessment of tumor hypoxia in lung cancer with Cu-60-ATSM. Eur J Nucl Med Mol Imaging 2003;30:844–50.

[112] Hustinx R, Lemaire C, Jerusalem G, Moreau P, Cataldo D, Duysinx B, et al. Whole-body tumor imaging using PET and 2–18F-fluoro-L-tyrosine: preliminary evaluation and comparison with 18F-FDG. J Nucl Med 2003;44:533–9.

[113] Higashi K, Ueda Y, Matsunari I, Kodama Y, Ikeda R, Miura K, et al. C-11-acetate PET imaging of lung cancer: comparison with F-18-FDG PET and Tc-99m-MIBI SPET. Eur J Nucl Med Mol Imaging 2004; 31:13–21.

[114] Wallace WE, Gupta NC, Hubbs AF, Mazza SM, Bishop HA, Keane MJ, et al. Cis-4- F-18 fluoro-L-proline PET imaging of pulmonary fibrosis in a rabbit model. J Nucl Med 2002;43:413–20.

[115] Rusch V, Godwin J, Shuman W. The role of computed tomography scanning in the initial assessment and follow-up of malignant pleural mesothelioma. J Thorac Cardiovasc Surg 1988;96:171–7.

[116] Leung AN, Muller NL, Miller RR. CT in differential diagnosis of diffuse pleural disease. AJR Am J Roentgenol 1990;154:487–92.

[117] Heelan RT, Rusch VW, Begg CB, Panicek DM, Caravelli JF, Eisen C. Staging of malignant pleural mesothelioma: comparison of CT and MR imaging. AJR Am J Roentgenol 1999;172:1039–47.

[118] Erasmus JJ, McAdams HP, Rossi SE, Goodman PC, Coleman RE, Patz EF. FDG PET of pleural effusions in patients with non-small cell lung cancer. AJR Am J Roentgenol 2000;175:245–9.

[119] Falaschi F, Battolla L, Mascalchi M, Cioni R, Zampa V, Lencioni R, et al. Usefulness of MR signal intensity in distinguishing benign from malignant pleural disease. AJR Am J Roentgenol 1996;166:963–8.

[120] McVay PA, Toy PT. Lack of increased bleeding after paracentesis and thoracentesis in patients with mild coagulation abnormalities. Transfusion 1991;31: 164–71.

[121] McCartney JP, Adams 2nd JW, Hazard PB. Safety of thoracentesis in mechanically ventilated patients. Chest 1993;103:1920–1.

[122] Bartter T, Mayo PD, Pratter MR, Santarelli RJ, Leeds WM, Akers SM. Lower risk and higher yield for thoracentesis when performed by experienced operators. Chest 1993;103:1873–6.

[123] Collins T, Sahn S. Thoracocentesis. Clinical value, complications, technical problems, and patient experience. Chest 1987;91:817–22.

[124] Menzies R, Charbonneau M. Thoracoscopy for the diagnosis of pleural disease. Ann Intern Med 1991; 114:271–6.

[125] Patz Jr EF, Lowe VJ, Hoffman JM, Paine SS, Burrowes P, Coleman RE, et al. Focal pulmonary abnormalities: evaluation with F-18 fluorodeoxyglucose PET scanning. Radiology 1993;188:487–90.

[126] Price B. Analysis of current trends in United States mesothelioma incidence. Am J Epidemiol 1997;145: 211–8.

[127] Wang ZY, Reddy GP, Gotway MB, Higgins CB, Jablons DM, Ramaswamy M, et al. Malignant pleural mesothelioma: Evaluation with CT, MR imaging, and PET. Radiographics 2004;24:105–19.

[128] Marom EM, Erasmus JJ, Pass HI, Patz Jr EF. The role of imaging in malignant pleural mesothelioma. Semin Oncol 2002;29:26–35.

[129] Belhocine TZ, Daenen F, Duysinx B, Bury T, Rigo P. Typical appearance of mesothelioma on an F-18FDG positron emission tomograph. Clin Nucl Med 2000; 25:636.

[130] Benard F, Sterman D, Smith R, Kaiser L, Albelda S, Alavi A. Metabolic imaging of malignant mesothelioma with fluorine-18-deoxyglucose positron emission tomography. Chest 1998;114:713–22.

[131] Rusch VW, Venkatraman ES. Important prognostic factors in patients with malignant pleural mesothelioma, managed surgically. Ann Thorac Surg 1999; 68:1799–804.

[132] Schneider DB, Clary-Macy C, Challa S, Sasse KC, Merrick SH, Hawkins R, et al. Positron emission tomography with F18-fluorodeoxyglucose in the staging and preoperative evaluation of malignant pleural mesothelioma. J Thorac Cardiovasc Surg 2000;120: 128–33.

[133] Flores RM, Akhurst T, Gonen M, Larson SM, Rusch VW. Positron emission tomography defines metastatic disease but not locoregional disease in patients with malignant pleural mesothelioma. J Thorac Cardiovasc Surg 2003;126:11–6.

[134] Nanni C, Castellucci P, Farsad M, Pinto C, Moretti A, Pettinato C, et al. Role of F-18-FDG PET for evaluating malignant pleural mesothelioma. Cancer Biother Radiopharm 2004;19:149–54.

[135] Haberkorn U. Positron emission tomography in the diagnosis of mesothelioma. Lung Cancer 2004; 45(Suppl 1):S73–6.

[136] Benard F, Sterman D, Smith RJ, Kaiser LR, Albelda SM, Alavi A. Prognostic value of FDG PET imaging in malignant pleural mesothelioma. J Nucl Med 1999; 40:1241–5.

[137] Kramer H, Pieterman RM, Slebos DJ, Timens W, Vaalburg W, Koeter GH, et al. PET for the evaluation of pleural thickening observed on CT. J Nucl Med 2004;45:995–8.

[138] Mountain CF. Revisions in the International System for Staging Lung Cancer. Chest 1997;111:1710–7.

[139] Gupta NC, Rogers JS, Graeber GM, Gregory JL, Waheed U, Mullet D, et al. Clinical role of F-18 fluorodeoxyglucose positron emission tomography imaging in patients with lung cancer and suspected malignant pleural effusion. Chest 2002;122:1918–24.

[140] Bury T, Paulus P, Dowlati A, Corhay JL, Rigo P, Radermecker MF. Evaluation of pleural diseases with FDG-PET imaging: preliminary report. Thorax 1997;52:187–9.

[141] Carretta A, Landoni C, Melloni G, Ceresoli GL, Compierchio A, Fazio F, et al. 18-FDG positron emission tomography in the evaluation of malignant pleural diseases—a pilot study. Eur J Cardiothorac Surg 2000;17:377–82.

[142] Schaffler GJ, Wolf G, Schoellnast H, Groell R, Maier A, Smolle-Juttner FM, et al. Non-small cell lung cancer: evaluation of pleural abnormalities on CT scans with T-18 FDG PET. Radiology 2004;231:858–65.

[143] Duysinx B, Nguyen D, Louis R, Cataldo D, Belhocine T, Bartsch P, et al. Evaluation of pleural disease with 18-fluorodeoxyglucose positron emission tomography imaging. Chest 2004;125: 489–93.

[144] Alavi A, Gupta N, Alberini JL, Hickeson M, Adam LE, Bhargava P, et al. Positron emission tomography imaging in nonmalignant thoracic disorders. Semin Nucl Med 2002;32:293–321.

[145] Balogova S, Grahek D, Kerrou K, Montravers F, Younsi N, Aide N, et al. [18F]-FDG imaging in apparently isolated pleural lesions. Rev Pneumol Clin 2003;59:275–88.

ELSEVIER
SAUNDERS

Radiol Clin N Am 43 (2005) 23 – 33

RADIOLOGIC
CLINICS
of North America

Fluorodeoxyglucose-PET in the management of malignant melanoma

Rakesh Kumar, MD, Ayse Mavi, MD, Gonca Bural, MD, Abass Alavi, MD*

*Division of Nuclear Medicine, Department of Radiology, Hospital of the University of Pennsylvania, 110 Donner Building,
3400 Spruce Street, Philadelphia, PA 19104, USA*

Malignant melanoma is diagnosed in more than 40,000 patients annually in United States [1]. It is most common cause of death from cutaneous malignancies. The incidence of malignant melanoma is increasing when compared with other malignancies. In most cases, melanoma is curable by surgical excision if diagnosed in early stages of the disease. Six percent to 10% of patients, however, show detectable metastases at the time of diagnosis, and 16% of patients develop metastases over time [2,3]. Among the patients who develop metastases over the time, 70% initially develop regional metastases, whereas 30% progress directly to distant metastases [3]. The prognosis is linked directly to the initial stage at diagnosis. The patients who present with locally advanced or metastatic disease at the time of diagnosis have a poor prognosis, but the multidisciplinary treatment approach improves the prognosis. The 10-year survival after lymphadenectomy for palpable regional lymph node metastasis is 24% [2]. Therefore, early diagnosis and treatment of local lymph node and distant metastases improve the prognosis in patients with malignant melanoma. Centers for Medicare and Medicaid Services guidelines approve 2-fluorine-18, 2-fluoro-2-deoxy-D-glucose-PET (FDG-PET) for diagnosis, staging, and restaging of melanoma. For diagnosis of melanoma, noninvasive imaging modality is rarely required because the lesion is usually cutaneous and amenable

to diagnostic biopsy without much complication. Therefore no study has investigated the use of PET for the diagnosis of malignant melanoma. Little is known about the FDG uptake in benign pigmented lesions and atypical nevi. This review focuses on the role of FDG-PET imaging in staging and restaging in patients with malignant melanoma.

Initial staging of melanoma

Malignant melanoma has a well-known propensity for spreading to unusual sites. Therefore a baseline staging in patients with primary cutaneous malignant melanoma is routine. Melanoma staging is now based on the depth of invasion of the primary lesion. Ulceration upstages patients in each T-stage subgroup, the number of lymph nodes in N staging is significant, and stage IV metastatic disease is subclassified based on anatomic site and elevated serum lactate dehydrogenase. Most of the staging information in these patients is usually obtained from CT imaging. CT imaging has limitations, because lymph node size is a main diagnostic criterion of malignancy; CT scan defines only anatomy and is insufficient for the depiction of small volumes of tumor in normal-sized structures. Therefore, the accuracy of anatomic imaging modalities in the identification of disease in normal-sized lymph nodes or in the detection of nonmalignant disease within enlarged nodes is limited [4]. Unlike CT, FDG-PET imaging is based on increased glucose metabolism in malignant lesions. Wahl et al [5] showed high

---

* Corresponding author.
 E-mail address: alavi@rad.upenn.edu (A. Alavi).

intracellular concentration of FDG by melanoma cells using human tumor xenograft in nude mice.

Primary tumors

FDG-PET has no or little influence on staging of primary tumor because the highest stage (T4 = 4 mm) is beyond the practical spatial resolution of current PET scanners. Primary tumor staging of malignant melanoma is rarely required, because this assessment is made at the time of punch biopsy or surgical excision, which almost always occurs before the FDG-PET scanning. Spread of the disease in the skin can be readily detected by whole-body imaging at the early and later stages of the disease, however (Fig. 1).

Regional lymph node metastasis

Metastatic involvement of local and regional lymph nodes is an important prognostic criterion in patients with malignant melanoma. In the past, staging and treatment protocols have included full lymph node dissection of the likely nodal basin to identify sites of disease. In recent times, this approach has largely been replaced by sentinel lymph node (SLN) biopsy [6]. SLN biopsy has been established as a safe and accurate procedure for determining the presence or absence of disease spread to regional lymph node basin [7]. This technique, however, does not provide any information about possible distant metastases. Therefore FDG-PET has been evaluated for local-regional lymph node staging and detecting distant metastases.

When FDG-PET has been compared with SLN biopsy or lymph node dissection, the sensitivity of FDG-PET in detecting regional lymph node metastasis varies from 0 to 100% (Table 1.). Most of the earlier studies, which reported good accuracy of FDG-PET in evaluating regional lymph node status, were obtained in patients with clinical or imaging suspicion of metastatic lymph node involvement [8–12]. Recent reports have suggested that sensitivity of FDG-PET for assessment of regional nodes in these patients is much lower than initially reported [13–17]. This large variation in the reported sensitivity of FDG-PET results from the introduction of

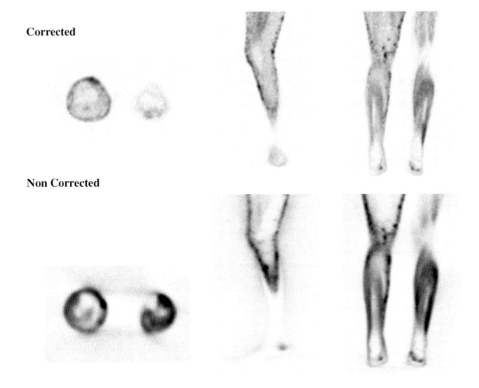

Corrected

Non Corrected

Fig. 1. This patient with a history of right ankle melanoma was treated with surgery and chemotherapy. FDG-PET scan was done 8 weeks after chemotherapy. The images show numerous small foci of increased FDG activity superficially in the right leg and right thigh on transverse, sagittal, and coronal slices. Skin lesions appear more prominent on noncorrected images (*lower row*) than on attenuation corrected images.

Table 1
Studies showing sensitivity and specificity of fluorodeoxy-glucose-PET and sentinel lymph node biopsy in detecting lymph node metastases in patients with melanoma

Study	No. of patients	Sensitivity (%)		Specificity	
		PET	SLNB	PET	SLNB (%)
Hafner et al, 2004 [17]	100	8	100	100	100
Fink et al 2004 [16]	48	13	100	—	—
Longo et al, 2003 [15]	25	22	100	—	—
Havenga et al, 2003 [14]	53	15	100	—	—
Acland et al, 2001 [13]	50	0	100	—	—
Crippa et al, 2000 [11]	38	95	—	84	—
		66	—	99	—
Wagner et al, 1999 [12]	70	17	94	96	100
MacFarlane et al, 1998 [10]	22	85	—	92	—
Wagner et al, 1997 [9]	11	100	—	100	—
Blessing et al, 1995 [8]	20	74	—	93	—

Abbreviation: SLNB, sentinel lymph node biopsy.

step sectioning and immunohistochemical staining that detect micrometastasis. FGD-PET can miss micrometastasis in lymph nodes, because there are fewer tumor cells, which may or may not have increased glucose metabolism, to be detected. In any case, FDG-PET and any other imaging modalities are expected to have a higher false-negative rate than SLN biopsy and histologic examination of tissues. In contrast to the variable sensitivity of FDG-PET, almost all studies have shown specificities higher than 90%, and there are reports of sensitivities approaching 1000% [8–12]. The high specificity of FDG-PET warrants its use in preoperative staging of patients with malignant melanoma, especially in patients with clinical suspicion of nodal involvement. FDG-PET also provides additional information about the extent of the disease (eg, metastases to skin, muscles, bones, bowel, omentum, and mesentery) (Fig. 2).

Blessing et al [8] reported a sensitivity of 74% and a specificity of 93% in 20 patients with clinically palpable lymph nodes. In another study of 11 patients with clinically nonpalpable nodes but a high likelihood of lymph node involvement, FDG-PET showed sensitivity and specificity of 100% [9]. In a similar study of 22 patients with clinical suspected or pathological proved lymph node metastases, FDG-PET showed sensitivity of 85% and specificity of 92% [10]. Crippa et al [11] correctly identified regional lymph node metastases in 35 of 37 patients (95%). All of these patients had clinical suspicion of lymph node metastases by physical examination, CT, or ultrasonography. When results for individual lymph nodes were analyzed, FDG-PET had a significantly lower sensitivity of 66%. In a study by Klein et al [18] of 17 patients with primary cutaneous melanoma, PET had an accuracy of 94% when compared with findings from SLN mapping. It has been shown that for PET to demonstrate disease in regional lymph nodes with 90% sensitivity, a 78-mm^3 volume of tumor must be present [19].

In contrast to initial studies, most of the recent studies compared FDG-PET and SLN biopsy in patients who had no clinical evidence of nodal spread of the disease. All these recent studies have found that PET is relatively less sensitive than SLN biopsy for detection of early nodal disease [14–17]. Wagner et al [12] studied 89 patients with stage I, II, or III cutaneous melanoma and reported a sensitivity of 17% with PET as compared with SLN biopsy and surgical exploration. Acland et al [13] demonstrated similar results in 50 patients with clinically undetectable metastases: FDG-PET had a sensitivity of 0% as compared with 100% for SLN biopsy. Havenga et al [14] reported the value of SLN biopsy and FDG-PET in detecting metastases in 55 patients with primary cutaneous melanoma larger than 1.0 mm and clinically negative nodes. FDG-PET could detect metastases only in 2 of the 13 patients with SLN metastases. In a recent study, Fink et al [16] compared FDG-PET with histopathologic results of SNL biopsy to determine the value of FDG-PET in predicting regional lymph node involvement in patients with stage I and II primary malignant melanoma. Of the 48 patients included in the study, 8 (16.7%) had a positive SNL biopsy. PET was positive in only 1 patient with a positive SNL biopsy, yielding a sensitivity of 13%. Similarly, Hafner et al [17] studied the sensitivity and specificity of ultrasonography, FDG-PET, and SLN biopsy in the early detection of regional lymph node metastases or distant metastases. SLN biopsy was positive in 26 patients, whereas ultrasonography and PET detected 2 of 26 histologically tumor-positive sentinel nodes (sensitivity of 8%).

Distant metastasis

Melanoma can metastasize widely to the skin, muscles, bones, bowel, omentum, mesentery, and

Coronal Slices   **Projection Image**

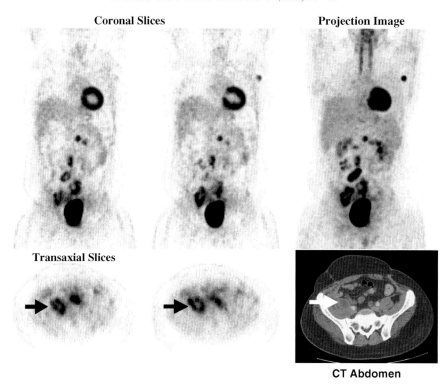

Transaxial Slices

CT Abdomen

Fig. 2. (*Top row*) PET images show several sites of abnormal FDG uptake in the mesenteric, common iliac, and para-aortic nodes in the abdomen. (*Bottom row left and middle*) A large lesion is seen in the right iliac fossa and exhibits central photopenia on transaxial images. (*Bottom row at right*) The contrast CT of pelvis shows bilateral multiple common iliac lymphadenopathy. The largest adenopathy in the common iliac region shows central necrosis corresponding to the photopenic area in the PET scan (*arrows*). In addition, a focus of abnormal FDG uptake is seen in the left axillary region. Arrows indicate metastis with central necrosis of right iliac lymph node.

other tissues. Therefore, FDG-PET has been shown to be more accurate than conventional modalities such as CT, MR imaging, ultrasonography, and physical examination for determining the presence and extent of metastatic disease (Figs. 3–5). Schwimmer et al [20] reviewed the literature and reported that PET has been found to be 92% sensitive and 90% specific for metastases. When PET is added to CT in evaluation of patients undergoing initial staging of high-risk primary melanoma, a change in patient care occurs in up to 90% of cases because unsuspected sites of disease are detected [18]. To the authors' best knowledge and in their literature review, only one study reported detection of more lesions with CT than with FDG-PET [21], but the histopathologic diagnosis was not obtained in most of the cases. CT has also been reported to be more sensitive than PET in detecting lung metastases in patients with malignant melanoma [22,23]. This superiority of CT to FDG-PET in detecting in pulmonary lesions is expected, because

CT has high resolution and high contrast between pulmonary tumor and surrounding lung tissue.

Nine studies compared the sensitivity and specificity FDG-PET to conventional diagnostic modalities in evaluating regional and distant metastases (Table 2). The sensitivity of FDG-PET for metastatic lesions or abnormal regions ranged from 78% to 100%. In a study of 33 patients with suspected metastases, the sensitivity of FDG-PET was 92%; the specificity for reading the PET images was 77% without clinical information and 100% with clinical information [24]. Initial reports of 100 patients by Damian et al [25] suggest that FDG-PET may offer greater diagnostic accuracy and versatility than conventional modalities in staging patients with metastatic melanoma. FDG-PET showed a sensitivity of 93% (388/415) in evaluation of metastatic lesions. In 20 patients, PET detected 24 metastases up to 6 months earlier than conventional imaging or physical examination. In another study of 100 patients, the

Coronal images

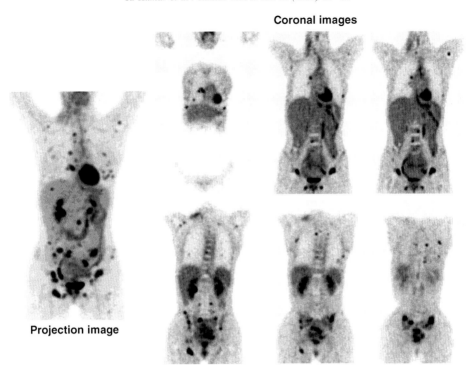

Projection image

Fig. 3. This patient with malignant melanoma demonstrates multiple small foci of intense uptake throughout the body, a finding that is consistent with advanced metastatic disease. The projection image (*left*) and the coronal slices (*right*) show the distribution of the metastatic sites.

Sagittal　　　**Coronal**

Transaxial

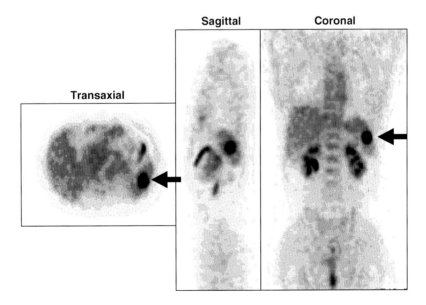

Fig. 4. This patient underwent a PET examination for metastatic melanoma. The FDG-PET images show a focus of intense FDG activity in the spleen (*arrows*), a finding that is consistent with metastasis. No FDG activity was visualized in the known small lung nodules seen on CT. FDG-PET has limited sensitivity in detecting small lung nodules. Arrows indicate splenic metastasis.

Coronal images

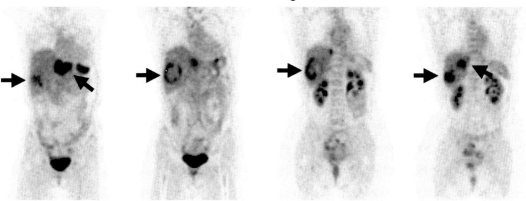

Fig. 5. The FDG-PET scan of this patient with malignant melanoma shows multiple foci of intense FDG uptake in the liver. The largest lesion in the right lobe of liver appears with central necrosis (*arrows*), whereas several other metastases are seen throughout the liver (*arrows*).

sensitivity of PET was 100%, and the specificity was 94%, whereas conventional modalities demonstrated a lower specificity (80%) at primary diagnosis of malignant melanoma [22]. The accuracy of FDG-PET was 100% on the basis of patients and 92% on the basis of single metastases, whereas conventional modalities had accuracy of 77.1% on the basis of patients and only 55.7% on the basis of single metastases. For the detection of melanoma metastases, Holder et al [26] reported a significantly higher sensitivity of 94.2% and a specificity of 83.3% for PET scanning compared with a sensitivity of 55.3% and a specificity of 84.4%, for CT scanning. The causes of false-positive PET scans were papillary carcinoma of the thyroid (1 case), bronchogenic carcinoma (1 case), inflamed epidermal cyst (1 case), Warthin's tumor of the parotid gland (1 case), surgical wound inflammation (2 cases), leiomyoma of the

uterus (1 case), suture granuloma (1 case), and endometriosis (1 case). Eigtved et al [27] also demonstrated the lower sensitivity and specificity of conventional modalities as compared with FDG-PET in 38 patients. Tyler et al [28] reported the identification of 144 of the 165 (87.3%) metastatic lesions using FDG-PET [28]. There were 39 false-positive lesions, of which 13 could be attributed to recent surgery, 3 to arthritis, 3 to infection, 2 to superficial phlebitis, 1 to a benign skin nevus, and 1 to a colonic polyp. Acland et al [29] reported a lower sensitivity with FDG-PET, especially in patients with stage I and stage II disease. PET scanning had an overall sensitivity of 78% and specificity of 87%. In a retrospective cohort review of 104 patients with primary or recurrent melanoma, 157 FDG-PET scans and 70 CT scans were analyzed, with a median patient follow-up of 24 months [30]. Metastases were

Table 2

Studies showing sensitivity and specificity of fluorodeoxyglucose-PET and conventional modalities for detecting metastatic disease in patients with melanoma

Study	No. of patients	Sensitivity (%)		PET	Specificity conventional modalities (%)
		PET	Conventional modalities		
Finkelstein et al, 2004 [31]	18	79	76	87	87
Swetter et al, 2002 [30]	104	84	58	97	70
Acland et al, 2000 [29]	44	78	—	87	—
Tyler et al, 2000 [28]	95	87	—	44	—
Eigtved et al, 2000 [27]	38	97	62	56	22
Holder Jr et al, 1998 [26]	76	94	55	83	84
Rinne et al, 1998 [22]	100	100	85	96	68
Damian et al, 1996 [24]	100	93	—	—	—
Steinert et al, 1995 [25]	33	92	—	77	—

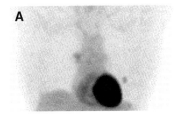
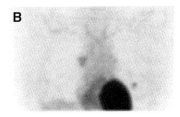

Fig. 6. This patient with history of melanoma underwent dual time point FDG-PET imaging. A focus of FDG uptake in the region of left lower lung is visible. Another irregular focus of increased FDG uptake is seen in the right hilum (*A*). Uptake in both lesions becomes more prominent over time as noted on the repeated image (*B*). Both mean and maximum standardized uptake values (SUVs) increase on delayed images.

confirmed with positive histology (87.5%) or documented disease progression (12.5%). PET demonstrated sensitivity of 84% and specificity of 97%, whereas CT showed sensitivity of 58% and specificity of 70%. In a recent study, Finkelstein et al [31] studied 94 lesions in 18 patients who underwent preoperative assessment, metastasectomy, and long-term follow-up (median, 24 months). In lesion-by-lesion analysis, conventional modalities demonstrated a sensitivity of 76% and a specificity of 87%. FDG-PET demonstrated a sensitivity of 79% and a specificity of 87%. For FDG-PET plus conventional modalities, the sensitivity was 88%, specificity was 91%, positive predictive value was 91%, and negative predictive value was 88%. The authors believe that by performing dual time point imaging the sensitivity and the specificity of the FDG-PET imaging could improve in both primary and metastatic disease (Fig. 6).

Restaging of melanoma

FDG-PET is highly sensitive and specific for initial staging and identification of metastatic disease in patients with malignant melanoma. Therefore, FDG-PET can be used for surveillance after treatment in patients with high-risk stage III and IV melanoma (Fig. 7). Many surgeons advocate aggressive surgical excision of metastatic foci as they develop. In patients with known recurrence of melanoma, FDG-PET scanning has been shown to detect additional unsuspected sites of disease and to result in alteration of treatment planning in up to 20% of cases [20]. There have been three reports of the utility of FDG-PET for evaluating recurrent disease in melanoma patients [32–34]. Stas et al [32] analyzed 100 consecutive PET scans performed on 84 melanoma patients with regional or distant recurrence according to conventional modalities. FDG-PET scanning showed a sensitivity of 85%, a specificity of 90%, and an

accuracy of 88%. The similar values for conventional modalities were 81%, 87%, and 84%, respectively. Mijnhout et al [33] assessed the reproducibility and clinical impact of FDG-PET in 58 consecutive patients with suspected recurrent melanoma. The authors concluded that in problematical cases of suspected recurrent melanoma, FDG-PET had considerable impact on diagnostic understanding and management. Fuster et al [34] compared the accuracy of FDG-PET and standard conventional modalities in detecting recurrent melanoma in 156 patients. The sensitivity and specificity of PET for detecting lesions on an individual-patient basis were 74% and 86%, respectively, compared with respective values of 58% and 45% for conventional modalities alone. The overall accuracy for PET was 81%, compared with 52% for other methods. PET was more accurate (91% versus 67%) than clinical procedures in detecting locoregional disease and distant metastases (85% versus 55%).

Impact on patient management

Many authors have evaluated the impact of FDG-PET on the management of patients with malignant melanoma [24,28,29,32,33,35–37]. PET can affect therapeutic planning in many ways (Fig. 8). Damian et al [24] studied 100 patients and reported that surgical or medical management was specifically influenced by PET findings in 22 patients and that PET was used to clarify another 12 cases in which CT findings were inconclusive. Tyler et al [28], in a prospective study of 106 scans in 95 patients with stage III regional disease, specifically evaluated the role of FDG-PET in the management of melanoma patients. The authors reported a change in management in 15% of cases (16 of 106 studies) with FDG-PET. FDG-PET detected previously unsuspected distant metastases leading to change in stage (stage IV). Similarly, Acland et al [29] reported

Bone Scan

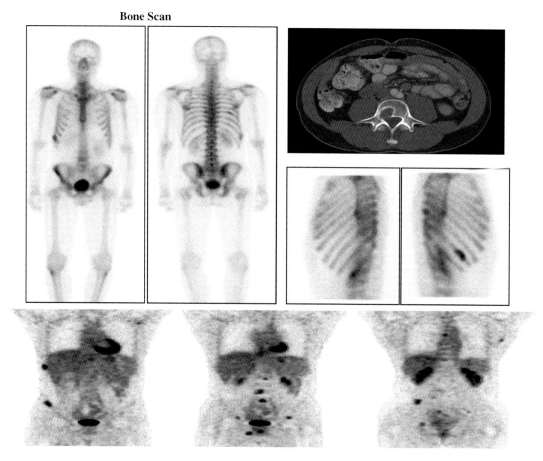

Fig. 7. In this patient with history of melanoma, anterior and posterior whole-body bone scans and lateral spot views reveal focal areas of increased uptake in the right tenth rib posterolaterally and at the right eighth rib posteriorly. On the transverse CT image, a metastatic lesion in the L4 vertebrae is also visualized. PET images demonstrate multiple sites of involvement of bone marrow including the pelvis, thoracic and lumbar spine, ribs, and left axilla. This finding indicates that early metastatic lesions in the marrow may not result in reactive bone formation adequate for visualization by conventional planar bone scanning.

detection of distant metastases using FDG-PET in 28% of patients with stage III disease. Therefore the management was altered in a significant number of patients.

Jadvar et al [35] assessed the effect of FDG-PET on the treatment in 38 patients with malignant melanoma. Compared with PET, the extent of disease was underestimated by CT in 5 patients (13%). Planned surgical resection of metastases was canceled in 2 of these patients. In another patient, surveillance PET detected an unsuspected jejunal metastatic melanoma. Overall, PET influenced surgical management in 3 patients (8%), but it did not affect the wait-and-watch strategy or the decision to initiate immunotherapy in the others. Stas et al [32] retrospectively analyzed 100 PET scans of melanoma patients with suspected regional or distant recurrence.

PET scans provided information in addition to that obtained by conventional modalities leading to upstaging in 10 cases and to downstaging in 24 cases and depicted more lesions within the same stage of disease in 15 cases. The overall therapeutic impact reached 26%: 17 of 71 cases (24%) with regional recurrence, 1 of 18 cases (5.5%) with distant metastasis, and 8 of 11 cases (73%) with suspicion of recurrence where conventional modalities remained doubtful. Wong et al [36] studied the impact of FDG-PET on patient stage and management from the referring physician's perspective. A questionnaire was sent to referring physicians to investigate whether and how PET altered clinical decisions in the treatment of melanoma patients. Referring physicians indicated that FDG-PET changed the clinical stage in 15 of 51 patients (29%) (two thirds were

Projection Images   **Coronal images**

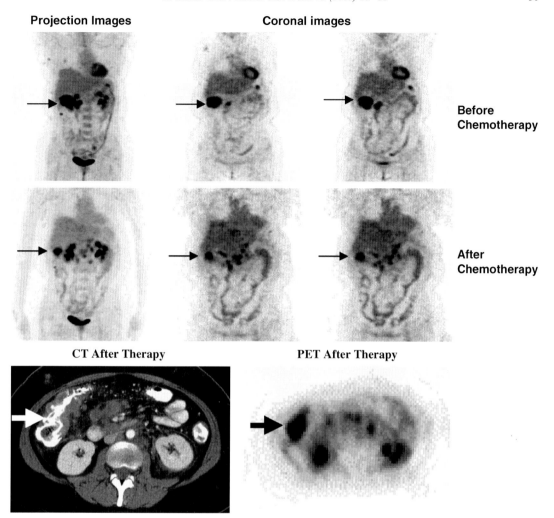

Fig. 8. This patient with malignant melanoma underwent two FDG-PET examinations, one before and the other after the chemotherapy. (*Top row*) On the baseline study, PET images showed a large focus with intense FDG uptake in the region of hepatic flexure of colon with irregular borders (*arrows*). (*Lower row*) After therapy, the repeat PET scan revealed interval development of new foci of intense FDG uptake in the celiac region (*arrows*). The intensity of FDG uptake in the region of the hepatic flexure has decreased compared with the prior scan, however. Abdominal CT with intravenous and oral contrast showed thickened hepatic flexors and multiple retroperitoneal mesenteric lymphadenopathies consistent with active disease following therapy.

upstaged and one third were downstaged). The PET findings resulted in intermodality management changes in 15 of 51 patients (29%) and intramodality management changes in 9 patients (18%). Mijnhout et al [33] assessed the clinical impact of FDG-PET in 58 consecutive patients with suspected recurrent melanoma. Diagnostic understanding and choice of therapy by referring physicians were evaluated before, directly after, and 6 months after PET. FDG-PET improved diagnostic understanding in 33 cases

(57%). In 6 patients (10%), diagnostic understanding was based solely on PET information. PET contributed to a positive change in planned treatment in 23 patients (40%) and increased confidence in the chosen treatment in 23 (40%). In patients who had undergone CT scans of the chest, abdomen, and pelvis and MR imaging of the brain, Gulec et al [37] identified more metastatic sites using FDG-PET in 27 of 49 patients (55%). In 6 of those 27 patients, PET detected disease outside the fields of CT and MR imaging. Among these 49 patients, 51 lesions were resected surgically. Forty-four of these lesions were pathologically confirmed to be melanoma. The results of PET led to treatment changes in 24 patients (49%).

Summary

FDG-PET is of limited use in patients with early-stage disease without nodal or distant metastases (stage I–II), because sentinel node biopsy is much more sensitive in detecting microscopic lymph node metastases. Because of the high tumor-to-background ratio, FDG-PET can highlight metastases at unusual sites that are easily missed with conventional imaging modalities. PET has been shown to have a strong role in detecting metastatic disease. FDG-PET is more sensitive than CT for detecting metastatic lesions in skin, lymph nodes, and abdomen, but CT is equivalent to or more sensitive than FDG-PET for detecting small pulmonary lesions. FDG-PET identifies the location and number of metastatic lesions in stage III and IV disease and therefore is important for surgical planning. Most of the false-negative FDG-PET results are caused by micrometastases and lesion smaller than 10 mm. Postsurgical inflammation, other inflammatory lesions, and some benign tumors cause some false-positive FDG-PET results.

References

[1] American Cancer Society. Cancer facts and figures 2002, American Cancer Society surveillance research. Available at: www.cancer.org. Accessed February 13, 2004.

[2] Balch CM, Soong SJ, Gershenwald JE, et al. Prognostic factor analysis of 17 600 melanoma patients: validation of the American Joint Committee on Cancer melanoma staging system. J Clin Oncol 2001;19: 3622–34.

[3] Meier F, Will S, Ellwanger U, et al. Metastatic pathways and time courses in the orderly progression of cutaneous melanoma. Br J Dermatol 2002;147:62–70.

[4] Vinnicombe SJ, Reznek RH. Computerised tomography in the staging of Hodgkin's disease and non-Hodgkin's lymphoma. Eur J Nucl Med Mol Imaging 2003;30(Suppl 1):S42–55.

[5] Wahl RL, Kaminski MS, Ethier SP, et al. The potential of 2-deoxy-2[18F]fluoro-D-glucose (FDG) for the detection of tumor involvement in lymph nodes. J Nucl Med 1990;31(11):1831–5.

[6] Gershenwald JE, Thompson W, Mansfield PF, et al. Multi-institutional melanoma lymphatic mapping experience: the prognostic value of sentinel lymph node status in 612 stage I or II melanoma patients. J Clin Oncol 1999;17:976–83.

[7] Topping A, Dewar D, Rose V, et al. Five years of sentinel node biopsy for melanoma: the St George's Melanoma Unit experience. Br J Plast Surg 2004; 57(2):97–104.

[8] Blessing C, Feine U, Geiger L, et al. Positron emission tomography and ultrasonography. A comparative retrospective study assessing the diagnostic validity in lymph node metastases of malignant melanoma. Arch Dermatol 1995;131(12):1394–8.

[9] Wagner JD, Schauwecker D, Hutchins G, et al. Initial assessment of positron emission tomography for detection of nonpalpable regional lymphatic metastases in melanoma. J Surg Oncol 1997;64(3):181–9.

[10] Macfarlane DJ, Sondak V, Johnson T, et al. Prospective evaluation of 2-[18F]-2-deoxy-D-glucose positron emission tomography in staging of regional lymph nodes in patients with cutaneous malignant melanoma. J Clin Oncol 1998;16(5):1770–6.

[11] Crippa F, Leutner M, Belli F, et al. Which kinds of lymph node metastases can FDG PET detect? A clinical study in melanoma. J Nucl Med 2000;41(9): 1491–4.

[12] Wagner JD, Schauwecker D, Davidson D, et al. Prospective study of fluorodeoxyglucose-positron emission tomography imaging of lymph node basins in melanoma patients undergoing sentinel node biopsy. J Clin Oncol 1999;17:1508–15.

[13] Acland KM, Healy C, Calonje E, et al. Comparison of positron emission tomography scanning and sentinel node biopsy in the detection of micrometastases of primary cutaneous melanoma. J Clin Oncol 2001;19: 2674–8.

[14] Havenga K, Cobben DC, Oyen WJ, et al. Fluorodeoxyglucose-positron emission tomography and sentinel lymph node biopsy in staging primary cutaneous melanoma. Eur J Surg Oncol 2003;29:662–4.

[15] Longo MI, Lazaro P, Bueno C, et al. Fluorodeoxyglucose-positron emission tomography imaging versus sentinel node biopsy in the primary staging of melanoma patients. Dermatol Surg 2003;29(3):245–8.

[16] Fink AM, Holle-Robatsch S, Herzog N, et al. Positron emission tomography is not useful in detecting metastasis in the sentinel lymph node in patients with primary malignant melanoma stage I and II. Melanoma Res 2004;14(2):141–5.

[17] Hafner J, Schmid MH, Kempf W, et al. Baseline staging in cutaneous malignant melanoma. Br J Dermatol 2004;150(4):677–86.

[18] Klein M, Freedman N, Lotem M, et al. Contribution of whole body F-18-FDG-PET and lymphoscintigraphy to the assessment of regional and distant metastases in cutaneous malignant melanoma: a pilot study. Nuklearmedizin 2000;39:56–61.

[19] Wagner JD, Schauwecker DS, Davidson D, et al. FDG-PET sensitivity for melanoma lymph node metastases is dependent on tumor volume. J Surg Oncol 2001;77: 237–42.

[20] Schwimmer J, Essner R, Patel A, et al. A review of the literature for whole-body FDG PET in the management of patients with melanoma. Q J Nucl Med 2000; 44:153–67.

[21] Krug B, Dietlein M, Groth W, et al. Fluor-18-fluorodeoxyglucose positron emission tomography (FDG-PET) in malignant melanoma. Diagnostic comparison with conventional imaging methods. Acta Radiol 2000;41(5):446–52.

[22] Rinne D, Baum RP, Hor G, et al. Primary staging and follow-up of high risk melanoma patients with whole-body 18F-fluorodeoxyglucose positron emission tomography: results of a prospective study of 100 patients. Cancer 1998;82(9):1664–71.

[23] Gritters LS, Francis IR, Zasadny KR, et al. Initial assessment of positron emission tomography using 2-fluorine-18-fluoro-2-deoxy-D-glucose in the imaging of malignant melanoma. J Nucl Med 1993;34(9): 1420–7.

[24] Steinert HC, Huch Boni RA, Buck A, et al. Malignant melanoma: staging with whole-body positron emission tomography and 2-[F-18]-fluoro-2-deoxy-D-glucose. Radiology 1995;195(3):705–9.

[25] Damian DL, Fulham MJ, Thompson E, et al. Positron emission tomography in the detection and management of metastatic melanoma. Melanoma Res 1996;6(4): 325–9.

[26] Holder Jr WD, White Jr RL, Zuger JH, et al. Effectiveness of positron emission tomography for the detection of melanoma metastases. Ann Surg 1998; 227(5):764–9.

[27] Eigtved A, Andersson AP, Dahlstrom K, et al. Use of fluorine-18 fluorodeoxyglucose positron emission tomography in the detection of silent metastases from malignant melanoma. Eur J Nucl Med 2000;27(1): 70–5.

[28] Tyler DS, Onaitis M, Kherani A, et al. Positron emission tomography scanning in malignant melanoma. Cancer 2000;89:1019–25.

[29] Acland KM, O'Doherty MJ, Russell-Jones R. The value of positron emission tomography scanning in the detection of subclinical metastatic melanoma. J Am Acad Dermatol 2000;42(4):606–11.

[30] Swetter SM, Carroll LA, Johnson DL, et al. Positron emission tomography is superior to computed tomography for metastatic detection in melanoma patients. Ann Surg Oncol 2002;9(7):646–53.

[31] Finkelstein SE, Carrasquillo JA, Hoffman JM, et al. A prospective analysis of positron emission tomography and conventional imaging for detection of stage IV metastatic melanoma in patients undergoing metastasectomy. Ann Surg Oncol 2004;11(8):731–8.

[32] Stas M, Stroobants S, Dupont P, et al. 18-FDG PET scan in the staging of recurrent melanoma: additional value and therapeutic impact. Melanoma Res 2002; 12(5):479–90.

[33] Mijnhout GS, Comans EF, Raijmakers P, et al. Reproducibility and clinical value of 18F-fluorodeoxyglucose positron emission tomography in recurrent melanoma. Nucl Med Commun 2002;23(5):475–81.

[34] Fuster D, Chiang S, Johnson G, et al. Is 18F-FDG PET more accurate than standard diagnostic procedures in the detection of suspected recurrent melanoma? J Nucl Med 2004;45(8):1323–7.

[35] Jadvar H, Johnson DL, Segall GM. The effect of fluorine-18 fluorodeoxyglucose positron emission tomography on the management of cutaneous malignant melanoma. Clin Nucl Med 2000;25(1):48–51.

[36] Wong C, Silverman DH, Seltzer M, et al. The impact of 2-deoxy-2[18F] fluoro-D-glucose whole body positron emission tomography for managing patients with melanoma: the referring physician's perspective. Mol Imaging Biol 2002;4(2):185–90.

[37] Gulec SA, Faries MB, Lee CC, et al. The role of fluorine-18 deoxyglucose positron emission tomography in the management of patients with metastatic melanoma: impact on surgical decision making. Clin Nucl Med 2003;28(12):961–5.

ELSEVIER
SAUNDERS

Radiol Clin N Am 43 (2005) 35 – 47

RADIOLOGIC
CLINICS
of North America

PET imaging for differentiating recurrent brain tumor from radiation necrosis

Roland Hustinx, MD[a],*, Michael Pourdehnad, BS[b], Bruno Kaschten, MD[c], Abass Alavi, MD[d]

[a]Division of Nuclear Medicine, University Hospital of Liège, Campus Universitaire du Sart Tilman,
B35 4000 Sart Tilman, Belgium
[b]Finch University of Health Science–Chicago Medical School, North Chicago, IL 60064, USA
[c]Department of Neurosurgery, University Hospital of Liège, Campus Universitaire du Sart Tilman,
B35 4000 Sart Tilman, Belgium
[d]Division of Nuclear Medicine, Department of Radiology, Hospital of the University of Pennsylvania, 110 Donner Building,
3400 Spruce Street, Philadelphia, PA 19104, USA

Brain tumors

In 2002, 17,000 patients in the United States were diagnosed with tumors of the central nervous system (CNS) [1]. The majority of these lesions occurred in the brain, because spinal cord locations represent only a small fraction of all CNS tumors. A wide variety of pathologic subtypes are represented, with gliomas accounting for 45% of all brain tumors. The World Health Organization (WHO) classification, revised in 1993, relies upon the cellular origin of the tumors [2]. Neuroepithelial tumors include astrocytomas, oligodendrogliomas, ependymomas, mixed gliomas, pineal tumors, choroids plexus tumors, and embryonal cell tumors. Other common tumors are meningiomas, pituitary tumors, nerve sheath tumors, and lymphomas. Astrocytomas are further classified according to specific pathologic criteria such as cell appearance, number of mitoses, vascular cell proliferation, and necrosis or presence of cell atypia. Low-grade astrocytomas include WHO grade I (pilocytic astrocytomas) and WHO grade II (astrocytomas) lesions. High-grade gliomas include WHO grade III (anaplastic astrocytomas) and WHO grade IV (glioblastoma multiforme) astrocytic tumors.

Treatment options greatly depend on the tumor type, its location, the age of the patient, and the symptoms [3]. Radiation therapy is frequently used, often in combination with surgery. For instance, high-grade gliomas are usually surgically resected, followed by involved-field radiotherapy. Low-grade gliomas are either resected (in a limited number of cases, because the lesions are large or involve critical regions of the brain) or receive radiation therapy. Treatment may be deferred in asymptomatic patients. Irradiation (stereotactic radiosurgery) is also part of therapeutic regimens for oligodendroglial tumors and, to some extent, for meningiomas. In all cases, radiation injuries are potential complications for which the diagnosis and management remain particularly challenging.

Radiation necrosis

Exposure of the brain to radiation may lead to injuries for which the severity and prognosis vary greatly (Table 1). Pathologic processes occurring after irradiation of the CNS in animal models are summarized in Table 2. Radiation damage to vascular endothelial cells and oligodendrocytes causes necrosis, axonal swelling, and reactive gliosis. Clinical manifestations can include personality changes, dementia, memory deficits, seizures, and motor im-

* Corresponding author.
E-mail address: rhustinx@chu.ulg.ac.be (R. Hustinx).

Table 1
Types of radiation injuries

Type of injury	Time interval after irradiation	Pathology	Prognosis
Acute	Hours to weeks	Tumor swelling	Good (reversible)
		Edema of the surrounding brain	
Early delayed	Weeks to months	Demyelination	Good (spontaneously reversible)
Late	Months to years	Liquefactive or coagulative necrosis	Usually irreversible
			Clinical severity variable

pairments. The term "radiation necrosis" has been loosely applied but should be reserved for the late-injury lesion in which necrosis actually occurs. The pattern of radiation necrosis may also vary, from diffuse, in which periventricular white matter is largely involved, to focal lesions that may be uni- or multifocal and localized in the vicinity of the tumor or occurring at distant sites [4,5]. The actual incidence of radiation necrosis is not well known. Few studies were performed in patients treated by irradiation only, and chemotherapy is known to increase the risk of radiation necrosis when both modalities are used. In addition, histopathologic proof of radiation necrosis, which is the only criterion standard, is not always available. The highest reported incidence of pathology-proven radiation necrosis is 24% [5,6]. In fact, irradiation protocols are constantly evolving to reduce the dose delivered to normal tissues while maintaining or even increasing the dose to the target lesion. Fractionation parameters and adaptation of the irradiated volume may decrease the incidence of radiation necrosis. Nevertheless, the stereotactic and intensity-modulated radiotherapy protocols currently used are still associated with this problem [7].

On MR imaging, edema, reactive gliosis, and radiation necrosis lesions appear as areas of increased signal intensity, best seen on the T2-weighted and fluid-attenuated inversion recovery sequences. Because of the disruption of the blood–brain barrier,

contrast enhancement is usually present on both MR imaging and CT. Therefore the appearances of radiation necrosis and of tumor regrowth are quite similar, and these entities cannot be distinguished based on CT or MR imaging alone. Dynamic susceptibility contrast MR imaging [8,9] and magnetic resonance spectroscopy [10,11] have been proposed with encouraging results, but definite data are lacking, and in most institutions these techniques are not used in routine clinical practice.

Fluorodeoxyglucose-PET imaging

Diagnosis of radiation necrosis/tumor recurrence

The rationale for using fluorodeoxyglucose-PET (FDG-PET) in differentiating radiation necrosis from tumor regrowth relies on the observation that the former shows decreased FDG uptake, whereas the later displays increased metabolism (Figs. 1–4). Such observations were first reported by Patronas et al [12] in 1982. Among five patients with similar clinical and CT presentations, two had radiation necrosis, and three had recurrent tumors. All were correctly identified by PET and confirmed at pathology. This initial report already poses an important methodologic question that is frequently encountered when analyzing the diagnostic performances of FDG-PET in this indication. Radiation necrosis was described as

Table 2
Time-course of the pathologic changes after irradiation of the central nervous system in animal models

Change	Hours	3–7 d	2 wk	4 wk	17 wk	24 wk
Vascular changes	Vasodilation	Edema	Vasoconstriction	Decreased permeability	Increased permeability, ischemia, hypoxia	Necrosis
Glial proliferation	Apoptosis	First inhibited then activated	Highly increased (peak)	Decreased	Increased (second phase)	

Data from Nieder C, Andratschke N, Price RE, et al. Innovative prevention strategies for radiation necrosis of the central nervous system. Anticancer Res 2002;22(2A):1017–23; and Shields AF. PET imaging with 18F-FLT and thymidine analogs: promise and pitfalls. J Nucl Med 2003;44(9):1432–4.

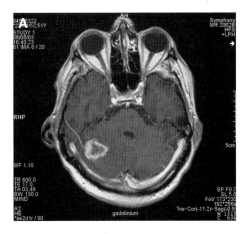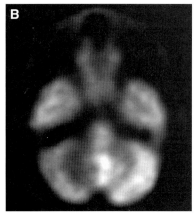

Fig. 1. Right cerebellar metastasis from a non–small cell lung cancer, treated by radiosurgery 2 years ago. T1-weighted MR imaging shows a right cerebellar necrotic lesion, with peripheral contrast enhancement and very limited edema. (*A*) FDG-PET shows an area of decreased uptake in the corresponding area, consistent with the diagnosis of radiation necrosis. (*B*) MR imaging remained unchanged 6 months later, without any treatment.

a cold spot as compared with adjacent cortex, and recurrent tumors were described as hot spots. The activity ratio, however, was 1.18 in a benign lesion and 1.25 in a tumor. It seems unlikely that lesions within such a limited range of FDG uptake could be differentiated as cold and hot. Metabolic rates were of no help, because there was a large overlap between the two types of lesion. Therefore the criteria used for positive and negative results remain an issue that is not yet fully resolved. Another concern raised by this initial presentation relates to the criterion standard. Although all five lesions were verified at pathology, only the initial diagnosis was given, including four low-grade gliomas that usually exhibit low metabolic rates. It is thus important to mention relevant pathologic results to assess the diagnostic performances of the test accurately, with regards to both the initial and the recurrent tumors (eg, biopsy soon after imaging). In the three cases reported by Patronas et al, the possibility that the recurrent tumors corresponded in fact to malignant transformation of astrocytomas must be considered.

Nevertheless, this initial report was highly encouraging and was further confirmed by larger series. Investigators from the same institution evaluated 95 patients with gliomas or brain metastases and found perfect sensitivity and specificity (both 100%) [13]. Doyle et al [14] reported 100% sensitivity and specificity in nine patients with high-grade tumors. The ratio of lesion to adjacent cortex activity ranged from 0.47 to 0.98 in radiation necrosis, as compared with 1.1 to 1.22 in recurrent tumors. The same group further studied 38 patients and found 81% sensitivity

with 88% specificity [15]. In this series, all patients also underwent rubidium-82–PET studies to localize the blood–brain barrier lesions, which were then coregistered with the FDG studies. This coregistration helped the authors identify and characterize lesions that may be difficult to delineate precisely from normal cortex. The regions of interest were visually analyzed and described as recurrent tumors when the activity was equal to or higher than that in the adjacent normal cortex. In a series of 35 patients, Davis et al [16] found a high concordance between gadolinium diethylenetriaminepentaacetic acid–enhancement on MR imaging and increased FDG uptake (defined as uptake higher than the uptake in the normal white matter) on PET. Most lesions were recurrent high-grade tumors, and there were three false-positive results with both PET and MR imaging. The false positives included two meningiomas, which are low-grade lesions, and one radiation necrosis. Kim et al [17] reported high sensitivity (80%) and specificity (93%) in 33 patients with various tumors. The same group found a 75% concordance between PET findings and pathologic analysis in a subgroup of 20 patients. The five patients misdiagnosed with PET had all previously undergone intensive radiotherapy, which prompted the authors to suggest that PET may not be suited for evaluating patients treated with such protocol. In this study the specificity was only 63%, with three false-positive results (the other two misdiagnoses were false negatives) [18]. The PET images were visually analyzed and deemed positive when the uptake was increased when compared with adjacent area or contralateral hemisphere.

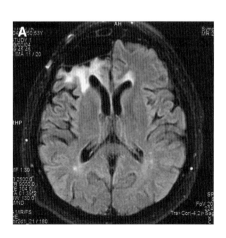
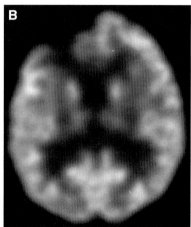
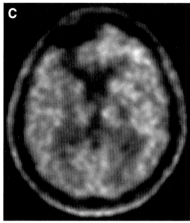

Fig. 2. Right frontal oligodendroglioma (WHO grade III) treated 2 years previously by surgery and radiotherapy. (*A*) T2-weighted MR imaging shows a hyperintense signal just behind the surgical site of resection. PET shows no uptake of FDG (*B*) or F-TYR (*C*) in this region, suggesting postradiation changes. A 9-month follow-up was negative.

The specificity was even lower in a study by Kahn et al [19], who compared 21 FDG-PET and thallium-201–single photon emission CT (^{201}Tl-SPECT) studies performed in 20 patients. Only two of five radiation necroses were correctly identified, and the observers disagreed on the interpretation of 24% of the PET studies. This disagreement further emphasizes the need for objective parameters to assess the metabolic activity of these lesions.

The diagnostic value of FDG-PET for differentiating radiation necrosis from recurrent tumors was questioned by several groups. Ricci et al [20] found a sensitivity of 73% and a specificity of 56% in 31 patients with a pathology-proven final diagnosis. These results were obtained using a semiquantitative visual score, according to which only lesions with uptake equal to or higher than the uptake in the cortex were considered as positive. Most recurrent tumors were high-grade lesions. Even though this study was subject to selection bias, because patients with negative PET findings are less likely to undergo surgical confirmation of their status, the negative predictive value was low: only 45% (5 of 11) of the hypometabolic areas correctly characterized the MR anomalies (ie, corresponded to radiation necrosis). Other studies questioned the sensitivity of the technique. In a limited series (15 patients), the sensitivity was only 43% (6 of 14 patients) and was a clearly function of the size of the lesion according to MR imaging: 75% of the lesions smaller than 6 cm^3 were missed by PET [21]. Nothing is said in this retrospective study regarding the methodology used for reading the PET studies, and this omission greatly limits the study's scientific value. FDG-PET was both

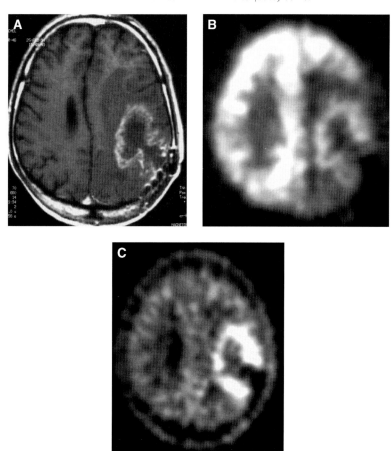

Fig. 3. Left fronto-parietal glioblastoma treated by surgery and radiotherapy 5 months previously. (*A*) T1-weighted MR imaging shows a rim on contrast enhancement around the operative cavity. PET shows increased uptake of both FDG (*B*) and MET (*C*), indicating tumor recurrence, which was confirmed by a second surgery. Note that the contrast between the tumor and normal cortex is much higher on the MET image than on the FDG study.

insensitive (one third of recurrences were detected) and nonspecific (uptake was increased in six of eight negative cases) in patients evaluated after stereotactic radiosurgery [22]. This series, however, was heterogeneous for tumor histology and lacked surgical confirmation, and once again, the methodology used for image analysis was poorly defined.

Other investigators emphasized the complementary use of physiologic and morphologic information from FDG-PET and MR imaging, respectively, in evaluating the results of stereotactic radiosurgery. In a series of 44 lesions, FDG-PET had a sensitivity of 75% (21 of 28) and a specificity of 81% (13 of 16) [23]. Diagnostic performances were better in patients with gliomas (n = 8, 86% sensitivity, 100% specificity) than in those with metastases (n = 36; sensitivity 71%, specificity 80%). Moreover, in the subjects with

metastases, the sensitivity of PET alone was 65% but reached 86% when MR imaging and PET images were coregistered. Specificity remained unchanged at 80%. The authors emphasized sensitivity when reading the PET studies, because any area of uptake higher than the uptake in the adjacent white/gray matter was considered as suspicious, as was any FDG uptake in a region showing contrast enhancement on the coregistered MR images. Even so, the specificity remained fairly good (greater than 80%) in all subgroups of patients. Belohlavek et al [24] compared FDG-PET and MR imaging in 25 patients with a total of 57 brain metastases treated by stereotactic radiosurgery with the Leksell gamma knife (Elekta Instruments, Norcross, Georgia). They found PET to be useful in the group of patients with positive or nondiagnostic MR imaging. Sensitivity was better for

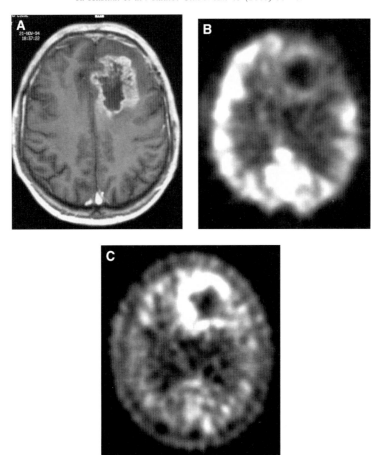

Fig. 4. Left frontal glioblastoma treated 5 months previously by surgery and radiotherapy. (*A*) T1-weighted MR imaging shows a left frontal lesion with a necrotic center and peripheral gadolinium enhancement, consistent with either tumor recurrence or radiation necrosis. PET shows mild uptake of FDG (*B*) and a very high uptake of MET (*C*), indicating a tumor recurrence. Tumor recurrence was confirmed by subsequent surgery.

MR imaging (100%) than for PET (75%), but only eight lesions progressed over a mean follow-up of 26 weeks, and only the foci with FDG uptake higher than the uptake in normal gray matter were considered positive, factors that promote specificity. Conversely, both the specificity and the accuracy were higher with PET (94% and 91%, respectively) than with MR imaging (65% and 70%, respectively).

Prognosis

The ability of FDG-PET to predict survival in patients with brain tumors, in particular those with gliomas, was demonstrated early on [25,26] and was recently confirmed in a large population [27]. Such ability was also shown in patients with suspected recurrent tumors and has prompted Di Chiro and

Fulham [28] to propose FDG-PET as a clinical criterion standard, actually better than pathology for predicting a patient's fate. Given the low specificity of even the most modern anatomic imaging techniques, the invasiveness of biopsy procedures (which are also subject to sampling errors and are difficult to interpret because of the tumor heterogeneity), and the changes over time in the histologic nature of gliomas (most low-grade tumors eventually transform into malignant lesions), there may indeed be an important role for metabolic imaging methods.

Patronas et al [29] evaluated 45 patients with malignant gliomas treated by various combinations of surgery, irradiation, or chemotherapy. All had CT findings suggestive of recurrent/persistent tumor. Those with a low FDG uptake (activity ratio with the opposite brain <1) had a mean survival of

19 months, as compared with 5 months in lesions with high FDG uptake. Similar results were obtained in a more recent study using MR imaging anomalies consistent with tumor recurrence as an inclusion criterion [30]. All 55 patients had a previous history of high-grade glioma and were treated with various schemes that included radiation therapy. FDG-PET was an independent predictive factor in multivariate analysis. Median survival was 10 months in patients with lesions showing FDG uptake greater than or equal to the uptake in the adjacent cortex, whereas it was 20 months in patients with a lower uptake. The intensity of FDG uptake also had a strong predictive value in patients with brain metastases treated by stereotactic irradiation [24,31,32].

It is common to note areas of cortical and other gray matter hypometabolism both adjacent to and distant from the tumor sites (Fig. 5). There is much controversy about the cause of this observation. Some investigators have attributed this phenomenon to radiation necrosis and therefore consider it an irreversible complication of treatment. The authors of this article have noted that, significant evidence for white matter edema adjacent to the sites of hypometabolism on PET images can be demonstrated on MR or CT images [33]. Edema, which is associated with acute and early-delayed radiation injury as well as with breakdown in the blood–brain barrier caused by tumor itself, therefore seems to play a major role in the pathology seen in patients with brain tumors. On the other hand, the authors found that radiation necrosis correlated to less extensive areas of cortical suppression. Recently they were able to reproduce similar data in a larger series of patients [34]. The data generated included quantitative correlation between the extent of edema as demonstrated by MR imaging and the degree of hypometabolism as assessed by PET images.

Because there is a clear correlation between the presence of edema and hypometabolism in the adjacent cortex and other gray matter structures, this phenomenon seems to be reversible and does not indicate permanent damage to the cortex as a result of radiation necrosis. The cause of such a decline in cortical function is unclear. These findings may be secondary to edema causing both mass effect and direct toxicity to axons, blood vessel damage from radiation (particularly in areas which lack collaterals), or deafferentation. The authors believe that edema is the causative factor in most patients.

Implications of this hypometabolism and resulting dysfunction are significant and should be taken into consideration in interpreting these scans, particularly when the edema extends to the visual cortex (Fig. 5).

This edema usually results in significant loss of function in the affected visual cortex, and therefore homonymous hemianopsia is a serious consequence of this complication. Often the edema is previously undiagnosed, and the observation made on PET is subsequently confirmed by clinical examination of the visual field. Dysfunction in the rest of the affected brain also correlates with clinical findings in these patients.

FDG uptake is commonly significantly decreased in the contralateral cerebellum. This cerebellar diaschisis is caused by the loss of function of the affected neurons that connect the cortical structures to the contralateral side (Fig. 6) [35]. This decreased uptake is seen with many supratentorial disorders, regardless of cause, including stroke and head injury. The impact of such information on patient management has not yet been elucidated. PET may be prognostic for brain injury from radiation as well as for tumor recurrence and progression.

Even though the initial studies were published 20 years ago, few data are available about the impact of FDG-PET on patient management. Evaluating the clinical impact of a new imaging technique is a challenging task. The choice of the methodology (eg, prospective, randomized studies or cost-effectiveness modeling) remains highly controversial. This evaluation becomes particularly difficult when the tumor to be studied is relatively infrequent and is highly heterogeneous with a wide variety of pathologic subtypes. Some authors found the usefulness of PET to be limited, either because MR imaging performed well, as reported by Olivero et al [36] in an heterogeneous series of 39 patients, or simply because of the high concordance rate between MR imaging and PET [16]. In a series of 75 patients with gliomas, in which the majority (87%) of the cases were evaluated for tumor recurrence versus radiation necrosis, FDG-PET helped define the therapeutic approach in 90% of the cases [16]. Treatment was initiated in 31% and withheld in 59% of the cases. The therapeutic decision was based on PET results alone in 28% of the patients, a percentage that is rather high for a single test and will vary depending on experience. In a series of 50 patients with suspected tumor progression, PET findings had a major impact on the treatment of the patients who did not undergo surgical confirmation of the diagnosis [37]. Treatment was changed in 14 of 30 cases (47%), and PET contributed to the management in 24 of 30 cases (80%).

No study, however, has been specifically designed to evaluate the impact of FDG-PET in patients with suspected tumor recurrence in a fashion that would

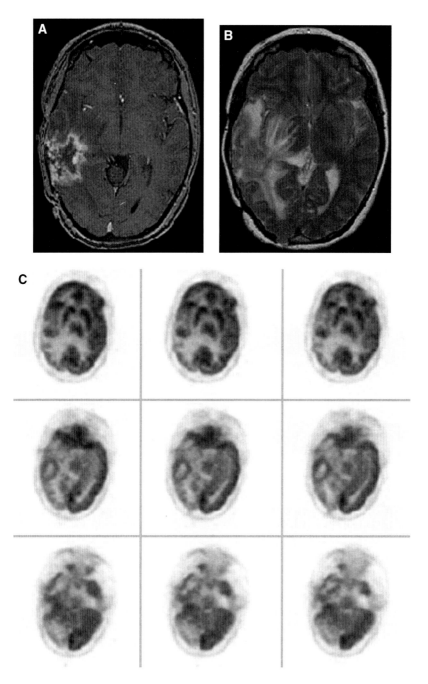

Fig. 5. Anaplastic astrocytoma grade 3 brain tumor treated with radiation, then removed surgically. Following surgery, the patient received another course of radiation therapy and subsequent chemotherapy. (*A*) Contrast-enhanced T1-weighted image demonstrates a donut-shaped area of enhancement located in the right temporal lobe. (*B*) T2-weighted image reveals significant edema, which seems to involve most of the right hemisphere extending to the visual cortex. (*C*) Corresponding FDG-PET images demonstrate a metabolically active tumor corresponding to the areas of enhancement in shape and size. In addition, the entire cortex and the adjacent gray matter structures appear hypometabolic. Note the loss of function in the ipsilateral visual cortex, which frequently is associated with homonymous hemianopsia.

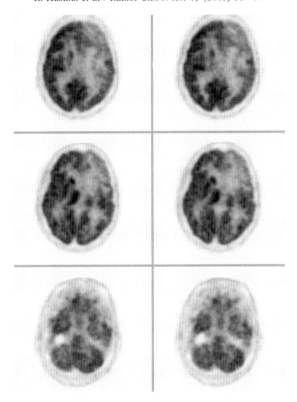

Fig. 6. Patient with anaplastic astrocytoma after resection. FDG-PET images demonstrate tumor recurrence in left frontal lobe with decreased metabolism in the ipsilateral adjacent cortex, ipsilateral basal ganglia, and the contralateral cerebellum. This figure is an example of commonly seen cerebellar diaschisis.

be fully acceptable by the standards of evidence-based medicine.

PET imaging with alternative tracers

Considering the mechanisms of the FDG uptake, the encouraging results reported here could seem quite surprising. Both sensitivity and specificity are indeed a concern from a theoretic perspective. The high, and highly variable, uptake by normal cortex makes it difficult to distinguish tumors from adjacent normal gray matter, especially when no significant edema surrounds the lesion. In addition, low-grade gliomas usually appear as hypometabolic when compared with normal cortex [38], limiting the potential of FDG-PET for detecting such recurrent lesions. Most patients evaluated in the various studies cited in the previous paragraphs suffered from either high-grade lesions or brain metastases. On the other hand, various non-neoplastic diseases that also dis-

play increased glucose metabolism are potential sources of false-positive results. For instance, brain abscesses can show increased FDG uptake [39,40]. Extremely high levels of uptake have also been reported in radiation necrosis, as Fischman et al [41], who observed the activity rations of lesion to gray matter and lesion to white matter to be 1.37 and 4.40, respectively, in a lesion totally devoid of tumor cells. In this case pathology revealed the presence of extensive reactive gliosis with limited foci of necrosis and chronic inflammation. Ricci and colleagues [20] also reported that 88% of their cases with radiation necrosis demonstrated increased FDG uptake. In some cases, recognition of a specific pattern of uptake may help identifying the lesions. For example, a rimlike uptake after intracavitary administration of radiolabeled antibodies as a treatment for primary brain tumor has been described independently of the presence of residual tumor cells [42]. Such a pattern was in fact related to macrophage infiltration, and only nodular uptake was associated with tumor recurrence. Because of these factors, no study has proved that quantitative methods are better than visual interpretation by the physician.

In many cases, however, discriminating tumor relapse from radiation necrosis is difficult based on FDG-PET alone. Although coregistering the PET and MR imaging or CT images is helpful, coregistration cannot be performed in all cases and does not solve all problems. There could thus be a role for a tracer that would show both increased tumor-to-background contrast and limited nonspecific uptake. Among these, amino acid analogues have been most widely investigated.

Radiolabeled amino acid analogues

Carbon-11–methyl-methionine ([11C]-MET) has been widely used for evaluating primary brain tumors, guiding stereotactic biopsies, or assessing prognosis [43–46]. To a large extent, the intensity of MET uptake is related to the grade of the tumor [43,47,48], but the uptake by the normal cortex is low, and most low-grade tumors are easily detected. Compared with FDG, MET allows a much better tumor delineation (see Figs. 3 and 4). Animal studies suggested a lower accumulation in inflammatory cells [49,50], but more recent studies as well as clinical studies in humans do not firmly establish any superiority of MET over FDG for tumor specificity [51,52]. In the particular setting of postradiation evaluation, animal experiments suggested that MET, and radiolabeled thymidine as well, perform better than FDG for detecting residual tumor after fractionated irradiation [53]. Although MET uptake reflects the level of amino acid transport and, to a lesser extent, protein synthesis, it is also highly affected by disruption of the blood–brain barrier, which may limit its value for evaluating contrast-enhancing lesions [54]. The major limitation of MET is the short physical half-life of the isotope, which prevents its use in centers without an on-site cyclotron.

MET has been available for 2 decades, but few studies were published regarding its performance for differentiating radiation necrosis from brain tumor recurrence. Ogawa et al [55] studied 15 patients with both FDG-PET and MET-PET. They found that all hypometabolic lesions on the FDG scan were radiation injury except for a false negative in one case of recurrent tumor. MET uptake was similar to the cortex background in radiation injuries, and it was increased in tumors. The authors conclude that the combination of both tracers could improve the overall diagnostic accuracy. Sonoda et al [56] compared MET-PET and 201Tl-SPECT in 12 patients, including five recurrent gliomas and seven radiation necroses.

MET-PET provided the accurate diagnosis in 11 of 12 cases (8 of 12 for 201Tl-SPECT), with five true-positive results and only one false-positive result. More recently, Tsuyuguchi et al [57] studied 21 patients with brain metastases treated by stereotactic radiosurgery. All had suspicious findings on MR studies. Nine patients had recurrent disease (all confirmed by pathologic examination), and 12 had radiation necrosis (based on follow-up in 10 of 12 cases). When analyzed visually, MET studies correctly identified seven of nine recurrences and 10 of 12 radiation injuries. Semiquantitative scores improved the diagnostic accuracy: a cut-off of 1.42 for the target-to-cortex activity ratios yielded 78% sensitivity and 100% and specificity. The activity ratios were more accurate than the standardized uptake values. MET-PET was also useful in a series of 10 patients with brain lymphoma evaluated after radiation therapy [58]. As reported for evaluating brain lesions before treatment [59], the combination of MET and FDG-PET studies is in fact probably superior to each test performed separately for evaluating posttherapeutic changes as well.

Other tracers have been proposed, such as 11C-tyrosine [60] or 1-aminocyclobutane-1- [11C]-carboxylic acid [61], but clinical results are scarce, and these compounds are limited by their short half-life.

The development of fluorinated amino acid analogues is a promising phenomenon: because of their more favorable half-life, such tracers could be made widely available and used in various indications. Among these, 2-(fluorine-18 [18F])fluoro-L-tyrosine (F-TYR) can be synthesized with both high yield and high specific activity [62]. It has been shown to accumulate in primary brain tumors, with a low uptake in the normal cortex [63]. In Liège, F-TYR has completely replaced MET and is used along with FDG, with similar clinical results. After a 30-minute uptake period, the activity ratios between tumors or foci of radiation necrosis and normal cortex are similar to those observed with MET. Other fluorinated compounds that could replace MET include O-(2-[18F]fluoroethyl)-L-tyrosine (FET) [64], 3,4-dihydroxy-6-[18F]fluoro-phenylalanine (FDOPA) [65], and 3-O-methyl-6-[18F]fluoro-L-DOPA (OMFD) [66].

Other tracers

3′-Deoxy-3′-[18F]fluorothymidine (FLT) is a proliferation marker [67], and it does not cross the blood–brain barrier. It has a high potential for imaging in this setting by taking advantage of tumor-associated breakdown in the blood–brain barrier

[68], although there is no report in the literature yet. Choline analogues labeled with ^{18}F or ^{11}C have also been tested in patients with brain tumors, with encouraging results [69,70]. These compounds have generated a great interest, but no superiority to FDG and MET has yet been demonstrated.

Summary

The exact incidence of true radiation necrosis is largely unknown. It is probably much less frequent than indicated by MR or CT findings. Differentiating radiation necrosis from recurrent tumor is a diagnostic challenge, however, and has important implications for the patient's management. Even though the first results were published 20 years ago, the total number of case studies using FDG-PET in this indication remains limited. Several reports are also hampered by methodologic limitations. The technique has been largely criticized, notably in articles that themselves were not completely free of methodological flaws. Overall however, FDG-PET seems to be a valuable clinical tool. As a general rule, suspicious lesions on MR imaging that show increased FDG uptake (ie, uptake equal to or great than that in normal cortex) are likely to represent tumor recurrence. Sensitivity is an issue, especially but not exclusively with low-grade gliomas. Although false-positive results may occur, specificity is usually high in routine clinical practice. Coregistration with MR imaging surely improves the diagnostic performances of FDG-PET because it helps delineate the suspicious area. Another important aspect is the prognostic value of FDG uptake, which is now well established. It seems clear that only the combination of FDG with a radiolabeled amino acid analogue (MET or a more recent fluorinated compound) can provide a comprehensive characterization of suspected brain tumor recurrence.

References

[1] Cancer facts and figures 2002. New York: American Cancer Society; 2002. p. 5.

[2] Smirniotopoulos JG. The new WHO classification of brain tumors. Neuroimaging Clin N Am 1999;9(4): 595–613.

[3] DeAngelis LM. Brain tumors. N Engl J Med 2001; 344(2):114–23.

[4] Plowman PN. Stereotactic radiosurgery. VIII. The classification of postradiation reactions. Br J Neurosurg 1999;13(3):256–64.

[5] Giglio P, Gilbert MR. Cerebral radiation necrosis. Neurologist 2003;9(4):180–8.

[6] Kumar AJ, Leeds NE, Fuller GN, et al. Malignant gliomas: MR imaging spectrum of radiation therapy- and chemotherapy-induced necrosis of the brain after treatment. Radiology 2000;217(2):377–84.

[7] Nieder C, Andratschke N, Price RE, et al. Innovative prevention strategies for radiation necrosis of the central nervous system. Anticancer Res 2002;22(2A): 1017–23.

[8] Aronen HJ, Perkio J. Dynamic susceptibility contrast MRI of gliomas. Neuroimaging Clin N Am 2002; 12(4):501–23.

[9] Wenz F, Rempp K, Hess T, et al. Effect of radiation on blood volume in low-grade astrocytomas and normal brain tissue: quantification with dynamic susceptibility contrast MR imaging. AJR Am J Roentgenol 1996; 166(1):187–93.

[10] Schlemmer HP, Bachert P, Herfarth KK, et al. Proton MR spectroscopic evaluation of suspicious brain lesions after stereotactic radiotherapy. AJNR Am J Neuroradiol 2001;22(7):1316–24.

[11] Rock JP, Hearshen D, Scarpace L, et al. Correlations between magnetic resonance spectroscopy and image-guided histopathology, with special attention to radiation necrosis. Neurosurgery 2002;51(4):912–9 [discussion: 919–20].

[12] Patronas NJ, Di Chiro G, Brooks RA, et al. Work in progress: [18F] fluorodeoxyglucose and positron emission tomography in the evaluation of radiation necrosis of the brain. Radiology 1982;144(4):885–9.

[13] Di Chiro G, Oldfield E, Wright DC, et al. Cerebral necrosis after radiotherapy and/or intraarterial chemotherapy for brain tumors: PET and neuropathologic studies. AJR Am J Roentgenol 1988;150(1):189–97.

[14] Doyle WK, Budinger TF, Valk PE, et al. Differentiation of cerebral radiation necrosis from tumor recurrence by [18F]FDG and 82Rb positron emission tomography. J Comput Assist Tomogr 1987;11(4): 563–70.

[15] Valk PE, Budinger TF, Levin VA, et al. PET of malignant cerebral tumors after interstitial brachytherapy. Demonstration of metabolic activity and correlation with clinical outcome. J Neurosurg 1988;69(6): 830–8.

[16] Davis WK, Boyko OB, Hoffman JM, et al. [18F]2-fluoro-2-deoxyglucose-positron emission tomography correlation of gadolinium-enhanced MR imaging of central nervous system neoplasia. AJNR Am J Neuroradiol 1993;14(3):515–23.

[17] Kim EE, Chung SK, Haynie TP, et al. Differentiation of residual or recurrent tumors from post-treatment changes with F-18 FDG PET. Radiographics 1992; 12(2):269–79.

[18] Janus TJ, Kim EE, Tilbury R, et al. Use of [18F]fluorodeoxyglucose positron emission tomography in patients with primary malignant brain tumors. Ann Neurol 1993;33(5):540–8.

[19] Kahn D, Follett KA, Bushnell DL, et al. Diagnosis of

recurrent brain tumor: value of 201Tl SPECT vs 18F-fluorodeoxyglucose PET. AJR Am J Roentgenol 1994;163(6):1459–65.

[20] Ricci PE, Karis JP, Heiserman JE, et al. Differentiating recurrent tumor from radiation necrosis: time for re-evaluation of positron emission tomography? AJNR Am J Neuroradiol 1998;19(3):407–13.

[21] Thompson TP, Lunsford LD, Kondziolka D. Distinguishing recurrent tumor and radiation necrosis with positron emission tomography versus stereotactic biopsy. Stereotact Funct Neurosurg 1999;73(1–4):9–14.

[22] Ross DA, Sandler HM, Balter JM, et al. Imaging changes after stereotactic radiosurgery of primary and secondary malignant brain tumors. J Neurooncol 2002;56(2):175–81.

[23] Chao ST, Suh JH, Raja S, et al. The sensitivity and specificity of FDG PET in distinguishing recurrent brain tumor from radionecrosis in patients treated with stereotactic radiosurgery. Int J Cancer 2001;96(3):191–7.

[24] Belohlavek O, Simonova G, Kantorova I, et al. Brain metastases after stereotactic radiosurgery using the Leksell gamma knife: can FDG PET help to differentiate radionecrosis from tumour progression? Eur J Nucl Med Mol Imaging 2003;30(1):96–100.

[25] Di Chiro G. Positron emission tomography using [18F] fluorodeoxyglucose in brain tumors. A powerful diagnostic and prognostic tool. Invest Radiol 1987;22(5):360–71.

[26] Alavi JB, Alavi A, Chawluk J, et al. Positron emission tomography in patients with glioma. A predictor of prognosis. Cancer 1988;62(6):1074–8.

[27] Padma MV, Said S, Jacobs M, et al. Prediction of pathology and survival by FDG PET in gliomas. J Neurooncol 2003;64(3):227–37.

[28] Di Chiro G, Fulham MJ. Virchow's shackles: can PET-FDG challenge tumor histology? AJNR Am J Neuroradiol 1993;14(3):524–7.

[29] Patronas NJ, Di Chiro G, Kufta C, et al. Prediction of survival in glioma patients by means of positron emission tomography. J Neurosurg 1985;62(6):816–22.

[30] Barker II FG, Chang SM, Valk PE, et al. 18-Fluorodeoxyglucose uptake and survival of patients with suspected recurrent malignant glioma. Cancer 1997;79(1):115–26.

[31] Mogard J, Kihlstrom L, Ericson K, et al. Recurrent tumor vs radiation effects after gamma knife radiosurgery of intracerebral metastases: diagnosis with PET-FDG. J Comput Assist Tomogr 1994;18(2):177–81.

[32] Ericson K, Kihlstrom L, Mogard J, et al. Positron emission tomography using 18F-fluorodeoxyglucose in patients with stereotactically irradiated brain metastases. Stereotact Funct Neurosurg 1996;66(Suppl 1):214–24.

[33] Powe JE, Alavi JB, Alavi A, et al. Cerebral metabolic changes in patients with brain tumors demonstrated by positron emission tomography. J Neuroimag 1992;2:1–7.

[34] Pourdehnad M, Duarte P, Okpaku AS, et al. Adverse effects of edema on adjacent gray matter function in patients with brain tumor as determined by FDG-PET imaging [abstract]. J Nucl Med 1999;40(5 Suppl S 453):112P.

[35] Kushner M, Alavi A, Reivich M, et al. Contralateral cerebellar hypometabolism following cerebral insult. Ann Neurol 1984;15(5):425–34.

[36] Olivero WC, Dulebohn SC, Lister JR. The use of PET in evaluating patients with primary brain tumours: is it useful? J Neurol Neurosurg Psychiatry 1995;58(2):250–2.

[37] Janus TJ, Kim EE, Tilbury R, et al. Use of [18F]fluorodeoxyglucose positron emission tomography in patients with primary malignant brain tumors. Ann Neurol 1993;33(5):540–8.

[38] Kim CK, Alavi JB, Alavi A, et al. New grading system of cerebral gliomas using positron emission tomography with F-18 fluorodeoxyglucose. J Neurooncol 1991;10(1):85–91.

[39] Meyer MA, Frey KA, Schwaiger M. Discordance between F-18 fluorodeoxyglucose uptake and contrast enhancement in a brain abscess. Clin Nucl Med 1993;18(8):682–4.

[40] Sasaki M, Ichiya Y, Kuwabara Y, et al. Ringlike uptake of [18F]FDG in brain abscess: a PET study. J Comput Assist Tomogr 1990;14(3):486–7.

[41] Fischman AJ, Thornton AF, Frosch MP, et al. FDG hypermetabolism associated with inflammatory necrotic changes following radiation of meningioma. J Nucl Med 1997;38(7):1027–9.

[42] Marriott CJ, Thorstad W, Akabani G, et al. Locally increased uptake of fluorine-18-fluorodeoxyglucose after intracavitary administration of iodine-131-labeled antibody for primary brain tumors. J Nucl Med 1998;39(8):1376–80.

[43] Kameyama M, Shirane R, Itoh J, et al. The accumulation of 11C-methionine in cerebral glioma patients studied with PET. Acta Neurochir (Wien) 1990;104(1–2):8–12.

[44] Derlon JM, Bourdet C, Bustany P, et al. [11C]L-methionine uptake in gliomas. Neurosurgery 1989;25(5):720–8.

[45] Pirotte B, Goldman S, David P, et al. Stereotactic brain biopsy guided by positron emission tomography (PET) with [F-18]fluorodeoxyglucose and [C-11] methionine. Acta Neurochir Suppl (Wien) 1997;68:133–8.

[46] De Witte O, Goldberg I, Wikler D, et al. Positron emission tomography with injection of methionine as a prognostic factor in glioma. J Neurosurg 2001;95(5):746–50.

[47] Bustany P, Chatel M, Derlon JM, et al. Brain tumor protein synthesis and histological grades: a study by positron emission tomography (PET) with C11-L-Methionine. J Neurooncol 1986;3(4):397–404.

[48] Kaschten B, Stevenaert A, Sadzot B, et al. Preoperative evaluation of 54 gliomas by PET with fluorine-18-fluorodeoxyglucose and/or carbon-11-methionine. J Nucl Med 1998;39(5):778–85.

[49] Kubota K, Kubota R, Yamada S, et al. Effects of radiotherapy on the cellular uptake of carbon-14 labeled L-methionine in tumor tissue. Nucl Med Biol 1995;22(2):193–8.

[50] Kubota R, Kubota K, Yamada S, et al. Methionine uptake by tumor tissue: a microautoradiographic comparison with FDG. J Nucl Med 1995;36(3): 484–92.

[51] Rau FC, Weber WA, Wester HJ, et al. *O*-(2-[18F]fluoroethyl)-L-tyrosine (FET): a tracer for differentiation of tumour from inflammation in murine lymph nodes. Eur J Nucl Med 2002;29(8):1039–46.

[52] Nettelbladt OS, Sundin AE, Valind SO, et al. Combined fluorine-18-FDG and carbon-11-methionine PET for diagnosis of tumors in lung and mediastinum. J Nucl Med 1998;39(4):640–7.

[53] Reinhardt MJ, Kubota K, Yamada S, et al. Assessment of cancer recurrence in residual tumors after fractionated radiotherapy: a comparison of fluorodeoxyglucose, L-methionine and thymidine. J Nucl Med 1997; 38(2):280–7.

[54] Roelcke U, Radu EW, von Ammon K, et al. Alteration of blood-brain barrier in human brain tumors: comparison of [18F]fluorodeoxyglucose, [11C]methionine and rubidium-82 using PET. J Neurol Sci 1995; 132(1):20–7.

[55] Ogawa T, Kanno I, Shishido F, et al. Clinical value of PET with 18F-fluorodeoxyglucose and L-methyl-11C-methionine for diagnosis of recurrent brain tumor and radiation injury. Acta Radiol 1991;32(3):197–202.

[56] Sonoda Y, Kumabe T, Takahashi T, et al. Clinical usefulness of 11C-MET PET and 201Tl SPECT for differentiation of recurrent glioma from radiation necrosis. Neurol Med Chir (Tokyo) 1998;38(6):342–7 [discussion: 347–8].

[57] Tsuyuguchi N, Sunada I, Iwai Y, et al. Methionine positron emission tomography of recurrent metastatic brain tumor and radiation necrosis after stereotactic radiosurgery: is a differential diagnosis possible? J Neurosurg 2003;98(5):1056–64.

[58] Ogawa T, Kanno I, Hatazawa J, et al. Methionine PET for follow-up of radiation therapy of primary lymphoma of the brain. Radiographics 1994;14(1): 101–10.

[59] Chung JK, Kim YK, Kim SK, et al. Usefulness of 11C-methionine PET in the evaluation of brain lesions that are hypo- or isometabolic on 18F-FDG PET. Eur J Nucl Med Mol Imaging 2002;29(2):176–82.

[60] Heesters MA, Go KG, Kamman RL, et al. 11C-tyrosine position emission tomography and 1H magnetic resonance spectroscopy of the response of brain gliomas to radiotherapy. Neuroradiology 1998;40(2): 103–8.

[61] Hubner KF, Thie JA, Smith GT, et al. Positron emission tomography (PET) with 1-aminocyclobutane-1-[(11)C]carboxylic acid (1-[(11)C]-ACBC) for detecting recurrent brain tumors. Clin Positron Imaging 1998;1(3):165–73.

[62] Lemaire C, Gillet S, Kameda M, et al. Enantioselective synthesis of 2-[18F]fluoro-L-tyrosine by catalytic phase-transfer alkylation. J Labelled Cpd Radiopharm 2001;44:S857–9.

[63] Wienhard K, Herholz K, Coenen HH, et al. Increased amino acid transport into brain tumors measured by PET of L-(2-18F)fluorotyrosine [see comments]. J Nucl Med 1991;32(7):1338–46.

[64] Weber WA, Wester HJ, Grosu AL, et al. O-(2-[18F] fluoroethyl)-L-tyrosine and L-[methyl-11C]methionine uptake in brain tumours: initial results of a comparative study. Eur J Nucl Med 2000;27:542–9.

[65] Becherer A, Karanikas G, Szabo M, et al. Brain tumour imaging with PET: a comparison between [18F]fluorodopa and [11C]methionine. Eur J Nucl Med Mol Imaging 2003;30(11):1561–7.

[66] Beuthien-Baumann B, Bredow J, et al. 3-O-methyl-6-[18F]fluoro-L-DOPA and its evaluation in brain tumour imaging. Eur J Nucl Med Mol Imaging 2003; 30(7):1004–8.

[67] Shields AF. PET imaging with 18F-FLT and thymidine analogs: promise and pitfalls. J Nucl Med 2003; 44(9):1432–4.

[68] Vander Borght T, Pauwels S, Lambotte L, et al. Brain tumor imaging with PET and 2-[carbon-11]thymidine. J Nucl Med 1994;35(6):974–82.

[69] Ohtani T, Kurihara H, Ishiuchi S, et al. Brain tumour imaging with carbon-11 choline: comparison with FDG PET and gadolinium-enhanced MR imaging. Eur J Nucl Med 2001;28(11):1664–70.

[70] Hara T, Kondo T, Kosaka N. Use of 18F-choline and 11C-choline as contrast agents in positron emission tomography imaging-guided stereotactic biopsy sampling of gliomas. J Neurosurg 2003;99(3):474–9.

**RADIOLOGIC
CLINICS**
of North America

ELSEVIER
SAUNDERS

Radiol Clin N Am 43 (2005) 49 – 65

The role of PET imaging in the management of patients with central nervous system disorders

Andrew B. Newberg, MD*, Abass Alavi, MD

*Division of Nuclear Medicine, Department of Radiology, Hospital of the University of Pennsylvania, 3400 Spruce Street,
110 Donner Building, Philadelphia, PA 19104, USA*

PET has been widely used in the study of various central nervous system (CNS) disorders. A number of different radiopharmaceuticals labeled with positron-emitting isotopes, such as carbon-11 ($[^{11}C]$), fluorine-18 ($[^{18}F]$), and nitrogen-13 ($[^{13}N]$), have been developed for measuring cerebral blood flow (CBF), cerebral metabolism, and neurotransmitter systems [1,2]. In fact, virtually every aspect of brain physiology can be evaluated by a PET radiopharmaceutical. Perhaps the most commonly used radiopharmaceutical for both research and clinical purposes is $[^{18}F]$-fluorodeoxyglucose (FDG). FDG-PET allows for the evaluation of cerebral glucose metabolism and has physical characteristics that make it relatively easy to produce and use, and provide high-resolution images of cerebral metabolism (Fig. 1). PET, along with its available radiotracers, has been used to study many pathologic states in the brain and assist with the management of these disorders. Specific CNS disorders in which PET studies may influence the management of the patient include seizures, brain tumors, movement disorders [3,4], dementia [5], head trauma, and depression.

Alzheimer's disease

Perhaps the most important use for PET imaging in the work-up of the dementia patient is to aid in making an accurate diagnosis as early in the course of Alzheimer's disease (AD) as possible. The criteria for the diagnosis of AD were defined by the Working Group of the National Institute of Neurological and Communicative Disorders and Stroke and the Alzheimer's Disease and Related Disorders Association in 1984 [6] and require evidence of progressive, chronic cognitive deficits in middle-aged and elderly patients with no identifiable underlying cause. Unfortunately, although it is possible to make an accurate diagnosis of dementia in most patients with severe disease, it is very difficult to differentiate between AD and other dementing disorders in patients with mild cognitive impairment [7,8]. It is believed that functional imaging studies, such as PET, might help in making the diagnosis of AD and elucidating the mechanisms underlying the disorder.

Since 1980, a large number of studies have used PET in the assessment of patients with AD. Initial $[^{18}F]$-FDG PET studies, comparing CMRGlc in patients with AD with age-matched, healthy controls, showed that there is a 20% to 30% decrease in whole-brain CMRGlc values in patients with AD when compared with healthy age-matched controls [9]. Other studies showed that patients with AD have decreased whole brain glucose metabolism (CMRGlc), whereas the bilateral parietal and temporal lobes are particularly affected [10 – 13]. This parietal hypometabolism (Fig. 2) is often referred to as representing the typical pattern of AD and may be particularly pronounced in patients with an age less than 65 years [14]. Although the bilateral parietal pattern is highly predictive of AD [15,16], the pattern is not pathognomic for AD and may be seen in patients with

* Corresponding author.
E-mail address: newberg@rad.upenn.edu (A.B. Newberg).

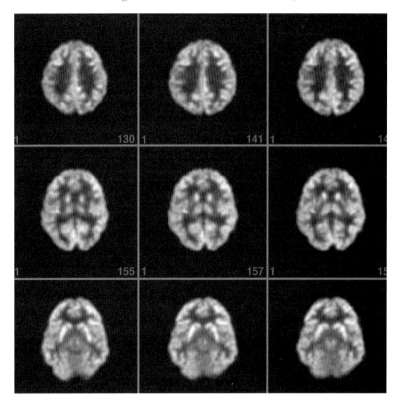

Fig. 1. FDG-PET image of normal subject using a high-resolution gadolinium orthosilacte PET camera. The resolution of 2.5 to 3mm is superior to prior PET cameras and demonstrates significant cortical and subcortical detail.

Parkinson's disease (PD), bilateral parietal subdural hematomas, bilateral parietal stroke, and bilateral parietal radiation therapy ports [17].

In patients with AD of varying severity, the magnitude and extent of hypometabolism correlates with the severity of the dementia symptoms [18–20]. Usually, there are only minor decreases in the parietal lobes in patients with early mild AD. Moderately affected patients show significantly decreased metabolism in the left midfrontal lobes, bilateral parietal

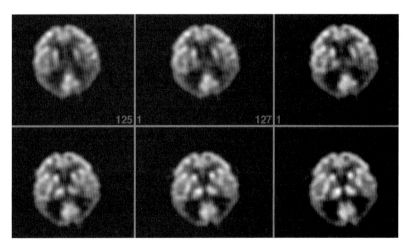

Fig. 2. FDG-PET scan of a patient with moderately advanced Alzheimer's disease. The findings demonstrate significant bilateral temporoparietal hypometabolism.

lobes, and the superior temporal regions. In patients with severe AD, the same regions are affected, but the hypometabolism is much more pronounced with sparing only of the sensorimotor, visual, and subcortical areas (Fig. 3). Longitudinal studies have shown that CMRGlc values decrease more rapidly over time in patients with AD than age-matched control subjects and particularly affect the temporal, parietal, and frontal lobes [21]. The authors' research group has also developed a semiquantitative subjective scoring system designed to assess for disease severity in AD patients [18]. Such a scoring system, which weighs metabolic values according to the areas particularly involved in AD, such as the parietal, temporal, and frontal lobes, may be beneficial for routine clinical use and future research studies of therapeutic interventions.

PET imaging also provides the ability to measure changes in neurotransmitter systems that might be affected in AD. One study demonstrated significant decreases in acetylcholinesterase activity in the neocortex, hippocampus, and amygdala of all patients with AD, suggesting a loss of cholinergic innervation in the basal forebrain [22]. The temporal and parietal cortices were the most affected, although reductions were relatively uniform in the cerebral neocortex. PET can also play an important role in the evaluation of therapeutic interventions for AD. The relatively recent development of several pharmaceuticals for

AD provides an important area for PET imaging. For example, patients treated with donepezil were found to have relatively similar cerebral metabolism at 24 weeks compared with the placebo group that was observed to have a 10% decline [23]. In terms of the exact pharmacologic mechanism, one PET study explored how donepezil affected acetylcholinesterase activity [24]. Donepezil hydrochloride reportedly provides nearly complete inhibition of cerebral cortical acetylcholinesterase activity in patients with AD. This study, however, demonstrated an average of only 27% inhibition of acetylcholinesterase activity. More recent studies have suggested that the therapeutic response of drugs, such as donepezil and rivastigmine, is associated with acetylcholinesterase activity primarily in the frontal lobes [25].

PET continues to play a major role in the study and diagnosis of AD. It has the ability to aid in the diagnosis and the determination of the course and severity of the disease. With improved methods for quantitative analysis of specific regions, such as the hippocampus, PET may help further unravel the pathophysiologic changes in AD. The role of PET imaging will be significantly enhanced as successful therapeutic interventions evolve in the treatment of AD. This is of particularly great importance in the management of patients with early AD.

Pick's disease

Pick's disease is a neurodegenerative dementia with a predilection for the frontal and temporal lobes where Pick's bodies are noted on histopathologic examination. The disease is associated with cognitive and language dysfunction, and behavioral changes. The most common finding in PET images (Fig. 4) is hypometabolism in the frontal and anterior temporal lobes bilaterally [26,27]. This pattern of anterior hypometabolism is consistent with the findings on histopathologic examination, and frontal and temporal lobe atrophy on CT and MR images [28]. The small number of studies reported in the literature may not allow determination of the accuracy of [18F]-FDG PET imaging in the diagnosis of Pick's disease. Furthermore, there are disorders, such as other frontal lobe dementias and schizophrenia, that also may have a pattern of frontal lobe hypometabolism, and these should be considered in the differential diagnosis. Clinical findings, however, are significantly different between these two disorders. At the present time, there are no clear therapeutic interventions for Pick's disease and PET imaging is

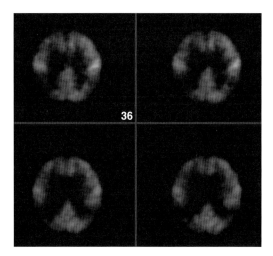

Fig. 3. FDG-PET scan of a patient with advanced Alzheimer's disease. The findings demonstrate significant bilateral temporoparietal hypometabolism in addition to frontal lobe hypometabolism. The sensorimotor areas, visual cortex, and cerebellum are relatively preserved.

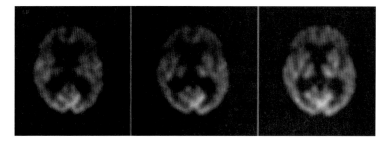

Fig. 4. FDG-PET scan of a patient with Pick's disease demonstrating moderately decreased metabolism in the frontal lobes including the anterior cingulate gyrus. The temporoparietal, occipital, and subcortical areas have relatively preserved metabolism.

less likely to have a role in the long-term management of such patients.

Brain tumors

Primary intracranial tumors comprise approximately 5% to 9% of all cancers and carry a median survival of approximately 1 year. Further, gliomas represent 50% of all intracranial tumors. PET can play an important role in the evaluation and management of patients with brain tumors, including the grading of tumors, determination of prognosis, and the differentiation of recurrent tumor from radiation necrosis [29,30].

Many of the studies of brain tumors with PET have been performed using FDG, although studies have been reported in which tracers, such as carbon-11–L-methionine ($[^{11}C]$- L-MET; reflecting neutral

amino acid transport), have been used [31,32]. Most FDG studies have concluded that high-grade tumors are hypermetabolic, whereas low-grade tumors are hypometabolic. In a study by DiChiro et al on 72 patients, the mean CMRGlc, measured with FDG, for low-grade tumors was 4 ± 1.8 mg glucose/100 g/min, whereas high-grade tumors had a CMRGlc of 7.4 ± 3.5 mg glucose/100 g/min. Other groups [33,34] have corroborated the finding of hypermetabolism in high-grade tumors and hypometabolism in low-grade tumors. One distinction from this typology is juvenile pilocytic astrocytomas, which typically have a high glucose metabolism despite their benign nature [35,36]. It should be noted that PET does not differentiate between primary lymphomas of the CNS, brain secondaries, or malignant gliomas, because all of these may be hypermetabolic [37]. In fact, a PET study of brain metastases from small cell lung cancer indicated increased rCMRglu, rCBF, and

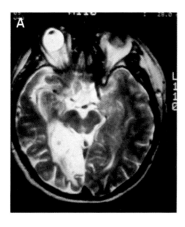
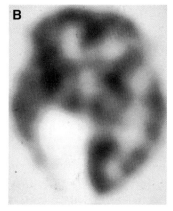

Fig. 5. (*A*) Patient with a history of right temporal lobe astrocytoma status post–radiation therapy presenting with worsening symptoms and an MR imaging abnormality that could not categorized as either radiation necrosis or recurrent tumor. (*B*) FDG-PET scan demonstrates hypometabolism in the same region with no foci of increased activity where the MR imaging abnormality was noted. This finding indicates that there is radiation necrosis and no evidence of recurrent tumor.

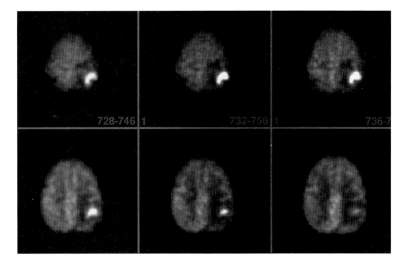

Fig. 6. FDG-PET scan of a patient with astrocytoma in the right parietal lobe status post–surgical resection and radiation therapy now with clinical concern for recurrence. The scan demonstrates a large area of intensely increased metabolism in the right parietal lobe consistent with recurrent tumor.

regional cerebral blood volume (rCBV) in tumor tissue even though there was a high degree of variability in these measures [38]. No correlation between survival and metabolic or hemodynamic parameters, however, could be demonstrated.

Although [^{18}F]-FDG–PET seems to be useful in grading brain tumors and determining their prognosis, PET also has another advantage over anatomic imaging. Unlike CT or MR imaging, PET can distinguish radiation necrosis from tumor recurrence [39,40]. The sensitivity for making this determination may be as high as 86% with a specificity as high as 56% [41]. Others, however, have questioned how useful this approach may be in distinguishing necrosis from active tumor [42]. In general, areas of radiation necrosis are hypometabolic (Fig. 5), whereas tumor recurrence appears hypermetabolic on FDG-PET (Fig. 6). One study showed that radiation necrosis was associated with hypometabolism in the white matter only, whereas necrosis caused by chemotherapy was associated with gray matter changes in addition to white matter abnormalities. These investigators were also able to distinguish an area of tumor recurrence among necrotic changes. Further, they found no false-positive or false-negative results in this study.

Parkinson's disease

PD is caused by loss of the pigmented neurons in the substantia nigra and the locus coeruleus and is characterized by the triad of bradykinesia, tremor, and rigidity. The loss of pigmented neurons is associated with decreased production of dopamine, decreased storage of dopamine, and nigrostriatal system dysfunction. It is believed that initially there is an upregulation of dopamine receptors [43] followed by a down-regulation that occurs as the disease progresses. Eventually, PD can lead to dementia in 20% to 30% of the patients. PET offers the ability not only to study cerebral metabolism, but the dopamine transmitter receptor system, which may prove extremely useful in the diagnosis of PD and the determination of the pathophysiology of this disease [44,45].

Several groups have reported hypermetabolism in the basal ganglia in early, untreated PD [46,47]. Similarly, hemiparkinsonism is associated with hypermetabolism in the contralateral basal ganglia [48]. Another group [49] reported decreases in glucose metabolism in the basal ganglia contralateral to the side of the symptoms in patients with hemiparkinsonism–hemiatrophy syndrome. PD patients have been shown to have mild diffuse cortical hypometabolism compared with controls. Further, this hypometabolism correlates with the severity of bradykinesia, but is unrelated to the duration of the disease.

Regarding therapy, one study demonstrated that hypometabolism in the striatum and inferior thalamus in the side contralateral to the predominant parkinsonian signs was associated with L-dopa unresponsiveness, whereas hypermetabolism in the striatum and inferior thalamus contralateral to the predominant side were found in L-dopa–responsive patients [50].

Blesa et al [51] reported a reversal of pallidal hyper-metabolism with levodopa therapy. Another study by Jenkins et al [52] indicated that PD patients had improved activation in the supplementary motor cortex during a motor function task when akinesia was reversed with apomorphine infusion (a dopamine agonist).

Dementia in PD seems to be associated with a uniform cerebral hypometabolism. Severe dementia in PD may be indistinguishable from AD on PET images, however, both showing significant bilateral parietal hypometabolism [53]. Peppard et al [54] showed that PD patients with dementia differed from PD patients without dementia in that the former had hypometabolic perirolandic and angular gyrus regions. PD patients with dementia, however, did not have significantly different CMRGlc values than AD patients [55]. Further, the parietal cortex:caudate-thalamus ratio negatively correlated with the severity and duration of the disease in PD patients and in AD patients. The results from these studies indicate that PD patients with dementia may suffer from an underlying Alzheimer-type process or may have a dementia specifically associated with the PD that affects the frontal lobes. The dopaminergic system may also play a role in the dementia symptoms of PD because reduced presynaptic dopamine activity in the caudate is associated with impairment in neuro-psychologic tests measuring verbal fluency, working memory, attentional functioning, and somatosensory discrimination [56–58].

PET imaging in PD has also been performed with [18F] fluorodopa to evaluate presynaptic dopaminer-gic function, and has shown abnormalities in the nigrostriatal dopaminergic projection [59,60] and reduced basal ganglia activity, particularly in the posterior putamen (Fig. 7) [61]. Others have argued that the limited spatial resolution of PET with fluorodopa may result in substantial underestimation of the true rate of fluorodopa uptake and metabolism in vivo, and may also obscure regional heterogeneity in the neurochemical pathology of PD [62]. Garnett et al [63] showed that in hemiparkinsonism, there is a marked decrease in activity in the contralateral basal ganglia. There is also decreased activity, although to a lesser extent, in the ipsilateral basal ganglia.

Fluorodopa studies have been used to investigate clinical course and the effects of therapy in patients with PD. For example, in patients with mild PD, levodopa infusion decreased dopa influx in the putamen, whereas in patients with advanced PD, levodopa induced significant up-regulation of dopa influx [64]. This study might explain the less graded clinical response to levodopa in advanced PD and potentially explain the pathogenesis underlying motor fluctuations. More recent PET studies have demonstrated that although loss of putamen dopamine storage predisposes PD patients to motor complications, it cannot be the only factor determining when such motor symptoms arise clinically [65]. Additional PET studies suggest that loss of striatal dopamine storage capacity along with pulsatile exposure to exogenous L-dopa results in pathologically raised synaptic dopamine levels and deranged basal ganglia opioid transmission. This, rather than altered dopamine receptor binding, may be the cause of inap-

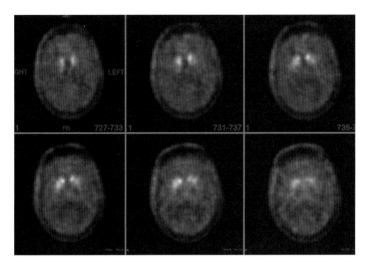

Fig. 7. [18F]-fluorodopa scan of a patient with moderately severe Parkinson's disease shows uptake in the caudate but little uptake in the putamen. More severe cases may show little uptake throughout the striatum.

propriate overactivity of basal ganglia-frontal projections, resulting in breakthrough involuntary movements [66].

Imaging with postsynaptic dopamine receptor tracers has also provided important information regarding the disease pathogenesis and course. [^{11}C]–N-methylspiperone (a postsynaptic D2 receptor antagonist) has shown variable results in activity early in the disease and decreased tracer binding in advanced PD [67,68]. It should also be noted that PET imaging with [^{11}C]–N-methylspiperone in hemiparkinsonism patients has shown bilateral variability in striatal uptake [69]. [^{11}C]-raclopride has also been used to investigate D2 receptors in PD patients. An increase in [^{11}C]-raclopride activity (receptor up-regulation) has been observed in the striatum contralateral to hemiparkinsonian symptoms in early disease corroborating the notion of initial up-regulation of dopamine receptors followed by subsequent down-regulation as the disease progresses [70].

A number of new surgical techniques have been developed for the treatment of PD and their effect has been observed with PET. For example, pallidotomy has been associated with increased activation of premotor areas and reduced hyperactivity of the lentiform nucleus [71,72]. Pallidal and subthalamic stimulation also increase activation of premotor areas but decrease activation in the primary motor area [73,74]. Suppression of unilateral tremor with thalamic stimulation has been shown to be associated with a reduction in CBF. These findings corroborate the general notion that increased activity in the subthalamic-pallidal projection is directly implicated in the pathophysiology of PD, and that surgical techniques that block these output nuclei lead to partial restoration of cortical physiology. The changes associated with transplantation of fetal tissue for PD has demonstrated inconsistent findings, with some studies showing increased fluorodopa uptake and others no significant changes [75,76].

Cerebrovascular disease

Cerebrovascular disease is the third leading cause of death in the United States and affects approximately half a million people. Stroke is often associated with a poor outcome, however, in part because of the lack of understanding of the mechanisms that underlie stroke and the process by which recovery may take place. PET imaging has been of great benefit in advancing the understanding of the pathophysiology of cerebrovascular disorders. PET imaging allows for the detection of stroke earlier and

with higher sensitivity than anatomic imaging with either MR imaging or CT. Further, PET imaging has been useful in evaluating the extent of the functional damage, because areas not immediately affected by the infarct may show hypometabolism or decreased blood flow. Initial stroke severity has been shown to correlate with the initially affected volume as determined by PET, whereas neurologic deterioration during the first week after stroke correlates with the proportion of the initially affected volume that infarcted, and functional outcome correlates with the final infarct volume [77].

In patients who have suffered a stroke, there is a characteristic uncoupling between CBF and metabolism in the infarcted area [78,79]. Several studies using [^{15}O]-H$_2$O have described "misery perfusion" in and near areas of infarct within the first hours to days after a stroke. This misery perfusion is described as a relative decrease in regional CBF compared with the regional glucose metabolism or oxygen metabolism. Further studies have shown that there is a marked increase in the regional oxygen extraction fraction (rOEF) in response to the diminished blood flow [80,81]. A recent study, however, showed no correlation between the degree of misery perfusion and angiographic findings in patients with carotid artery occlusion [82].

A recent study demonstrated that the oxygen consumption significantly decreased between the acute and chronic phases of stroke, but that acute-stage mesial-prefrontal metabolism was significantly correlated with neurologic recovery [83]. This study also showed that there was a delayed intrahemispheric remote hypometabolism that developed while the patient was clinically recovering and seems to be related to infarct size. Neurologic recovery was not a function of thalamic hypometabolism, but appeared to be influenced by mesial-prefrontal metabolism, possibly because this region is part of a network that has an important compensatory role in motor recovery.

Approximately 1 week after infarct "luxury perfusion" occurs, which is a relative increase of rCBF compared with cerebral metabolism [84]. Wise et al [85] found that rCBF increased compared with rCMRO2 over several days postinfarct. Further, there was a subsequent decrease in the rOEF in the infarcted area 18 hours to 7 days after the infarct. This is believed to reflect mitochondrial dysfunction and energy failure of the damaged tissue. In addition to the infarcted area, there exists a penumbral zone, a hypometabolic and presumably ischemic area that surrounds the infarct core [86]. This area also has increased rOEF suggesting that this area has decreased perfusion relative to the necessary oxygen requirements. If blood flow to this ischemic area is restored before irreversible damage occurs, then the tissue will likely recover and resume normal function [87].

Distant from the ischemic and the stroke sites, there are regions that also show alterations in metabolism despite being normal on anatomic imaging studies, such as CT or MR imaging [88,89]. It is not completely certain, however, what are the clinical consequences of these distant hypometabolic regions [83]. The most distinctive and characteristic example of such remote effects is crossed cerebellar diaschisis, first described by Baron et al [90]. Crossed cerebellar diaschisis (Fig. 8) refers to hypometabolism and hypoperfusion in the cerebellar cortex contralateral to the site of the infarct in the cortex and usually occurs during the first 2 months after infarction [91]. It is believed that this is caused by an interruption of the cerebro–ponto–cerebellar pathways as a result of the stroke. Interestingly, patients with persistent cerebellar diaschisis have a decrease in oxygen consumption that is less than the decrease in glucose use [92]. This

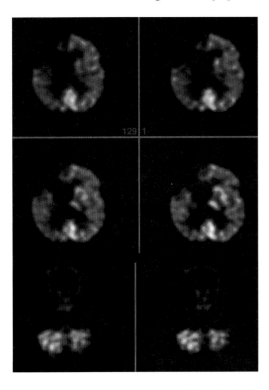

Fig. 8. FDG-PET scan of a patient after embolic stroke in the distribution of the right anterior cerebral artery. There is severely decreased metabolism in the right frontal lobe extending to the midline. There is also crossed cerebellar diaschisis with decreased metabolism in the left cerebellum.

uncoupling of oxygen consumption and glucose use may reflect a change in brain metabolism caused by deafferentation. Another study did demonstrate that the degree of neurologic improvement was worse in the patients with cerebellar diaschisis, which may be simply reflective of more severe and widespread ischemia resulting in the diaschisis [93]. There are also other areas that are hypometabolic after a cortical infarct [94]. These areas include the ipsilateral thalamus; the ipsilateral caudate nucleus; and the ipsilateral primary visual cortex (if the infarct is in the anterior visual pathways). A recent study also demonstrated a decline in oxygen metabolism in the unaffected hemisphere from the acute to the subacute stage, which suggests a delayed effect from transcallosal fiber degeneration [95].

PET studies have also been investigated the presence of chronic ischemia to determine the risk of stroke in these patients. Gibbs et al [96] found increased rCBV with normal rCBF and rCMRO2 ipsilateral to occlusion of the internal carotid artery. The increase in rCBV is likely caused by the vasodilation that occurs in response to the decreased perfusion pressure. When the compensatory vasodilator response is at maximum, any further decrease in perfusion pressure may result in a decreased rCBF with the high likelihood of ischemia and eventually stroke. Because rCBF remains relatively constant until the maximum rCBV is attained, the rCBF:rCBV ratio (which correlates well with rOEF) decreases by autoregulation before ischemia develops. Similar findings were reported by Sette et al [97], in which patients with cerebrovascular disease had evidence of normal autoregulation and an increase in rOEF in response to decreased perfusion pressure.

PET studies have not been shown to be as successful in assessing risk of stroke or the potential outcome of surgical intervention in patients with carotid artery disease [98,99]. Count-based PET measurement of OEF without arterial sampling has been shown accurately to predict the risk of stroke in patients with carotid artery occlusion [100]. This is corroborated somewhat by another study that demonstrated a lower frequency of hemodynamic abnormalities in asymptomatic patients [101]. In an earlier study of patients with carotid artery disease being treated with antithrombotic medication, there was no difference in the incidence of stroke in patients with normal and those with abnormal hemodynamics. The same group found no correlation between the degree of carotid artery stenosis and the hemodynamic measures of the cerebral circulation in 19 patients with significant carotid artery occlusion. In patients before and after extracranial-intracranial bypass surgery, however, decreases in rCBV and normalization of the rCBF:rCBV ratio were found after surgery [102]. Despite this finding, Powers et al [103] noted that 3 of 21 patients who underwent bypass surgery suffered ipsilateral stroke within 1 year. Further, none of the 23 patients who did not have surgery, but had PET findings similar to those in the surgical group, had a stroke. The conclusion from this study was that the PET results of the hemodynamic status of patients with carotid artery disease could not adequately predict which patients would benefit from bypass surgery.

There have been several studies correlating the functional recovery in patients with stroke to functional changes on PET scans [104]. Cerebral metabolic rates of glucose measured early after stroke have shown that receptive language disorders best correlate with metabolism in the left superior temporal cortex, and word fluency best correlates with metabolism in the left prefrontal cortex [105]. A PET study of patients with left inferior frontal gyrus strokes and resulting aphasia demonstrated a stronger-than-normal response in the homologous right inferior frontal gyrus [106]. Although the level of activation in the right inferior frontal gyrus did not correlate with verbal performance, increased activity in the perilesional area occurred in the two patients who gave the best performance in certain verbal tasks and who also showed the most complete recovery from aphasia. Similar results were described in several other studies of patients with aphasia secondary to stroke that demonstrated increased right temporal lobe activity as a mechanism to compensate for the impaired left hemispheric function [107,108]. The best degree of speech restoration, however, has been found in those patients with at least some preservation of activity in the left temporal lobe that can ultimately be incorporated into the functional language network [109,110]. Another study measuring CBF associated with passive elbow movement showed that hemiplegic stroke initially activated the bilateral inferior parietal cortex, contralateral sensorimotor cortex, and ipsilateral dorsolateral prefrontal cortex, supplementary motor area, and cingulate cortex, but later included activation of the ipsilateral premotor area [111]. These results suggested that recovery from hemiplegia is accompanied by changes of brain activation in sensory and motor systems.

PET studies have also been used to monitor the success of various treatment regimens. PET has been used to evaluate the effects of thrombolytic therapy in acute stroke and has found that critically hypoperfused tissue can be preserved by early reperfusion and that large infarcts can be prevented by early reperfusion to misery perfused but viable tissue [112]. Imaging of benzodiazepine receptors by flumazenil PET has been found to distinguish between irreversibly damaged and viable penumbra tissue early after acute stroke [113]. In the future, functional imaging modalities that could eventually include tracers for neuronal integrity might be used to help in the selection of patients for thrombolytic therapy possibly permitting the extension of the critical time period for inclusion of patients to aggressive stroke management strategies [114]. Hakim et al [115] found that stroke patients treated with nimodipine had a greater increase in the rCBF in the ischemia core (7 days after the infarct) than did patients receiving placebo. There was also an increase in rCBF in the penumbral zone in the nimodipine group compared with the placebo group (but these results were not statistically significant). Another study using [^{18}F]-FDG PET found that patients on nimodipine had greater increases in glucose metabolism in the affected areas compared with controls [116].

Head trauma

There have been a limited number of studies using PET in the evaluation of patients with head trauma. One of the problems with the use of PET in these cases is that PET cannot distinguish between structural damage and cerebral dysfunction because these may all result in areas of decreased metabolism [117]. It is helpful to compare PET with anatomic images, such as those obtained by MR imaging or CT, especially because cerebral dysfunction can extend beyond the boundary of anatomic lesions [118] and may even appear in remote locations from the trauma.

Lesions, such as cortical contusions, intracranial hematoma, and resultant encephalomalacia, have metabolic effects that are confined primarily to the site of injury. Subdural and epidural hematomas, however, often cause widespread hypometabolism and may even affect the contralateral hemisphere [119]. Another entity, diffuse axonal injury, has been found to cause diffuse cortical hypometabolism with particularly marked decrease in metabolism in the parietal occipital cortex (Fig. 9) [120]. Further, crossed cerebellar diaschisis, and ipsilateral cerebellar hypometabolism, has been found in head-injury patients with supratentorial lesions [121].

Alavi et al [118] found a good correlation between the severity of head trauma as measured by the Glasgow Coma Scale and the extent of whole brain hypometabolism. Another study demonstrated that persistent symptoms in minor head-injury patients

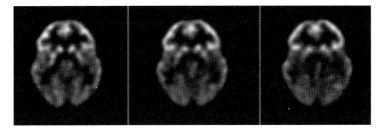

Fig. 9. FDG-PET scan of a patient with traumatic brain injury showing decreased metabolism in the parietal and occipital cortices consistent with diffuse axonal injury.

may be associated with corresponding deficits in both neuropsychologic testing and cerebral metabolism [122]. Another study demonstrated that regionally decreased glucose metabolism was observed in 88% of patients [123]. The prevalence of global cortical CMRglc reduction was higher in severely head-injured patients (86% versus 67% mild-moderate), although the absolute values were similar across the injury severity spectrum. As many as half of head-injury patients may also have increased glucose metabolism as early as 1 week after injury [124]. This hyperglycolysis may occur either regionally or globally and also suggests that the metabolic state of the traumatically injured brain should be defined differentially in terms of glucose and oxygen metabolism. PET imaging may not be as helpful in determining overall prognosis in head-injury patients, however, particularly children and adolescents, with respect to rehabilitation [125].

It has also been found that after head injury, even though a patient may be in a persistent vegetative state, their brain actually responds to the emotional attributes of sound or speech. This was determined using PET to measure CBF changes when a story was told by a patient's mother [126]. During auditory presentation, there was increased activity in the rostral anterior cingulate, right middle temporal, and right premotor cortices.

Epilepsy and other seizure disorders

Epilepsy affects 0.5% to 1% of the population, can cause focal or generalized seizures, and usually begins in childhood. In general, during an epileptic seizure cerebral metabolism and blood flow are markedly increased. The focus of partial seizures can be identified using [18F]-FDG PET because these areas have increased metabolism during the seizure and decreased metabolism in the interictal period [127,128]. It has been shown that single hypometabolic regions can be identified in 55% to 80% of

patients with focal EEG abnormalities [129,130]. Performing ictal PET studies is somewhat impractical, however, because of the short half-life of the positron emitters and other logistical reasons. One of the most effective treatments for partial epilepsy, refractory to medical intervention, is surgical removal of the involved area. Using high-resolution PET images, accurate localization of seizure foci can be achieved to aid in selecting the appropriate surgical intervention [131]. It also seems that certain clinical features affect the metabolic and CBF findings [132]. The degree of asymmetry in the region of the seizure focus seems greater with increasing duration of the seizure disorder. Cerebral glucose metabolism seems to have a greater rate of increase in asymmetry than CBF. These results indicate an uncoupling of cerebral metabolism and blood flow that is progressive and results from the differential response of glucose metabolism and blood flow to chronic seizure activity. The type of seizure preceding the PET study may also affect the metabolic landscape such that hypometabolism is limited to the epileptogenic zone if the preceding seizure is focal limbic, whereas patients with widespread limbic seizures have hypometabolism that included one or several additional areas of the limbic cortex [133].

Another important aspect of seizure studies is how to distinguish those patients who will do well postoperatively from those who will be less likely to benefit from temporal lobectomy. Several PET studies did not find any correlation between the severity of abnormal temporal lobe activity and the frequency of postoperative seizures [134]. Other studies have shown that in those patients with hypometabolism only in the affected temporal lobe, there is a higher likelihood of a successful outcome [135–137]. It has also been shown that patients with a greater degree of hypometabolism in the temporal lobe (ie, a more distinct asymmetry) tended to have a better outcome than those with a lesser degree of asymmetry [138,139]. It may be that those patients without significant hypometabolism of the affected temporal lobe (ie, minimal asymmetry between the temporal lobes) might have extratemporal or bitemporal seizure foci. These patients may be less amenable to surgical resection. This is corroborated by other studies that have shown that patients with hypometabolism detected in the opposite hemisphere to the epileptic focus on EEG may be more likely to have postoperative seizures [140] and those patients with extratemporal hypometabolism tend to have a higher likelihood of postoperative seizures [141]. The authors have recently reported that the FDG-PET finding of thalamic hypometabolism may be an important added measure in the evaluation of patients with temporal lobe epilepsy with regard to postoperative seizure outcome [142]. Compared with patients with no thalamic asymmetry, patients with ipsilateral thalamic hypometabolism had a slightly higher risk, and those with contralateral hypometabolism had a markedly increased risk, for having postoperative seizures.

The temporal lobe is the most common focus of partial epilepsy (Fig. 10). Studies show that the sensitivity of PET in detecting temporal lobe epilepsy foci is over 70% in patients with partial complex seizures using FDG [143–145]. One FDG-PET study showed ipsilateral hypometabolism of the seizure focus in the temporal pole, but relatively increased metabolism in the ipsilateral mesiobasal region [146]. Contralateral to the seizure focus, metabolism was increased in the lateral temporal cortex and mesiobasal regions. A study using statistical parametric mapping (SPM) compared hemispheric asymmetry on FDG-PET images in patients with mesial temporal lobe epilepsy with controls [147]. When the SPM

program was used to detect temporal interhemispheric asymmetry, hypometabolism was identified on the side chosen for resection in most cases (sensitivity, 71%; specificity, 100%) and was predictive of favorable postsurgical outcome in 90% of the patients.

The other major site of seizure focus in partial epilepsy is the frontal lobe. Because many of these seizures begin in the medial or inferior aspects of the frontal lobe, scalp EEG readings do not provide adequate localization of foci [148]. Franck et al [149] used [^{18}F]-FDG PET to study 13 patients with presumed frontal lobe epilepsy and found PET to be the best modality for localizing seizure foci in this location. Additionally, the authors suggested that PET might help in determining the site of surgical excision or suggest a contraindication to surgical intervention in patients with multiple or bilateral foci. One study of 180 surgical specimens from patients with frontal lobe epilepsy found a high correlation between hypometabolic regions on PET images and structural, histopathologic changes in the surgical specimens, again demonstrating the value of PET in detecting seizure foci [150].

Performing ictal PET studies is somewhat impractical because of the relatively short half-life of positron-emitting isotopes, such as fluorine-18, and other logistical reasons [151]. Several ictal PET studies have been reported in the literature, however, which have been successful in detecting seizure foci in patients with partial seizures as hypermetabolic areas [152]. Complex partial seizures are associated with bilaterally increased CBF in a number of cortical areas, particularly the temporal and frontal lobes

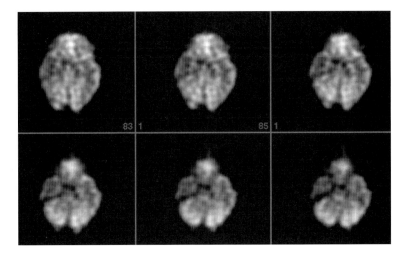

Fig. 10. Interictal FDG-PET scan of a patient with temporal lobe seizures refractory to medical treatment. The scan demonstrates moderate hypometabolism in the right temporal lobe consistent with a seizure focus.

[153]. In addition, these patients also had increased blood flow to the subcortical nuclei, which are activated during ictus.

Summary

PET will continue to play a critical role in both clinical and research applications with regard to CNS disorders. PET is useful in the initial diagnosis of patients presenting with CNS symptoms and can help clinicians determine the best course of therapy. PET studies can also be useful for studying the response to therapy. From the research perspective, the various neurotransmitter and other molecular tracers currently available or in development will provide substantial information about pathophysiologic process in the brain. As such applications become more widely tested, their introduction into the clinical arena will further advance the use of PET imaging in the evaluation and management of CNS disorders.

References

[1] Kung HF. Overview of radiopharmaceuticals for diagnosis of central nervous disorders. Crit Rev Clin Lab Sci 1991;28:269–86.

[2] Maziere B, Maziere M. Positron emission tomography studies of brain receptors. Fundam Clin Pharmacol 1991;5:61–91.

[3] Therapeutic and Technology Assessment Subcommittee of the American Academy of Neurology. Assessment: positron emission tomography. Neurology 1991;41:163–7.

[4] Shtern F. Positron emission tomography as a diagnostic tool: a reassessment based on literature review. Invest Radiol 1992;27:165–8.

[5] The Workshop Panel. Advances in clinical imaging using positron emission tomography. National Cancer Institute workshop statement. Arch Intern Med 1990; 150:735–9.

[6] McKhann G, Drachman D, Folstein M, et al. Clinical diagnosis of Alzheimer's disease: report of the NINCDS-ADRDA Work Group under the auspices of Department of Health and Human Services Task Force on Alzheimer's Disease. Neurol 1984; 34:939–44.

[7] Tierney MC, Gisher RH, Lewis AJ, et al. The NINCDS-ADRDA Workgroup criteria for the clinical diagnosis of probable Alzheimer's disease: a clinical pathological study of 57 cases. Neurology 1988; 38:359–64.

[8] Joachim CL, Morris JH, Selkow DJ. Clinical diagnosed Alzheimer's disease: autopsy results in 150 cases. Ann Neurol 1988;24:50–6.

[9] Alavi A, Reivich M, Ferris S, et al. Regional cerebral glucose metabolism in aging and senile dementia as determined by 18F-deoxyglucose and positron emission tomography. In: Hoyer S, editor. The aging brain: physiological and pathophysiological aspects. Berlin: Springer-Verlag; 1982. p. 87–195.

[10] Jamieson DG, Chawluck JB, Alavi A, et al. The effect of disease severity on local cerebral glucose metabolism in Alzheimer's disease [abstract]. J Cereb Blood Flow Metab 1987;7:S410.

[11] Kumar A, Schapiro MB, Grady C, et al. High-resolution PET studies in Alzheimer's disease. Neuropsychopharmacology 1991;4:35–46.

[12] Faulstich ME, Sullivan DC. Positron emission tomography in neuropsychiatry. Invest Radiol 1991; 26:184–94.

[13] Bonte FJ, Hom J, Tinter R, et al. Single photon tomography in Alzheimer's disease and the dementias. Semin Nucl Med 1990;20:342–52.

[14] Ichimiya A, Herholz K, Mielke R, et al. Difference of regional cerebral metabolic pattern between presenile and senile dementia of the Alzheimer type: a factor analytic study. J Neurol Sci 1994;123:11–7.

[15] Frackowiak R, Pozilli C, Legg N, et al. Regional cerebral oxygen supply and utilization in dementia: a clinical and physiological study with oxygen-15 and positron emission tomography. Brain 1981;104: 753–88.

[16] Foster NL, Mann U, Mohr E, et al. Focal cerebral glucose hypometabolism in definite Alzheimer's disease. Ann Neurol 1989;26:132–3.

[17] Mazziotta JC, Frackowiak RSJ, Phelps ME. The use of positron emission tomography in the clinical assessment of dementia. Semin Nucl Med 1992;22: 232–46.

[18] Newberg A, Cotter A, Udeshi M, et al. Metabolic imaging severity rating scale (MISRS) for the assessment of patients with cognitive impairment. Clin Nucl Med 2003;28:565–70.

[19] Cutler NR, Haxby J, Duara R, et al. Clinical history, brain metabolism, and neurophysiological function in Alzheimer's disease. Ann Neurol 1985;18:298–309.

[20] Friedland RP, Jagust WJ, Huesman RH, et al. Regional cerebral glucose transport and utilization in Alzheimer's disease. Neurology 1989;39:1427–34.

[21] Alexander GE, Chen K, Pietrini P, et al. Longitudinal PET evaluation of cerebral metabolic decline in dementia: a potential outcome measure in Alzheimer's disease treatment studies. Am J Psychiatry 2002;159:738–45.

[22] Shinotoh H, Namba H, Fukushi K, et al. Brain acetylcholinesterase activity in Alzheimer disease measured by positron emission tomography. Alzheimer Dis Assoc Disord 2000;14(Suppl 1):S114–8.

[23] Tune L, Tiseo PJ, Ieni J, et al. Donepezil HCl (E2020) maintains functional brain activity in patients with Alzheimer disease: results of a 24-week, double-blind, placebo-controlled study. Am J Geriatr Psychiatry 2003;11:169–77.

[24] Kuhl DE, Minoshima S, Frey KA, et al. Limited donepezil inhibition of acetylcholinesterase measured with positron emission tomography in living Alzheimer cerebral cortex. Ann Neurol 2000;48: 391–5.

[25] Kaasinen V, Nagren K, Jarvenpaa T, et al. Regional effects of donepezil and rivastigmine on cortical acetylcholinesterase activity in Alzheimer's disease. J Clin Psychopharmacol 2002;22:615–20.

[26] Salmon E, Maquet P, Sadzot B, et al. Positron emission tomography in Alzheimer's and Pick's disease. J Neurol 1988;235:S1.

[27] Lieberman AP, Trojanowski JQ, Lee VM, et al. Cog, neuroimaging, and pathological studies in a patient with Pick's disease. Ann Neurol 1998;43:259–65.

[28] Wechsler AF, Verity MA, Rosenchein S, et al. Pick's disease: a clinical computed tomographic, and histologic study with Golgi impregnation observations. Arch Neurol 1982;39:287–90.

[29] Wilson CB. Metabolic imaging of human brain tumors. Semin Neurol 1989;9:388–93.

[30] DiChiro G. Positron emission tomography using (18F) fluorodeoxyglucose in brain tumors: a powerful diagnostic and prognostic tool. Invest Radiol 1986; 22:360–71.

[31] DiChiro G, DeLaPaz RL, Brooks RA, et al. Glucose utilization of cerebral gliomas measured by 18F fluorodeoxy-glucose and positron emission tomography. Neurology 1982;32:1323–9.

[32] O'Tuama LA. Methionine transport in brain tumors. J Neuropsychiatry 1989;1(Suppl 1):S37–44.

[33] Alavi JB, Alavi A, Chawluk J, et al. Positron emission tomography in patients with glioma: a predictor of prognosis. Cancer 1988;62:1074–8.

[34] Delbeke D, Meyerowitz C, Lapidus RL, et al. Optimal cutoff levels of F-18 fluorodeoxyglucose uptake in the differentiation of low-grade from high-grade brain tumors with PET. Radiology 1995;195: 47–52.

[35] Katschten B, Stevenaert A, Sadzot B, et al. Preoperative evaluation of 54 gliomas by PET with fluorine-18-fluorodexyglucose and/or carbon-11-methionine. J Nucl Med 1998;39:778–85.

[36] Fulham MJ, Melisi JW, Nishimiya J, et al. Neuroimaging of juvenile pilocytic astrocytomas: an enigma. Radiology 1993;189:221–5.

[37] Roelcke U, Leenders KL. Positron emission tomography in patients with primary CNS lymphomas. J Neurooncol 1999;43:231–6.

[38] Lassen U, Andersen P, Daugaard G, et al. Metabolic and hemodynamic evaluation of brain metastases from small cell lung cancer with positron emission tomography. Clin Cancer Res 1998;4:2591–7.

[39] De Witte O, Levivier M, Violon P, et al. Prognostic value positron emission tomography with [18F] fluoro-2-deoxy-D-glucose in the low-grade glioma. Neurosurgery 1996;39:470–6.

[40] Rozental JM, Levine RL, Nickles RJ, et al. Changes in glucose uptake by malignant gliomas: preliminary study of prognostic significance. J Neurooncol 1991; 10:75–83.

[41] Ricci PE, Karis JP, Heiserman JE, et al. Differentiating recurrent tumor from radiation necrosis: time for reevaluation of positron emission tomography? AJNR Am J Neuroradiol 1998;19:407–13.

[42] Olivero WC, Dulebohn SC, Lister JR. The use of PET in evaluating patients with primary brain tumors: Is it useful? J Neurol Neurosurg Psychiatry 1995;58: 250–2.

[43] Marsden CD. The mysterious motor function of the basal ganglia. Neurology 1982;32:514–39.

[44] Eidelberg D. Positron emission tomography studies in parkinsonism. Neurol Clin 1992;10:421–33.

[45] Guttman M. Dopamine receptors in Parkinson's disease. Neurol Clin 1992;10:377–86.

[46] Rougemont D, Baron JC, Collard P, et al. Local cerebral glucose utilization in treated and untreated patients with Parkinson's disease. J Neurol Neurosurg Psychiatry 1984;47:824–30.

[47] Eidelberg D, Moeller JR, Dhawan V, et al. The metabolic anatomy of Parkinson's disease: complementary (18F) fluorodeoxyglucose and (18F) fluorodopa positron emission tomographic studies. Mov Disord 1990;5:203–13.

[48] Martin WRW, Stoessel A, Adam MJ, et al. Positron emission tomography in Parkinson's disease: glucose and dopa metabolism. Adv Neurol 1987;45:95–8.

[49] Przedborski S, Goldman S, Giladi N, et al. Positron emission tomography in hemiparkinsonism-hemiatrophy syndrome. Adv Neurol 1993;60:501–5.

[50] Dethy S, Van Blercom N, Damhaut P, et al. Asymmetry of basal ganglia glucose metabolism and dopa responsiveness in parkinsonism. Mov Disord 1998; 13:275–80.

[51] Blesa R, Blin J, et al. Levodopa-reduced glucose metabolism in striatopallidothalamocortico circuit in Parkinson's disease. Neurology 1991;41:359.

[52] Jenkins IH, Fernandez W, Playford ED, et al. Impaired activation of the supplementary motor area in Parkinson's disease is reversed when akinesia is treated with apomorphine. Ann Neurol 1992;32: 749–57.

[53] Mazziotta JC. Movement disorders. In: Mazziotta JC, Gilman S, editors. Clinical brain imaging: principles and applications. Philadelphia: Davis; 1992. p. 244–93.

[54] Peppard RF, Martin WR, Clark CM, et al. Cortical glucose metabolism in Parkinson's and Alzheimer's disease. J Neurosci Res 1990;27:561–8.

[55] Kuhl DE, Metter EJ, Benson DF, et al. Similarities of cerebral glucose metabolism in Alzheimier's and Parkinsonian dementia [abstract]. J Nucl Med 1985; 26:P69.

[56] Rinne JO, Portin R, Ruottinen H, et al. Cog impairment and the brain dopaminergic system in Parkinson disease: [18F]fluorodopa positron emission tomographic study. Arch Neurol 2000;57:470–5.

[57] Weder BJ, Leenders KL, Vontobel P, et al. Impaired

somatosensory discrimination of shape in Parkinson's disease: association with caudate nucleus dopaminergic function. Human Brain Map 1999;8:1–12.

[58] Holthoff-Detto VA, Kessler J, Herholz K, et al. Functional effects of striatal dysfunction in Parkinson disease. Arch Neurol 1997;54:145–50.

[59] Brooks DJ, Ibanez V, Sawle GV, et al. Differing patterns of striatal (18F)-dopa uptake in Parkinson's disease, multiple system atrophy, and progressive supranuclear palsy. Ann Neurol 1990;28:547–55.

[60] Nahmias C, Garnett ES, Firnau G, et al. Striatal dopamine distribution in Parkinsonian patients during life. J Neurol Sci 1985;69:223–30.

[61] Leenders KL, Salmon EP, Tyrrell P, et al. The nigrostriatal dopaminergic system assessed in vivo by positron emission tomography in healthy volunteer subjects and patients with Parkinson's disease. Arch Neurol 1990;47:1290–8.

[62] Rousset OG, Deep P, Kuwabara H, et al. Effect of partial volume correction on estimates of the influx and cerebral metabolism of 6-[(18)F]fluoro-L-dopa studied with PET in normal control and Parkinson's disease subjects. Synapse 2000;37:81–9.

[63] Garnett ES, Nahmias C, Firnau G. Central dopaminergic pathways in hemiparkinsonism examined by positron emission tomography. Can J Neurol Sci 1984;11:174–9.

[64] Torstenson R, Hartvig P, Langstrom B, et al. Differential effects of levodopa on dopaminergic function in early and advanced Parkinson's disease. Ann Neurol 1997;41:334–40.

[65] Brooks DJ. PET studies and motor complications in Parkinson's disease. Trends Neurosci 2000;23(Suppl 10): S101–8.

[66] Brooks DJ, Piccini P, Turjanski N, et al. Neuroimaging of dyskinesia. Ann Neurol 2000;47(4 Suppl 1): S154–8.

[67] Shinotoh H, Hirayama K, Tateno Y. Dopamine D1 and D2 receptors in Parkinson's disease and striatonigral degeneration determined by PET. Adv Neurol 1993;60:488–93.

[68] Sawle GV, Brooks DJ, Ibanez V, et al. Striatal D2 receptor density is inversely proportional to dopa uptake in untreated hemi-Parkinson's disease. J Neurol Neurosurg Psychiatry 1990;53:177.

[69] Wijnand A, Rutgers F, Lakke JPW, et al. Tracing of dopamine receptors in hemiparkinsonism with positron emission tomography (PET). J Neurol Sci 1987; 80:237–48.

[70] Antonini A, Schwarz J, Oertel WH, et al. Long-term changes of striatal dopamine D2 receptors in patients with Parkinson's disease: a study with positron emission tomography and [11C]raclopride. Mov Disord 1997;12:33–8.

[71] Henselmans JM, de Jong BM, Pruim J, et al. Acute effects of thalamotomy and pallidotomy on regional cerebral metabolism, evaluated by PET. Clin Neurol Neurosurg 2000;102:84–90.

[72] Eidelberg D, Moeller JR, Ishikawa T, et al. Regional

metabolic correlates of surgical outcome following unilateral pallidotomy for Parkinson's disease. Ann Neurol 1996;39:450–9.

[73] Limousin P, Greene J, Pollak P, et al. Changes in cerebral activity pattern due to subthalamic nucleus or internal pallidum stimulation in Parkinson's disease. Ann Neurol 1997;42:283–91.

[74] Davis KD, Taub E, Houle S, et al. Globus pallidus stimulation activates the cortical motor system during alleviation of parkinsonian symptoms. Nat Med 1997; 3:671–4.

[75] Piccini P, Lindvall O, Bjorklund A, et al. Delayed recovery of movement-related cortical function in Parkinson's disease after striatal dopaminergic grafts. Ann Neurol 2000;48:689–95.

[76] Hauser RA, Freeman TB, Snow BJ, et al. Long-term evaluation of bilateral fetal nigral transplantation in Parkinson disease. Arch Neurol 1999;56:179–87.

[77] Read SJ, Hirano T, Abbott DF, et al. The fate of hypoxic tissue on 18F-fluoromisonidazole positron emission tomography after ischemic stroke. Ann Neurol 2000;48:228–35.

[78] Lenzi G, Frackowiak R, Jonres T. Cerebral oxygen metabolism and blood flow in human cerebral ischemic infarction. J Cereb Blood Flow Metab 1982;2:321–35.

[79] Kuhl DE, Phelps M, Kowell A, et al. Effects of stroke on local cerebral metabolism and perfusion: mapping by emission tomography of 18FDG and 12NH3. Ann Neurol 1980;8:47–69.

[80] Baron J, Rougemont D, Bousser M, et al. Local interrelationships of cerebral oxygen consumption and glucose utilization in normal subjects and in ischemic stroke patients. J Cereb Blood Flow Metab 1984;4:140–9.

[81] Wise R, Bernardi S, Frackowiak R, et al. Serial observations on the pathophysiology of acute stroke: the transition from ischemia to infarction as reflected in regional oxygen extraction. Brain 1983; 106:197–222.

[82] Derdeyn CP, Shaibani A, Moran CJ, et al. Lack of correlation between pattern of collateralization and misery perfusion in patients with carotid occlusion. Stroke 1999;30:1025–32.

[83] Iglesias S, Marchal G, Viader F, et al. Delayed intrahemispheric remote hypometabolism: correlations with early recovery after stroke. Cerebrovasc Dis 2000;10:391–402.

[84] Lassen N. The luxury perfusion syndrome and its possible relation to acute metabolic acidosis localized within the brain. Lancet 1966;2:1113–5.

[85] Wise R, Bernardi S, Frackowiak R, et al. Serial observations on the pathophysiology of acute stroke: the transition from ischemia to infarction as reflected in regional oxygen extraction. Brain 1983;106:197–222.

[86] Marchal G, Evans A, Dagher A, et al. The evolution of cerebral infarction with time. A PET study of the ischemia penumbra. J Cereb Blood Flow Metab 1987; 7(Suppl 1):S99.

[87] Baron J, Bousser M, Rey A, et al. Reversal of focal "misery-perfusion syndrome" by extra-intracranial arterial bypass in hemodynamic cerebral ischemia. Stroke 1981;12:454–9.

[88] Kushner M, Alavi A, Reivich M, et al. Contralateral cerebellar hypometabolism following cerebral insult: a positron emission tomographics study. Ann Neurol 1984;15:425–34.

[89] Herholz K, Heindel W, Rackl A, et al. Regional cerebral blood flow in leukoaraiosis and atherosclerotic carotid disease. Arch Neurol 1990;47:392–7.

[90] Baron J, Bousser M, Comar D, et al. Crossed cerebellar diaschisis in human supratentorial brain infarction. Trans Am Neurol Assoc 1980;105:459–61.

[91] Baron J, Bousser MG, Comar D. Crossed cerebellar diaschisis: a remote functional depression secondary to supratentorial infarction in man. J Cereb Blood Flow Metab 1981;1:S500–1.

[92] Yamauchi H, Fukuyama H, Nagahama Y, et al. Uncoupling of oxygen and glucose metabolism in persistent crossed cerebellar diaschisis. Stroke 1999; 30:1424–8.

[93] De Reuck J, Decoo D, Lemahieu I, et al. Crossed cerebellar diaschisis after middle cerebral artery infarction. Clin Neurol Neurosurg 1997;99:11–6.

[94] Broich K, Alavi A, Kushner M. Positron emission tomography in cerebrovascular disorders. Semin Nucl Med 1992;22:224–32.

[95] Iglesias S, Marchal G, Rioux P, et al. Do changes in oxygen metabolism in the unaffected cerebral hemisphere underlie early neurological recovery after stroke? A positron emission tomography study. Stroke 1996;27:1192–9.

[96] Gibbs J, Wise R, Leenders K, et al. Evaluation of cerebral perfusion reserve in patients with carotid-artery occlusion. Lancet 1984;1:310–4.

[97] Sette G, Baron J, Mazoyer B, et al. Local brain hemodynamics and oxygen metabolism in cerebrovascular disease. Brain 1989;112:931–51.

[98] Powers W, Press G, Grubb R, et al. The effect of hemodynamically significant carotid artery disease on the hemodynamic status of the cerebral circulation. Ann Intern Med 1987;106:27–35.

[99] Powers W, Grubb R, Raichle M. Clinical results of extracranial-intracranial bypass-surgery in patients with hemodynamic cerebrovascular disease. J Neurosurg 1989;70:61–7.

[100] Derdeyn CP, Videen TO, Simmons NR, et al. Count-based PET method for predicting ischemic stroke in patients with symptomatic carotid arterial occlusion. Radiology 1999;212:499–506.

[101] Derdeyn CP, Yundt KD, Videen TO, et al. Increased oxygen extraction fraction is associated with prior ischemic events in patients with carotid occlusion. Stroke 1998;29:754–8.

[102] Samson Y, Baron J, Bousser M. Effects of extraintracranial arterial bypass on cerebral blood flow and oxygen metabolism in humans. Stroke 1985;16: 609–16.

[103] Powers W, Tempel L, Grubb R. Influence of cerebral hemodynamics on stroke risk: one-year follow-up of 38 medically treated patients. Ann Neurol 1989;25: 325–30.

[104] Heiss WD, Kessler J, Karbe H, et al. Cerebral glucose metabolism as a predictor of recovery from aphasia in ischemic stroke. Arch Neurol 1993;50:958–64.

[105] Karbe H, Kessler J, Herholz K, et al. Long-term prognosis of poststroke aphasia studied with positron emission tomography. Arch Neurol 1995;52:186–90.

[106] Rosen HJ, Petersen SE, Linenweber MR, et al. Neural correlates of recovery from aphasia after damage to left inferior frontal cortex. Neurology 2000;55: 1883–94.

[107] Ohyama M, Senda M, Kitamura S, et al. Role of the nondominant hemisphere and undamaged area during word repetition in poststroke aphasics: a PET activation study. Stroke 1996;27:897–903.

[108] Karbe H, Thiel A, Weber-Luxenburger G, et al. Brain plasticity in poststroke aphasia: what is the contribution of the right hemisphere? Brain Lang 1998;64: 215–30.

[109] Heiss WD, Kessler J, Thiel A, et al. Differential capacity of left and right hemispheric areas for compensation of poststroke aphasia. Ann Neurol 1999; 45:430–8.

[110] Warburton E, Price CJ, Swinburn K, et al. Mechanisms of recovery from aphasia: evidence from positron emission tomography studies. J Neurol Neurosurg Psychiatry 1999;66:155–61.

[111] Nelles G, Spiekramann G, Jueptner M, et al. Evolution of functional reorganization in hemiplegic stroke: a serial positron emission tomographic activation study. Ann Neurol 1999;46:901–9.

[112] Heiss WD, Grond M, Thiel A, et al. Tissue at risk of infarction rescued by early reperfusion: a positron emission tomography study in systemic recombinant tissue plasminogen activator thrombolysis of acute stroke. J Cereb Blood Flow Metab 1998;18: 1298–307.

[113] Heiss WD, Grond M, Thiel A, et al. Permanent cortical damage detected by flumazenil positron emission tomography in acute stroke. Stroke 1998; 29:454–61.

[114] Heiss WD, Graf R, Grond M, et al. Quantitative neuroimaging for the evaluation of the effect of stroke treatment. Cerebrovasc Dis 1998;8(Suppl 2):23–9.

[115] Hakim A, Evans A, Berger L, et al. The effect of nimodipine on the evolution of human cerebral infarction studies by PET. J Cereb Blood Flow Metab 1989;9:523–34.

[116] Heiss W, Holthoff V, Pawlik G, et al. Effect of nimodipine on regional cerebral glucose metabolism in patients with acute ischemic stroke as measured by positron emission tomography. J Cereb Blood Flow Metab 1990;10:127–32.

[117] Langfitt TW, Obrist WD, Alavi A, et al. Computerized tomography, magnetic resonance imaging, and positron emission tomography in the study of brain

trauma. Preliminary observations. J Neurosurg 1986; 64:760–7.

[118] Alavi A, Fazekas T, Alves W, et al. Positron emission tomography in the evaluation of head injury [abstract]. J Cereb Blood Flow Metab 1987;7:S646.

[119] George JK, Alavi A, Zimmerman RA, et al. Metabolic (PET) correlates of anatomic lesions (CT/MRI) produced by head trauma [abstract]. J Nucl Med 1989;30:802.

[120] Alavi A. Functional and anatomic studies of head injury. J Neuropsychiatry 1989;1:S45–50.

[121] Alavi A, Mirot A, Newberg A, et al. F-18 PET evaluation of crossed cerebellar diaschisis in head injury. J Nucl Med 1997;38:1717–20.

[122] Ruff RM, Crouch JA, Troster AI, et al. Selected cases of poor outcome following minor brain trauma: comparing neuropsychological and positron emission tomography assessment. Brain Inj 1994;8:297–308.

[123] Bergsneider M, Hovda DA, Lee SM, et al. Dissociation of cerebral glucose metabolism and level of consciousness during the period of metabolic depression following human traumatic brain injury. J Neurotrauma 2000;17:389–401.

[124] Bergsneider M, Hovda DA, Shalmon E, et al. Cerebral hyperglycolysis following severe traumatic brain injury in humans: a positron emission tomography study. J Neurosurg 1997;86:241–51.

[125] Worley G, Hoffman JM, Paine SS, et al. 18-Fluorodeoxyglucose positron emission tomography in children and adolescents with traumatic brain injury. Dev Med Child Neurol 1995;37:213–20.

[126] de Jong BM, Willemsen AT, Paans AM. Regional cerebral blood flow changes related to affective speech presentation in persistent vegetative state. Clin Neurol Neurosurg 1997;99:213–6.

[127] Engel Jr J, Kuhl DE, Phelps ME, et al. Comparative localization of the epileptic foci in partial epilepsy by PCT and EEG. Ann Neurol 1982;12:529–37.

[128] Theodore WH, Brooks R, Sato S, et al. The role of positron emission tomography in the evaluation of seizure disorders. Ann Neurol 1984;15:S1176–9.

[129] Henry TR, Sutherling WW, Engel Jr J, et al. Interictal cerebral metabolism in partial epilepsies of neocortical origin. Epilepsy Res 1991;10:174–82.

[130] Duncan R. Epilepsy, cerebral blood flow, and cerebral metabolic rate. Cerebrovasc Brain Metab Rev 1992; 4:105–21.

[131] Utsubo H, Chuang SH, Hwang PA, et al. Neuroimaging for investigation of seizures in children. Pediatr Neurosurg 1992;18:105–16.

[132] Breier JI, Mullani NA, Thomas AB, et al. Effects of duration of epilepsy on the uncoupling of metabolism and blood flow in complex partial seizures. Neurology 1997;48:1047–53.

[133] Savic I, Altshuler L, Baxter L, et al. Pattern of interictal hypometabolism in PET scans with fludeoxyglucose F 18 reflects prior seizure types in patients with mesial temporal lobe seizures. Arch Neurol 1997;54:129–36.

[134] Theodore WH, Gaillard WD, Sato S, et al. Positron emission tomographic measurement of cerebral blood flow and temporal lobectomy. Ann Neurol 1994; 36:241–4.

[135] Manno EM, Sperling MR, Ding X, et al. Predictors of outcome after anterior temporal lobectomy: positron emission tomography. Neurol 1994;44:2331–6.

[136] Radtke RA, Hanson MW, Hoffman JM, et al. Temporal lobe hypometabolism on PET: predictor of seizure control after temporal lobectomy. Neurol 1993;43:1088–92.

[137] Wong C-Y, Geller EB, Chen EQ, et al. Outcome of temporal lobe epilepsy surgery predicted by statistical parametric PET imaging. J Nucl Med 1996; 37:1094–100.

[138] Theodore WH, Sato S, Kufta C, et al. Temporal lobectomy for uncontrolled seizures: the role of positron emission tomography. Ann Neurol 1992;32:789–94.

[139] Delbeke D, Lawrence SK, Abou-Khalil BW, et al. Postsurgical outcome of patients with uncontrolled complex partial seizures and temporal lobe hypometabolism on 18FDG-positron emission tomography. Invest Radiol 1996;31:261–6.

[140] Benbadis SR, So NK, Antar MA, et al. The value of PET scan (and MRI and Wada test) in patients with bitemporal epileptiform abnormalities. Arch Neurol 1995;52:1062–8.

[141] Swartz BE, Tomiyasu U, Delgado-Escueta AV, et al. Neuroimaging in temporal lobe epilepsy: test sensitivity and relationships to pathology and postoperative outcome. Epilepsia 1992;33:624–34.

[142] Newberg A, Alavi A, Sperling M, et al. Thalamic metabolic asymmetry on FDG-PET scans as a determinant of seizure outcome after temporal lobectomy. J Nucl Med 1997;38:92P.

[143] Markand ON, Salanova V, Worth R, et al. Comparative study of interictal PET and ictal SPECT in complex partial seizures. Acta Neurol Scand 1997; 95:129–36.

[144] Salanova V, Markand O, Worth R, et al. FDG-PET and MRI in temporal lobe epilepsy: relationship to febrile seizures, hippocampal sclerosis and outcome. Acta Neurol Scand 1998;97:146–53.

[145] Knowlton RC, Laxer KD, Ende G, et al. Presurgical multimodality neuroimaging in electroencephalographic lateralized temporal lobe epilepsy. Ann Neurol 1997;42:829–37.

[146] Rubin E, Dhawan V, Moeller JR, et al. Cerebral metabolic topography in unilateral temporal lobe epilepsy. Neurol 1995;45:2212–23.

[147] Van Bogaert P, Massager N, Tugendhaft P, et al. Statistical parametric mapping of regional glucose metabolism in mesial temporal lobe epilepsy. Neuroimage 2000;12:129–38.

[148] Quesney LF, Olivier A, Andermann F, et al. Preoperative EEG investigation in patients with frontal lobe epilepsy: trends, results and pathophysiological considerations. J Clin Neurophysiol 1987;4:208–9.

[149] Franck G, Maquet P, Sadzot B, et al. Contribution of positron emission tomography to the investigation of epilepsies of frontal lobe origin. Adv Neurol 1992; 57:471–85.

[150] Robitaille Y, Rasmussen T, Dubeau F, et al. Histopathology of nonneoplastic lesions in frontal lobe epilepsy: review of 180 cases with recent MRI and PET correlations. Adv Neurol 1992;57:499–511.

[151] Alavi A, Hirsch LJ. Studies of central nervous system disorders with single photon emission computed tomography and positron emission tomography: evolution over the past 2 decades. Semin Nucl Med 1991;21:58–81.

[152] Chugani HT, Rintahaka PJ, Shewmon DA. Ictal patterns of cerebral glucose utilization in children with epilepsy. Epilepsia 1994;35:813–22.

[153] Theodore WH, Balish M, Leiderman D, et al. Effect of seizures on cerebral blood flow measured with 15O-H_2O and positron emission tomography. Epilepsia 1996;37:796–802.

ELSEVIER
SAUNDERS

Radiol Clin N Am 43 (2005) 67–77

RADIOLOGIC
CLINICS
of North America

PET imaging in the assessment of normal and impaired cognitive function

Daniel H.S. Silverman, MD[a,b,c,*], Abass Alavi, MD[d]

[a]Neuroimaging Section, University of California at Los Angeles Medical Center, Los Angeles, CA, USA
[b]University of California at Los Angeles Alzheimer's Disease Center Imaging Core, Los Angeles, CA, USA
[c]Ahmanson Biological Imaging Division, Department of Molecular and Medical Pharmacology,
David Geffen School of Medicine, University of California at Los Angeles Medical Center, CHS AR-144, MC694215,
Los Angeles, CA 90095-6942, USA
[d]Division of Nuclear Medicine, Department of Radiology, Hospital of the University of Pennsylvania, 110 Donner Building,
3400 Spruce Street, Philadelphia, PA 19104, USA

The past three decades have witnessed the introduction of a series of powerful imaging modalities that have allowed detailed analysis of structure/function relation in a multitude of diseases and disorders. Interestingly, performance of these modern modalities were first tested by acquiring images of a variety of central nervous system disorders before they were employed for assessing diseases of the other organs. Brain images in general, appear with high resolution and lend themselves well to quantitative analysis because of the favorable geometry of the head and minimal motion during data acquisition. For the same reason, coregistration of PET and structural images can be readily accomplished with modern algorithms that have been perfected for this purpose. Recent developments in small animal imaging that allow reconstruction of PET images with an extraordinary resolution (1–2 mm) has resulted in designing and building instruments for examining the brain with exquisite detail [1–6]. By employing modern crystals (lutetium oxyorthosilicate [LSO] and gadolinium orthosilicate [GSO]) as a multidetector assembly, attempts have been made to generate human brain images with a resolution that approaches 3 mm [7–9]. This degree of high-resolution imaging cannot be achieved elsewhere in the body. It is expected that the approved indications for PET imaging for central nervous system disorders will expand in the future and therefore, the interest for using dedicated brain imaging instruments may gain strength toward the end of this decade. This may improve the quality of the images generated and further enhance the impact of this modality in managing patients who have brain disorders.

With the introduction of several novel drugs to treat patients who have Alzheimer's disease (AD), accurate and early diagnosis of the disease is paramount for success of this type of therapeutic intervention. Because the disease is initiated in the molecular and the cellular levels early on in the course of AD, metabolic imaging would appear to be the modality of choice for screening patients who have memory loss. At the early stages of the disease, functional imaging with flow tracers (by employing single photon emmission computed tomography, PET, or perfusion studies with MR imaging) may not be sensitive enough to detect evidence of the disease. Likewise, structural images will remain negative for an indefinite period. However, as the disease progresses, changes in blood flow to the affected regions can be detected by the above described techniques. In advanced disease, significant cortical atrophy and ventricular enlargement will be noted. Obviously, this would imply an irreversible process.

* Corresponding author. Nuclear Medicine Clinic, David Geffen School of Medicine at the University of California at Los Angeles, CHS AR-144, MC694215, Los Angeles, CA 90095-6942.
E-mail address: dsilver@ucla.edu (D.H.S. Silverman).

0033-8389/05/$ – see front matter © 2004 Elsevier Inc. All rights reserved.
doi:10.1016/j.rcl.2004.09.012

Presence of atrophy should be taken into consideration in the interpretation of the PET images. In patients with normal structural studies and abnormal fluorine-18–fluorodeoxyglucose-PET ([18F]-FDG–PET) scans, metabolic changes accurately reflect the degree of functional impairment in the cortex or any other gray matter. However, presence of cortical atrophy adversely affects accurate measurement of regional metabolism in patients who have AD. Because the cerebrospinal fluid has no metabolic activity and cannot be completely resolved spatially from the cortical structures on PET images, the presence of cerebral atrophy artificially lowers the measured metabolic activity of the adjacent cortex. Therefore, in such circumstances, the measured metabolic rate should be corrected for the corresponding degree of atrophy [10–13]. This would require precise coregistration of PET and anatomic images and accurate calculation of the amount of the cerebrospinal fluid in the regions of interest assigned to the PET images. It is interesting that in the advanced stages of the disease, when metabolic rates are corrected for atrophy, the remaining cortex appears to have levels of activity comparable to those of age-matched controls. Therefore, it is essential that changes that are noted on PET images are carefully correlated with the structural abnormalities seen on either CT or MR imaging scans. This is particularly true when such studies are performed for research purposes.

Studies of normal brain

Cerebral metabolism

The most commonly performed PET studies of the brain are performed with FDG as the imaged radiopharmaceutical (Fig. 1). In the clinical arena, the resulting scans are typically interpreted qualitatively through visual analysis. This involves the reader examining the relative distribution of FDG throughout the patient's brain and comparing it with the distribution expected for a normal subject of similar age. The patient's age is relevant because of changes in cerebral metabolism that are known to occur in the course of normal development and aging (see below). Other factors that can influence scans of normal subjects—either with respect to regional activity or to

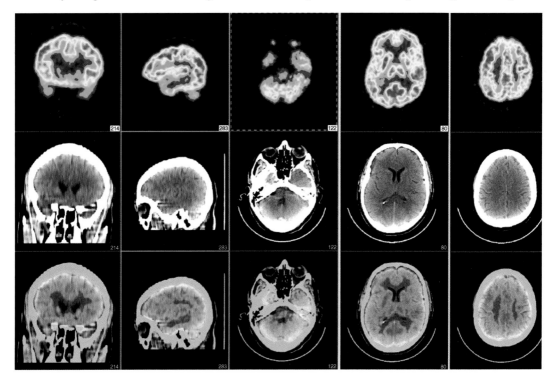

Fig. 1. PET/CT scan demonstrating normal brain scan in a 58-year-old man. PET data are displayed in a rainbow color scale related to radioactive counts per second per pixel overlying gray-scale CT data acquired during the same imaging session. Planes represent coronal (*column 1*), sagittal (*column 2*), and transaxial slices through low (*column 3*), mid- (*column 4*), and high (*column 5*) axial levels through the brain.

overall count rates—include sex, handedness, sensory environment, level of alertness, mood, drug effects, serum glucose levels, and head fraction (the portion of administered tracer that passes into the brain).

Visual analysis is also used in some research studies, but often the results of semiquantitative or absolute quantitative analyses are reported in addition to or instead of visual interpretation. In this context, *semiquantitative* refers to results that are based on regional concentrations of measured radioactivity, normalized to some internal reference standard—for example, a reference region of the brain, the whole brain activity, or the average whole-body concentration before excretion and decay-corrected to the actual time of imaging (ie, standardized uptake value). Those results turn out to be adequate for most clinical applications, as well as for many research applications. In contrast, *absolute quantitative* values are derived from biologically based mathematical models that reflect the partitioning of radioactivity into compartments that can reflect both physiologic boundaries (eg, the vascular space, the blood–brain barrier, the plasma membrane of neurons) and biochemical processes (enzymatic anabolism and degradation, transport molecules). These

models necessarily represent substantial simplifications of the actual biologic environment, but nevertheless have proven capable of yielding quantitative estimates in good agreement with similar measures obtained by more invasive methods. In the case of FDG studies, the biologic parameter that is being estimated is the rate of regional glucose use, based on a method described by Sokoloff and colleagues [14], originally developed with (unfluorinated) carbon-14 ($[^{14}C]$)-labeled 2-deoxyglucose. Early measures of regional glucose use rates in the human brain [15–19] yielded estimates of global cerebral metabolism of approximately 5.5 mg glucose/min/100 g, which ranged from 3.6 to 5.2 mg glucose/min/100 g in white matter structures to 5.8 to 10.3 mg glucose/min/100 g in gray matter structures. Regional values that have been more recently published (Table 1) [20–23], reflecting measurements using instruments and techniques with improved imaging capabilities, are in substantial agreement with these initially reported values. A recent study by Yamaji and colleagues [23] is notable for having obtained regional standardized uptake value measurements (see Table 1; values in parentheses) in the same group of subjects in whom absolute quantitative values were obtained,

Table 1
Rates of regional glucose use determined with fluorodeoxyglucose-PET in normal subjects

Region	Study				
	Minoshima et al, 1995 [20] 64 ± 8 y (n = 22)	Moeller et al, 1996 [21]		Ishii et al, 1998 [22] 67 ± 6 y (n = 21)	Yamaji et al, 2000 [23] 68 ± 6 y (n = 18)
		<50 y (n = 58)	50 y (n = 72)		
Frontal cortex	7.9	—	—	—	7.9 (7.7)
Inferior	—	—	—	7.7	—
Middle	—	—	—	7.6	—
Superior	—	—	—	7.2	—
Anterior	—	—	—	7.2	—
Medial	—	8.8	7.9	—	—
Lateral	—	9.1	8.4	—	—
Sensorimotor strip	7.7	8.7	8.0	7.6	8.1 (7.8)
Parietal cortex	7.8	—	—	—	7.8 (7.7)
Inferior	—	8.9	8.2	7.7	—
Superior	—	—	—	7.4	—
Temporal cortex	6.8	—	—	—	7.1 (7.0)
Anterior	—	—	—	6.3	—
Posterior	—	—	—	7.3	—
Medial	—	6.8	6.5	5.1	—
Lateral	—	6.6	6.1	—	—
Occipital cortex	8.1	—	—	—	7.8 (7.7)
Medial	—	8.5	8.1	8.0	—
Lateral	—	8.1	7.9	7.6	—
Basal ganglia	—	9.7	9.2	8.4	—
Thalamus	8.7	8.8	8.9	7.6	—
Cerebellum	—	5.6	6.9	6.7	—

All values are expressed in mg/min/100 g, except for numbers in parentheses, which are standardized uptake values.

with remarkably close correspondence of the two types of measures seen in the healthy brain.

Cerebral blood flow

In the healthy brain, cerebral blood flow is normally tightly coupled with local metabolic needs of brain tissue, through vasoconstrictive/vasodilatory autoregulation of blood supply. Thus, within a vascular territory, measures of cerebral blood flow and glucose metabolic rate co-vary nearly linearly. Between different vascular territories, however, different constants of proportionality can pertain. For example, because most of the lateral neocortex is supplied by the middle cerebral artery branch of the carotid circulation, the pattern of distribution of the blood flow tracer oxygen-15–labeled water ($H_2^{15}O$) closely parallels that of the metabolic tracer FDG throughout most of the cortical surface. However, dissociations also occur. The cerebellum, despite its lower metabolic activity relative to neocortex, is more richly perfused, being supplied by arterial branches of the vertebrobasilar circulation. Also, in certain pathologic circumstances (see later discussion regarding stroke), the normal coupling between metabolism and perfusion can be disturbed, such that a consistent relationship may not exist even within a vascular territory.

Images of regional cerebral activity can be obtained with $H_2^{15}O$ (or $^{15}O_2$), as with FDG. In the case of these former tracers, however, the short physical half-life (2 minutes) of the ^{15}O nuclide makes them especially suitable for acquiring multiple data sets from the same individual over a relatively brief period. This allows for statistical analyses of changes observed in regional cerebral activity (measured quantitatively or semiquantitatively, as described for FDG) during varying experimental conditions, such as resting versus motor, sensory, or cognitive activities; predrug versus postdrug and withdrawal states; waking versus various stages of sleeping; comfort versus discomfort or pain; and emotional calm versus induced sadness, anxiety, sexual arousal, fear, or anger. This paradigm for studying brain function, referred to as an *activation study*, has now been used in thousands of investigations, for the purpose of identifying cerebral correlates of normal and pathologic processes involved in mentation and behavior.

Efforts over the years to quantify cerebral blood flow in absolute units (generally mL/min/100 g) with PET have yielded values varying much more widely than corresponding efforts to quantify glucose metabolism (see previous discussion). Factors contributing to this variability include the radiopharmaceuticals used, the evolving spatial resolution of scanning

systems, whether and how volume corrections are performed, and whether one-compartment or two-compartment models are employed [24]. For example, an early report of cerebral blood flow measurements [25] in seven subjects with a mean age of 27 years, using $H_2^{15}O$-PET without correction for blood volume, estimated mean gray matter flow at 39 ± 7 mL/min/100 g. A later study [26] employing a one-compartment model and MR-based partial-volume corrections in 18 subjects with a mean age of 28 years, estimated cortical flow at 62 ± 10 mL/min/100 mL. In a recent systematic methodologic study [24], 64 $H_2^{15}O$ scans were acquired from eight subjects in whom the investigators found a two-compartment model to be superior to a one-compartment model for their imaging data. Using that model with partial-volume correction yielded values of gray matter flow at 107 ± 11 mL/min/100 g (substantially higher than their estimate using the same data set, but with a one-compartment model). Given that the standard deviations for "absolute" flow determinations within investigations are typically 10% to 20%, but that between investigations can vary by more than 100%, the need for each study to define a baseline or control range, maintaining a consistent methodology across both experimental and control groups or conditions is clear.

Functional development and aging

How PET-based measurements of normal brain function can be expected to change during the course of development and healthy aging is an important issue. It becomes especially pertinent in the clinical interpretation of scans (where no age-matched explicit control group typically exists) in deciding whether scan findings fall beyond the bounds of what is to be expected for a patient of a given age.

Because of understandable ethical concerns surrounding experimental radiation exposure of healthy children, few PET data are available to address normal changes at the young end of the developmental spectrum. Much of what is known in this regard comes from the seminal work of Chugani and colleagues [27–29]. Based on measurements of local cerebral metabolic rate for glucose in infants who had suffered transient neurologic events—but who were judged to be "nearly normal" at the time of PET and neurodevelopmentally normal throughout a subsequent follow-up period—the following picture has emerged. In the newborn, glucose metabolism is highest in the primary sensorimotor cortex, cingulate cortex, hippocampal region, thalamus, cerebellar vermis, and midbrain. During the first 3 months of life, the most prominent increases occur in the cerebellar cortex, basal ganglia, and parietal, temporal, and primary visual cortical areas. In later infancy, increases in glucose use are most noticeable in the frontal cortex, such that by the end of the first year, the relative distribution of glucose metabolism approximates that of the adult brain. In terms of absolute rates of glucose use, however, developmental changes occur throughout childhood. Initially lower than in adults, the absolute rate increases throughout the first 3 to 4 years of life, at which time global glucose use by the cerebral cortex is actually 2 to 3 times greater than the adult level. This level remains near-constant until 8 to 10 years of age, after which a gradual decline subsequently occurs, over approximately 8 years, when adult levels are reached. A similar developmental course has been observed with respect to PET measures of cerebral blood flow and oxygen metabolism [30]. In absolute terms, those rates are lower at birth than in adults and increase significantly during early childhood. The highest levels of cerebral blood flow throughout the brain are reached by 8 years, after which they decline toward adult levels, while the developmental time course of oxygen use shows more variation among regions. Serotonin synthesis capacity has also been reported to be greatest in early childhood years, and subsequently to decline to adult levels [31], though this remains less established.

At the other end of the age spectrum, effects of normal aging on brain function of adults have also been examined with PET. In a recent study of 37 healthy adults ranging in age from 19 to 50 years [32], the most significant age-related decline in cerebral blood flow was found in the mesial frontal cortex, encompassing the anterior cingulate cortex, and extending rostrally into the supplementary motor area. In an independent study of 27 healthy adults ranging from 19 to 76 years of age [26], the most significant age-related decline was found in the medial orbito-frontal cortex, and this was the only regional effect to remain significant after correction for partial volume effects of cerebral atrophy. Likewise, recent measures of metabolism using FDG have also identified an age-related decline in healthy adults [21], most consistently in frontal cortex; nevertheless, as has been reviewed previously [33], studies of carefully selected subjects find declines to be minimal in glucose metabolism throughout most of the brain in normal aging.

Alzheimer's disease and other dementing illnesses

Decreasing mortality, with consequent progressive aging of the mature adult population, has led to a rising prevalence of senile dementia. The condition is tremendously costly to patients, their families, and society in general. AD affects over 4 million people in the United States alone, incurring associated yearly expenses of nearly $70 billion. When indirect costs such as the lost productivity of caregivers are taken into account, total annual expenditures approximate $100 billion. As the baby boomers approach senior citizen status in the twenty-first century, it is estimated that over 14 million Americans will suffer from AD by 2050 [34–37].

PET studies of dementia, and of brain disorders in general, can be grouped into two broad categories: (1) those aimed at elucidating neurologic substrates, either of fundamental pathophysiology or of observed associations between disease and various other factors; and (2) those directly aimed at improving diagnosis, prognostic assessment, or therapeutic management of neurologically based disorders. With respect to dementia, examples of studies belonging to the first group include those that have examined associations of genetic or environmental risk factors with the presence or later development of AD. Epidemiologic studies indicate that lack of education is a major risk factor for AD [38,39]. Several studies implementing functional brain imaging have shed light on the effect of education on the clinical expression of AD. Using the xenon-133 (^{133}Xe) technique to quantify regional cerebral blood flow and approximate the pathophysiologic severity of AD, it was shown that among individuals with probable AD, those who have a high level of education have greater parietotemporal perfusion deficit than those who have a low level of education [40]. Similarly, it has been demonstrated that individuals who have occupations associated with higher interpersonal skills experience greater parietal perfusion deficit for a given level of cognitive function [41]. Using PET to assess cerebral glucose metabolism, Alexander and colleagues [42] compared AD patients matched for demographic characteristics and dementia severity but differing in estimated premorbid intellectual ability, as defined by demographics-based IQ estimates, as well as by performance on a test of word reading. They found that estimated premorbid intellectual ability was inversely correlated with cerebral metabolism in the prefrontal, premotor, and left superior parietal regions.

In addition to low education level, genetic risk factors for AD have been identified. The ε4 allele of the apolipoprotein E gene is associated with a significantly increased risk of developing AD of senile onset; overall, those with the ε4/ε3 or ε4/ε4 genotype are more than twice as likely to have AD compared with individuals with the ε3/ε3 genotype [43]. FDG-PET studies have linked the ε4 allele to hypometabolism in posterior cingulate, parietal, and temporal cortex, and have identified greater metabolic asymmetry in nondemented relatives of individuals with probable AD [44–47]. Furthermore, significant metabolic decline in these regions has been longitudinally observed in those who have inherited the ε4 allele as measured by repeating PET in the same subjects over a two-year interval [46].

With regard to the second broad category, investigations into clinical applications of PET with dementia patients stem from numerous studies that have found that many neurodegenerative diseases produce significant alterations in brain function detectable with PET. The use of PET in this regard has been under study since the early 1980s [48–51] and has been extensively reviewed in more recent years [52–57]. Thousands of patients with clinically diagnosed—and, in some cases, histopathologically confirmed—causes of dementia from many independent laboratories have been studied using PET measures of cerebral blood flow, glucose metabolism, or oxygen use. The best-studied application of this type is the use of FDG-PET to evaluate AD. Sensitivity of FDG-PET in this context has been consistently high, even in patients with mild impairment, suggesting that by the time a patient presents with symptoms of a neurodegenerative dementia, substantial alteration of cortical metabolic function generally has occurred. The associated decreases in glucose metabolism in certain brain areas are readily detectable on FDG images, and identification of the particular brain areas of involvement can be valuable

in the differential diagnosis of dementia. Some visually evident differences between scans of patients with different dementing illnesses are seen in Fig. 2.

Assessment of the diagnostic accuracy of PET had until recently been hindered by the paucity of studies involving patients who undergo long-term clinical follow-up or subsequent pathologic diagnosis; the approach used in most previous clinical series had been the comparison of PET findings to clinical assessments performed near the time of PET. The ability of the latter approach to assess diagnostic accuracy is unfortunately limited by the fact that clinical diagnosis can be inaccurate, particularly for patients presenting in the earliest stages of disease—a time when the opportunity for effective therapy and meaningful planning is at its greatest.

Studies comparing neuropathologic examination with imaging are thus most informative in assessing the diagnostic value of PET. In a pooled analysis [56] of three previously published studies [58–60], histopathologically confirmed sensitivity and specificity of PET for detecting the presence of AD were 92% and 71%, respectively. In the largest single-institution series, Hoffman and coworkers [61] found sensitivity and specificity of PET for AD to fall in the range of 88% to 93% and 63% to 67%, respectively. A subsequent multicenter study collected data from an international consortium of clinical facilities that had acquired both brain FDG-PET and histopathologic data for patients undergoing evaluation for dementia [62]. The PET results identified AD patients with a sensitivity and specificity of 94% and 73%, respec-

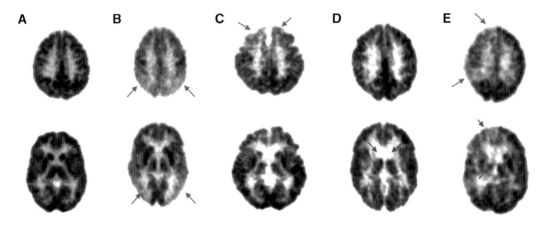

Fig. 2. Normal and abnormal patterns of FDG distribution. PET data are displayed in inverse gray scale, with darkness level of each pixel linearly related to radioactive counts per second. Planes are shown at high- (*top row*) and mid- (*bottom row*) transaxial levels for subjects with (*A*) normal metabolic pattern, (*B*) posterior (parietal, temporal, posterior cingulate) hypometabolism characteristic of early AD, (*C*) anterior hypometabolism characteristic of early frontal lobe dementia, (*D*) profound striatal hypometabolism characteristic of Huntington's disease, and (*E*) diffusely distributed foci of right-sided hypometabolism in cortical and subcortical structures, characteristic of multiple infarcts in tissue supplied by the right carotid artery.

tively. This latter study, which included over three times as many patients as the four previous studies combined, included a stratified examination of the subset of patients with documented early or mild disease. Performance of PET with respect to sensitivity (95%), specificity (71%), and overall accuracy (89%) was nearly the same. The above values are in accordance with the ranges found in a broader review of the PET literature which also included studies lacking neuropathologic confirmation of diagnoses [63], that reported sensitivities ranging from 90% to 96% and specificities ranging from 67% to 97%, as well as in a recent review of the PET literature reported by the AAN [64], in which it was concluded that "PET scanning appears to have promise for use as an adjunct to clinical diagnosis [of AD]," based on their review of published studies that demonstrated diagnostic accuracies of 86% to 100% for PET.

Regional cerebral metabolic changes associated with early AD can be detected with PET, even before the symptomatic manifestations of the disease become evident [62,65,66]. How accurately can FDG-PET be used in the evaluation of nondemented patients, who are in the earliest stages of cognitive impairment? The most recent FDG-PET neuroimaging studies involving patients classified as cognitively impaired nondemented (CIND) or having mild cognitive impairment (MCI), conducted or published between 2001 and 2003, were recently reviewed [53]. Studies were found through a PubMed search executed in July 2003 (keywords: positron emission tomography, cognitively impaired not demented, mild cognitive impairment) and by systematically checking through the bibliographies of relevant articles so identified. The major criterion for inclusion was the use of FDG-PET to evaluate cognitively impaired nondemented patients and patients having mild cognitive impairment as a specific subject subset in the study; investigations that did not involve FDG-PET were excluded. Overall accuracies achieved with use of FDG-PET were nearly as high in very mildly affected patients as in demented patients, generally exceeding 80%, and ranging from 75% to 100% in these recent studies. PET may be especially valuable in this clinical setting, considering the difficulty of distinguishing these patients from those with mild memory loss attributed to normal aging.

Prognosis

FDG-PET may also serve explicitly as a prognostic tool, to determine likelihood of deterioration of mental status in the period following the time of scanning. Relative hypometabolism of associative cortex can be accurately used to predict whether cognitive decline will occur at a rate faster than would be expected for normal aging, over the several years following a PET evaluation [65,67]. Moreover, the magnitude of decline over a 2-year period, for some standardized measures of memory, correlates with the initial degree of hypometabolism of inferior parietal, superior temporal, and posterior cingulate cortical regions [46]. As cognitive impairment caused by a neurodegenerative disease progresses, associated progression of regions of hypometabolism also occurs.

In a longitudinal evaluation of 170 patients who underwent brain PET, analyses were stratified according to presence of the most common comorbidities affecting cognitive function (other than primary neurodegenerative disease), depression and thyroid disease, and also according to scanner type [68]. Over one-third (65 of 170, 38%) of all patients were documented to have a history of depression at the time of PET, 18% had a history of thyroid disease, and 6% had a history of both. PET findings accurately predicted which patients would have a subsequent progressive course with a sensitivity of 91% (99 of 109). Patients having a subsequent nonprogressive course were identified with a specificity of 80% (49 of 61). Of the patients without a history of depression or thyroid disease, specificity of PET was nearly as high as its sensitivity (89%; 95% CI, 77%–100%), but tended to be lower for patients with a history of depression or thyroid disease (74%; 95% CI, 59%–88%) than in those without either condition. In contrast, sensitivity was unaffected by presence of those conditions (90%; 95% CI, 82%–98% vs. 92%; 95% CI, 84%–100%). While the prognosis of most subjects was correctly predicted by visual analysis of PET scans regardless of presence of depression or thyroid disease, specificity tended to be lower for patients with a history of those conditions, and the overall false positive rate of PET used in the prediction of a clinically progressive course of dementia was three times higher (3.5% [3 of 86] vs. 10.7% [9 of 84]) in patients with a history of depression or thyroid disease. It is thus suggested that physicians examining brain PET scans for dementia prognosis in cognitively impaired patients with depression and thyroid disease interpret positive scans with added caution because of the potentially confounding effects of those conditions on regional brain metabolism. Also of clinical pertinence is that because data collection occurred over a period of almost a decade, during that time there were changes in scanner type (eg, brain PET conducted on the older generation of scanners contained only 15 planes, while scans performed on the newer generation of scanners contained either 47 or 63 planes), so specificity tended to be higher for scans performed on the newer generation of scanners (87%; 95% CI, 73%–100%, vs. 76%; 95% CI, 63%–90%).

It is interesting to consider the mechanistic basis that may underlie at least some of the false positive associations. Bench and colleagues [69] reported that metabolism of certain cerebral regions are negatively correlated with mood symptoms and severity of psychomotor slowing in depression; these regions were found to include the inferior parietal and superior temporal cortex, areas also affected in AD. Effects of hypothyroidism on regional cerebral metabolism have also recently been described [70,71], involving relative reduction in parietal and temporal metabolism, which may further help explain the compromise in PET specificity associated with such conditions, particularly with older scanners lacking the resolution to distinguish characteristic patterns of regional involvement from similar but distinct regions.

With respect to incremental value of PET beyond conventional clinical assessment, it was recently found that among patients having clinical working diagnoses presuming nonprogressive etiologies for their cognitive complaints, those whose PET patterns were nevertheless indicative of progressive dementia were more than 18 times likelier to experience progressive decline than those with nonprogressive PET patterns [67]. When neurologists diagnosed their patients as having progressive dementia, they were correct in 84% of those cases. Adding a positive diagnosis from a PET scan boosted the accuracy of that prediction to 94%, and a negative PET scan made it 12 times more likely that the patient would remain cognitively stable.

Stroke

Application of PET to the study of cerebrovascular diseases enjoys a long history, extending back two decades [72,73]. PET has been used to directly quantify several parameters pertinent to the status of cerebral perfusion, including cerebral blood flow, cerebral blood volume, cerebral rate of oxygen metabolism, and cerebral glucose use. This methodology has allowed estimation of further relevant parameters through calculations based on the values derived from those measurements, including cerebrovascular mean transit time, cerebral perfusion pressure, oxygen extraction fraction, and stoichiometry of oxygen and glucose use. Each of these have been reported to change, in different ways, under circumstances stemming from the pathophysiologic events that occur during cerebrovascular compromise, and the evolution of stroke as well as its aftermath. To briefly summarize the most consistently reported findings:

1. In the early phase of cerebrovascular compromise, blood flow is maintained through autoregulated vasodilation, leading to an increase in blood volume.
2. As the compensatory capacity of autoregulation is exceeded, blood flow falls, while oxygen metabolism is maintained, corresponding to an increase in oxygen extraction fraction (the beginning of "misery perfusion").
3. Once oxygen extraction fraction has increased maximally, continued decline in blood flow leads to a decline in oxygen delivery and metabolism (the onset of ischemia).
4. Severe and prolonged compromise results in infarction of brain tissue, with decreased demand for oxygen metabolism, while vasodilation persists, leading to a decline in oxygen extraction fraction (and onset of "luxury perfusion"). As revascularization occurs, blood flow to the region increases, and the infarcted area typically remains in a state of luxury perfusion for days to weeks.

While there is a wealth of data supporting the sequence of events described above, there have been relatively few investigations directly assessing the clinical use of PET in the setting of cerebrovascular disease. The prognostic value of oxygen extraction fraction data, calculated from PET measures of regional oxygen metabolism and blood flow using $[^{15}O]$-gas and $[H_2^{15}O]$-water, was recently demonstrated in patients having a history of stroke or transient ischemic attack in the distribution of an occluded carotid artery [74]. The investigators divided 81 such patients studied by PET into two groups: 39 with elevated oxygen extraction fractions (operationally defined by asymmetry, through reference to a control group, approximately corresponding to exceeding the contralateral region by more than 8%), and 42 with normal (symmetric) oxygen extraction fractions. After adjusting for age, those in the first group had a sixfold higher risk of suffering a stroke (all but one occurring ipsilateral to the side with higher oxygen extraction fraction) than those in the second group. Shortly afterward, it was independently reported [75] that among 40 patients followed for 5 years after PET, increased hemispheric oxygen extraction (defined by a reference value derived from the mean and variance of the extraction fraction of a control group, corresponding to exceeding 53.3%) was associated with a sevenfold higher risk of suffering a stroke. A less significant difference was found between groups categorized according to asymmetry of oxygen extraction fraction. In the setting of acute stroke, Heiss and colleagues [76] measured cerebral blood flow with $H_2^{15}O$ in 12 patients before and after thrombolytic therapy with tissue plasminogen activator. Reperfusion, as documented by PET on the day of tissue plasminogen activator therapy, predicted clinical improvement assessed 3 weeks later. Marchal and colleagues [77] found that for 19 patients undergoing PET within 5 to 18 hours of onset of middle cerebral artery stroke, the extent of abnormally low cerebral blood flow or oxygen metabolism (but not blood volume, perfusion pressure, or oxygen extraction fraction) correlated with final infarct size and long-term clinical outcome.

Beyond investigation of these relatively well-studied hemodynamic parameters measurable with PET, recent studies with newer tracers (eg, those recognizing activated microglial cells or benzodiazepine receptors) are also showing promise of contributing clinically meaningful information to the assessment of patients who have cerebrovascular disease. It remains to be seen what impact any of these methods of using PET to assess various aspects of cerebral status will have on routine clinical management of patients with cerebrovascular disease, but well-controlled randomized trials have begun to be launched to rigorously examine this question [78].

Acknowledgments

The authors are indebted to Cecilia Yap and Betty Pio for their assistance with manuscript preparation.

References

[1] Cherry SR, Shao Y, Silverman RW, et al. Micropet—a high-resolution PET scanner for imaging small animals. IEEE Trans Nucl Sci 1997;44:1161–6.

[2] Surti S, Karp JS, Freifelder R, et al. Design Evaluation of A-PET: a high sensitivity animal PET camera. IEEE Trans Nucl Sci 2003;50:1357–63.

[3] Lecomte R, Cadorette J, Rodrigue S, et al. Initial results from the Sherbrooke avalanche photodiode positron tomograph. IEEE Trans Nucl Sci 1996;43: 1952–7.

[4] Chatziioannou AF, Cherry SR, Shao YP, et al. Performance evaluation of microPET: a high-resolution lutetium oxyorthosilicate PET scanner for animal imaging. J Nucl Med 1999;40:1164–75.

[5] Ziegler SI, Pichler BJ, Boening G, et al. A prototype high-resolution animal positron tomograph with avalanche photodiode arrays and LSO crystals. Eur J Nucl Med 2001;28:136–43.

[6] Lecomte R, Cadorette J, Richard P, et al. Design and engineering aspects of a high-resolution positron tomograph for small animal imaging. IEEE Trans Nucl Sci 1994;41:1446–52.

[7] Karp JS, Surti S, Freifelder R, et al. Performance of a GSO PET Camera. J Nucl Med 2003;44:1340–9.

[8] Bloomfield PM, Myers R, Hume SP, et al. Three-dimensional performance of a small-diameter positron emission tomograph. Phys Med Biol 1997;42:389–400.

[9] Ziegler SI, Pichler BJ, Boening G, et al. MadPET: high resolution animal pet with avalanche photodiode arrays and LSO crystals. J Nucl Med 2000;41:20P.

[10] Chawluk JB, Alavi A, Dann R, et al. Positron emission tomography in aging and dementia: effect of cerebral atrophy. J Nucl Med 1987;28(4):431–7.

[11] Chawluk JB, Dann R, Alavi A, et al. The effect of focal cerebral atrophy in positron emission tomographic studies of aging and dementia. Int J Rad Appl Instrum B 1990;17:797–804.

[12] Kohn MI, Tanna NK, Herman GT, et al. Analysis of brain and cerebrospinal fluid volumes with MR imaging. Part 1. Methods, reliability and validation. Radiology 1991;178:115–22.

[13] Tanna NK, Kohn MI, Horwich DN, et al. Analysis of brain and cerebrospinal fluid volumes with MR imaging: impact on PET data correction for atrophy. Part II. Aging and Alzheimer's dementia. Radiology 1991;178:123–30.

[14] Sokoloff L, Reivich M, Kennedy C, et al. The [^{14}C]deoxyglucose method for the measurement of local cerebral glucose utilization: theory, procedure and normal values in the conscious and anesthetized albino rat. J Neurochem 1977;28:897–916.

[15] Huang SC, Phelps ME, Hoffman EJ, et al. Noninvasive determination of local cerebral metabolic rate of glucose in man. Am J Physiol 1980;238:E69–E82.

[16] Kuhl DE, Phelps ME, Kowell AP, et al. Effects of stroke on local cerebral metabolism and perfusion: mapping local metabolism and perfusion in normal and ischemic brain by emission computed tomography of ^{18}FDG and ^{13}NH$_3$. Ann Neurol 1980;8:47–60.

[17] Mazziotta JC, Phelps ME, Miller J, et al. Tomographic mapping of human cerebral metabolism: normal unstimulated state. Neurology 1981;31:503–16.

[18] Phelps ME, Huang SC, Hoffman EJ, et al. Tomographic measurement of local cerebral glucose metabolic rate in humans with (F-18)2-fluoro-2-deoxyglucose: validation of method. Ann Neurol 1979;6: 371–88.

[19] Reivich N, Kuhl D, Wolf A, et al. The [^{18}F]fluorodeoxyglucose method for the measurement of local cerebral glucose utilization in man. Circ Res 1979; 44:127–37.

[20] Minoshima S, Frey KA, Burdette JH, et al. Interpretation of metabolic abnormalities in Alzheimer's

disease using three-dimensional stereotactic surface projections (3D-SSP) and normal database. J Nucl Med 1995;36:237P.

[21] Moeller JR, Ishikawa T, Dhawan V, et al. The metabolic topography of normal aging. J Cereb Blood Flow Metab 1996;16:385–98.

[22] Ishii K, Sakamoto S, Sasaki M, et al. Cerebral glucose metabolism in patients with frontotemporal dementia. J Nucl Med 1998;39:1875–8.

[23] Yamaji S, Ishii K, Sasaki M, et al. Evaluation of standardized uptake value to assess cerebral glucose metabolism. Clin Nucl Med 2000;25:11–6.

[24] Law I, Iida H, Holm S, et al. Quantitation of regional cerebral blood flow corrected for partial volume effect using O-15 water and PET: II. Normal values and gray matter blood flow response to visual activation. J Cereb Blood Flow Metab 2000;20:1252–63.

[25] Huang SC, Carson RE, Hoffman EJ, et al. Quantitative measurement of local cerebral blood flow in humans by positron computed tomography and ^{15}O-water. J Cereb Blood Flow Metab 1983;3:141–53.

[26] Meltzer CC, Cantwell MN, Greer PJ, et al. Does cerebral blood flow decline in healthy aging? A PET study with partial-volume correction. J Nucl Med 2000;41:1842–8.

[27] Chugani HT, Phelps ME. Maturational changes in cerebral function in infants determined by 18FDG positron emission tomography. Science 1986;231: 840–3.

[28] Chugani HT, Phelps ME, Mazziotta JC. Positron emission tomography study of human brain functional development. Ann Neurol 1987;22:487–97.

[29] Chugani HT. A critical period of brain development: studies of cerebral glucose utilization with PET. Prev Med 1998;27:184–8.

[30] Takahashi T, Shirane R, Sato S, et al. Developmental changes of cerebral blood flow and oxygen metabolism in children. AJNR Am J Neuroradiol 1999;20:917–22.

[31] Chugani DC, Muzik O, Behen M, et al. Developmental changes in brain serotonin synthesis capacity in autistic and nonautistic children. Ann Neurol 1999;45: 287–95.

[32] Schultz SK, O'Leary DS, Boles Ponto LL, et al. Age-related changes in regional cerebral blood flow among young to mid-life adults. Neuroreport 1999;10:2493–6.

[33] Mazziotta JC, Phelps ME. Positron emission tomography studies of the brain. In: Phelps M, Mazziotta J, Schelbert H, editors. Positron emission tomography and autoradiography: principles and applications for the brain and heart. New York: Raven Press; 1986. p. 493–579.

[34] Evans DA. Estimated prevalence of Alzheimer's disease in the US. Milbank Q 1990;68:267–89.

[35] Carr DB, Goate A, Phil D, et al. Current concepts in the pathogenesis of Alzheimer's disease. Am J Med 1997;103:3S–10S.

[36] Ernst RL, Hay JW. The US economic and social costs of Alzheimer's disease revisited. Am J Public Health 1994;84:1261–4.

[37] National Institute of Aging. Progress report on Alzheimer's disease. NIH Publication No. 96–4137. Bethesda (MD): National Institute of Aging; 1996.

[38] Zhang MY, Katzman R, Salmon D, et al. The prevalence of dementia and Alzheimer's disease in Shanghai, China: impact of age, gender, and education. Ann Neurol 1990;27:428–37.

[39] Katzman R. Education and the prevalence of dementia and Alzheimer's disease. Neurology 1993;43:13–20.

[40] Stern Y, Alexander GE, Prohovnik I, et al. Inverse relationship between education and parietotemporal perfusion deficit in Alzheimer's disease. Ann Neurol 1992;32:371–5.

[41] Stern Y, Alexander GE, Prohovnik I, et al. Relationship between lifetime occupation and parietal flow: implications for a reserve against Alzheimer's disease pathology. Neurology 1995;45:55–60.

[42] Alexander GE, Furey ML, Grady CL, et al. Association of premorbid intellectual function with cerebral metabolism in Alzheimer's disease: implications for the cognitive reserve hypothesis. Am J Psychiatry 1997;154:165–72.

[43] Evans DA, Beckett LA, Field TS, et al. Apolipoprotein E epsilon-4 and incidence of Alzheimer disease in a community population of older persons. JAMA 1997; 277:822–4.

[44] Small GW, Mazziotta JC, Collins MT, et al. Apolipoprotein E type 4 allele and cerebral glucose metabolism in relatives at risk for familial Alzheimer disease. JAMA 1995;273:942–7.

[45] Reiman EM, Caselli RJ, Yun LS, et al. Preclinical evidence of Alzheimer's disease in persons homozygous for the epsilon 4 allele for apolipoprotein E. N Engl J Med 1996;334:752–8.

[46] Small GW, Ercoli LM, Silverman DH, et al. Cerebral metabolic and cognitive decline in persons at genetic risk for Alzheimer's disease. Proc Natl Acad Sci U S A 2000;97:6037–42.

[47] Silverman DHS, Hussain SA, Ercoli LM, et al. Detection of differences in regional cerebral metabolism associated with genotypic and educational risk factors for dementia. In: Proceedings of the International Conference on Mathematics and Engineering Techniques in Medicine and Biological Sciences. Las Vegas: 2000. p. 422–7.

[48] Benson DF, Kuhl DE, Phelps ME, et al. Positron emission computed tomography in the diagnosis of dementia. Trans Am Neurol Assoc 1981;106:68–71.

[49] Farkas T, Ferris SH, Wolf AP, et al. ^{18}F-2-deoxy-2-fluoro-D-glucose as a tracer in the positron emission tomographic study of senile dementia. Am J Psychiatry 1982;139:352–3.

[50] Foster NL, Chase TN, Fedio P, et al. Alzheimer's disease: focal cortical changes shown by positron emission tomography. Neurology 1983;33:961–5.

[51] Frackowiak RS, Pozzilli C, Legg NJ, et al. Regional cerebral oxygen supply and utilization in dementia. A clinical and physiological study with oxygen-15 and positron tomography. Brain 1981;104:753–78.

[52] Devous Sr MD. Functional brain imaging in the dementias: role in early detection, differential diagnosis, and longitudinal studies. Eur J Nucl Med Mol Imaging 2002;29:1685–96.

[53] Silverman DH. Brain F-18-FDG PET in the diagnosis of neurodegenerative dementias: comparison with perfusion SPECT and with clinical evaluations lacking nuclear imaging. J Nucl Med 2004;45:594–607.

[54] Mazziotta JC, Frackowiak RSJ, Phelps ME. The use of positron emission tomography in the clinical assessment of dementia. Semin Nucl Med 1992;22:233–46.

[55] Herholz K. FDG PET and differential diagnosis of dementia. Alzheimer Dis Assoc Disord 1995;9:6–16.

[56] Silverman DHS, Small GW, Phelps ME. Clinical value of neuroimaging in the diagnosis of dementia: sensitivity and specificity of regional cerebral metabolic and other parameters for early identification of AD. Clin Positron Imaging 1999;2:119–30.

[57] Pietrini P, Alexander GE, Furey ML, et al. The neurometabolic landscape of cognitive decline: in vivo studies with positron emission tomography in AD. Int J Psychophysiol 2000;37:87–98.

[58] Mielke R, Schroder R, Fink GR, et al. Regional cerebral glucose metabolism and postmortem pathology in AD. Acta Neuropathol (Berl) 1996;91:174–9.

[59] Salmon E, Sadzot B, Maquet P, et al. Differential diagnosis of Alzheimer's disease with PET. J Nucl Med 1994;35:391–8.

[60] Tedeschi E, Hasselbalch SG, Waldemar G, et al. Heterogeneous cerebral glucose metabolism in normal pressure hydrocephalus. J Neurol Neurosurg Psychiatry 1995;59:608–15.

[61] Hoffman JM, Welsh-Bohmer KA, Hanson M, et al. FDG PET imaging in patients with pathologically verified dementia. J Nucl Med 2000;41:1920–8.

[62] Silverman DHS, Small GW, Chang CY, et al. Positron emission tomography in evaluation of dementia: regional brain metabolism and long-term outcome. JAMA 2001;286:2120–7.

[63] Gambhir SS, Czernin J, Schwimmer J, et al. A tabulated summary of the FDG PET literature. J Nucl Med 2001;42(5 Suppl):1S–93S.

[64] Knopman DS, DeKosky ST, Cummings JL, et al. Practice parameter: diagnosis of dementia (an evidence-based review). Report of the Quality Standards Subcommittee of the American Academy of Neurology. Neurology 2001;56:1143–53.

[65] Herholz K, Nordberg A, Salmon E, et al. Impairment of neocortical metabolism predicts progression in Alzheimer's disease. Dement Geriatr Cogn Disord 1999; 10:494–504.

[66] Minoshima S, Giordani B, Berent S, et al. Metabolic reduction in the posterior cingulate cortex in very early Alzheimer's disease. Ann Neurol 1997;42:85–94.

[67] Silverman DHS, Truong CT, Kim SK, et al. Prognostic value of regional cerebral metabolism in patients undergoing dementia evaluation: comparison to a quantifying parameter of subsequent cognitive performance and to prognostic assessment without PET. Mol Genet Metab 2003;80:350–5.

[68] Truong C, Czernin J, Chen W, et al. Improving specificity of PET for prognostic evaluation of dementia. J Nucl Med 2002;43(Suppl):62P.

[69] Bench CJ, Friston KJ, Brown RG, et al. Regional cerebral blood flow in depression measured by positron emission tomography: the relationship with clinical dimensions. Psychol Med 1993;23:579–90.

[70] Silverman DHS, Geist CL, Van Herle K, et al. Abnormal regional brain metabolism in patients with hypothyroidism secondary to Hashimoto's disease. J Nucl Med 2002;43(5 Suppl):254P.

[71] Bauer M, Marseille DM, Geist CL, et al. Effects of thyroid hormone replacement therapy on regional brain metabolism. J Nucl Med 2002;43(5 Suppl):254P.

[72] Ackerman RH, Correia JA, Alpert NM, et al. Positron imaging in ischemic stroke disease using compounds labeled with oxygen-15. Initial results of clinicophysiologic correlations. Arch Neurol 1981;38:537–43.

[73] Baron JC, Bousser MG, Rey A, et al. Reversal of focal "misery-perfusion syndrome" by extra-intracranial arterial bypass in hemodynamic cerebral ischemia: a case study with ^{15}O positron tomography. Stroke 1981;12:454–9.

[74] Grubb Jr RL, Derdeyn CP, Fritsch SM, et al. Importance of hemodynamic factors in the prognosis of symptomatic carotid occlusion. JAMA 1998;280: 1055–60.

[75] Yamauchi H, Fukuyama H, Nagahama Y, et al. Significance of increased oxygen extraction fraction in five-year prognosis of major cerebral arterial occlusive diseases. J Nucl Med 1999;40:1992–8.

[76] Heiss WD, Grond M, Thiel A, et al. Tissue at risk of infarction rescued by early reperfusion: a positron emission tomography study in systemic recombinant tissue plasminogen activator thrombolysis of acute stroke. J Cereb Blood Flow Metab 1998;18:1298–307.

[77] Marchal G, Benali K, Iglesias S, et al. Voxel-based mapping of irreversible ischaemic damage with PET in acute stroke. Brain 1999;122:2387–400.

[78] Powers WJ, Zazulia AR. The use of positron emission tomography in cerebrovascular disease. Neuroimaging Clin N Am 2003;13:741–58.

ELSEVIER
SAUNDERS

Radiol Clin N Am 43 (2005) 79–92

RADIOLOGIC
CLINICS
of North America

PET in seizure disorders

Andrew B. Newberg, MD*, Abass Alavi, MD

Division of Nuclear Medicine, Hospital of the University of Pennsylvania, 3400 Spruce Street,
110 Donner Building, Philadelphia, PA 19104, USA

Epilepsy affects 0.5% to 1% of the population and can cause focal, partial, generalized, and absence seizures and several unusual types. Seizure disorders often begin in childhood and are treated with a variety of pharmacologic or surgical interventions for those refractory to medical therapy. Functional imaging, with both PET and single-photon emission CT (SPECT), has been highly useful in the diagnosis, management, and follow-up of patients with seizure disorders (Fig. 1). The ability of functional imaging to provide important information about seizures derives from the fact that epileptic conditions result in significant physiologic alterations in the brain. These physiologic changes occur both during seizures and in the interictal state. Because generalized seizures affect a large part of the brain, it is typically more difficult to isolate the originating focus from other areas that are secondarily affected on functional imaging studies. For partial seizures and other types of seizures that originate from a specific focus, however, functional imaging can be useful for localizing the primary site. Functional imaging also helps in the understanding of the pathophysiology of seizure disorders.

PET imaging in particular has been used in the management of patients with seizure disorders over the past two decades. In general, during an epileptic seizure, cerebral metabolism and cerebral blood flow are markedly increased. During the interictal period, both cerebral metabolism and cerebral blood flow are decreased [1]. In patients with generalized seizures, interictal fluorine-18–fluorodeoxyglucose ([^{18}F]-

FDG) PET studies have revealed no focal areas of hypometabolism [2]. The focus of partial seizures (with or without secondary generalized seizures) can be identified using FDG-PET, however, because the seizure foci have increased metabolic activity during the seizure and decreased metabolic activity between seizures [3–8]. It has been shown that single hypometabolic regions can be identified in 55% to 80% of patients with focal surface electroencephalography (EEG) abnormalities [4,9–11]. These areas of decreased metabolism often appear more extensive in size than do anatomic abnormalities observed on MR imaging [1,12]. Interictal PET is also a useful technique in patients with an unlocalized surface ictal EEG seizure focus, and it can be used to reduce the number of invasive EEG studies [13,14].

Interictal PET imaging

Interictal PET scanning has been used in a variety of seizure disorders for diagnostic and research purposes. The most commonly studied disorders include temporal lobe epilepsy and frontal lobe seizures. For example, an interictal PET study [15] in patients with complex partial seizures compared cerebral glucose metabolism and blood flow with various clinical variables, such as duration of seizure disorder, age at seizure onset, frequency of complex partial seizures, history of secondary generalization, history of febrile seizures, and MR imaging evidence for mesial temporal sclerosis. In this study, only the duration of the seizure disorder correlated with the degree of interhemispheric asymmetry in glucose metabolism and blood flow. The degree of asymmetry was significantly greater for glucose uptake

* Corresponding author.
E-mail address: newberg@rad.upenn.edu (A.B. Newberg).

0033-8389/05/$ – see front matter © 2004 Elsevier Inc. All rights reserved.
doi:10.1016/j.rcl.2004.09.003

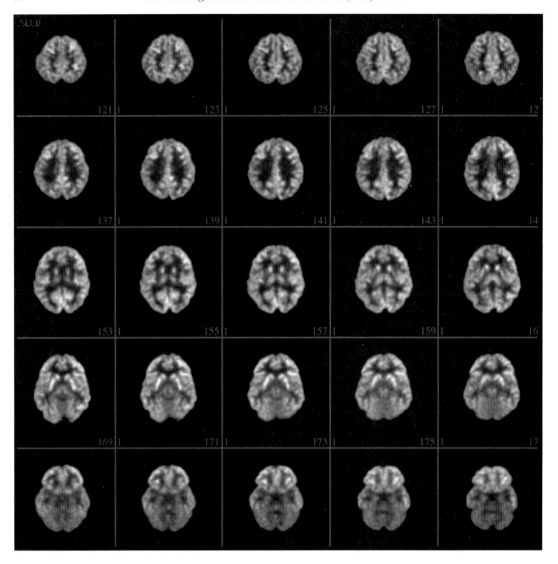

Fig. 1. Normal FDG-PET scan using a high-resolution bismuth germanate–dedicated head scanner. There is symmetric activity throughout the cortical gyri and subcortical structures.

than for blood flow suggesting that there is a relative uncoupling of metabolism and blood flow that is a progressive process. This uncoupling may result from the differential response of glucose metabolism and blood flow to chronic seizure activity. Another study of a single patient with bifrontal seizures demonstrated improvement in metabolic abnormalities after medical control of the seizures [16]. A study in contrast to the two reports described previously, however, did not find any association between complex partial seizure frequency and lifetime number of secondarily caused generalized seizures and hippocampal volume or metabolism [17]. These authors

concluded that the progression of metabolic or pathologic abnormalities may not be altered by adequate seizure control. Simply the presence of an epileptic focus might be associated with progressive neuronal injury even if the patient may be well-controlled medically.

A number of confounding clinical issues that may affect global or regional cerebral metabolism, such as the type of seizures, time since the most recent seizure, neuropsychiatric conditions such as depression (Fig. 2), and use of anticonvulsants (Fig. 3), require consideration in the evaluation of PET scans. Because it is not clear which factors play a role in the

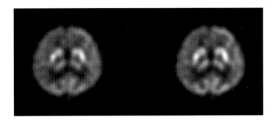

Fig. 2. FDG-PET study using a dedicated head PET of a subject with seizures demonstrating severely decreased metabolism throughout the entire cortex with relative preservation of the subcortical structures. This does not localize a seizure focus and is more consistent with depression or selected psychopharmacologic agents.

metabolic landscape of patients with complex partial seizures, Savic et al [18] investigated whether the metabolic pattern of interictal PET may be related to the EEG and clinical features of the seizure that preceded the scan. For this study, patients were classified into four groups: (1) focal limbic (characterized by auras or staring spells); (2) widespread limbic (including automatisms); (3) complex partial seizures with posturing; and (4) secondarily generalized seizures. The findings from this study showed that hypometabolism was limited to the epileptogenic zone if the preceding seizure was focal limbic, whereas patients with widespread limbic seizures had hypometabolism that included one or several additional areas of the limbic cortex. Patients with posturing were found to have hypometabolism in the extralimbic frontal lobe. Patients with secondarily generalized seizures were found to have significant cerebellar and parietal hypometabolism. The results of this study suggested that the mechanisms involved in the generation of a seizure that precedes a PET scan influences the interictal hypometabolic pattern and that it is important to consider the type of nonhabitual seizure that precedes a PET scan when interpreting images. A study by Barrington et al [19] addressed the application of simultaneous scalp EEG

during FDG administration to determine the exact ictal or interictal state of the patient with intractable seizures. This study demonstrated that seizures occur infrequently during FDG administration and that concurrent scalp EEG may not be necessary unless there is a significant problem with interpretation of the PET scan. Another study compared interictal regional slow activity as measured by scalp EEG with FDG-PET imaging and showed that the presence of such EEG activity had a high correlation with temporal lobe hypometabolism [20]. Interictal regional slow activity was not specifically related to mesial temporal sclerosis or any other pathology. The authors indicated that the findings from this study suggest that the hypometabolism observed on PET may delineate a field of reduced neuronal inhibition, which can receive interictal and ictal propagation.

Most patients with epilepsy respond to medical therapy. A certain number of patients, however, are found to be refractory to such treatments. One FDG-PET study in adolescents showed that detection of hypometabolism in the area of the seizure focus is associated with a poorer response to drug treatment compared with those without such findings [21].

One of the most effective treatments for partial epilepsy in patients refractory to medical interventions is surgical removal of the involved area, both in the pediatric and adult populations. Using high-resolution PET imaging, accurate localization of seizure foci can be achieved to help select appropriate candidates for surgical intervention [3–5,8,22]. Studies have also found that after surgical excision of the seizure foci, there is usually significant improvement in the function of the rest of the brain [23]. One study by Juhasz et al [24], however, suggested that it is the border zones of hypometabolic areas that may represent epileptogenic areas. Although somewhat contradictory to other studies, this finding helps to explain why some areas of hypometabolism miss seizure foci and still provides support for the notion that hypometabolic areas are related to seizure foci

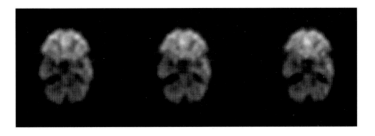

Fig. 3. Interictal FDG-PET study using a dedicated head PET of a subject with seizures. A specific seizure focus could not be identified, but there is bilaterally decreased metabolism in the cerebellum. This is a frequent finding in patients on antiseizure medications, such as phenytoin.

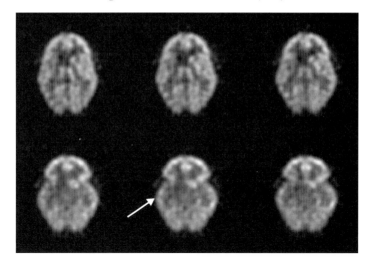

Fig. 4. Interictal PET images from a dedicated head PET of a subject with right temporal lobe seizure shown as decreased glucose metabolism in the right temporal lobe (*arrow*).

even though it may be the border zones that truly represent areas of seizure onset. Future studies are necessary to confirm these initial findings.

In terms of specific brain structures, the temporal lobe is the most common focus of partial epilepsy (Figs. 4 and 5). Initial studies showed that the sensitivity of PET in detecting temporal lobe epilepsy seizure focus is over 70% [25–37]. A later study by Sperling et al [38], however, has shown a positive finding on PET in only 44% of patients with temporal lobe epilepsy who had normal CT scans. Another study has shown that false lateralization can occur, reflected as hypometabolism of the temporal lobe

contralateral to the site of seizure focus as determined by EEG or MR imaging [39]. This is not a common phenomenon, however, as reflected in the sensitivity and specificity of PET for detecting seizure foci. PET imaging is also useful in detecting metabolic abnormalities in pediatric patients suggesting that focal functional deficits appear early in patients, especially those with medically refractory temporal lobe epilepsy [40]. PET imaging may help in the early identification of these patients.

Newer methods for analyzing PET images have also been explored, such as statistical parametric mapping in which each pixel represents a z-score

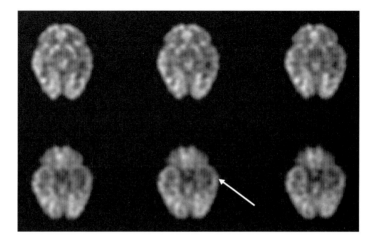

Fig. 5. Interictal PET images from a dedicated head PET of a subject with left temporal lobe seizure shown as decreased glucose metabolism in the left temporal lobe (*arrow*).

value determined by using the mean and standard deviation of count distribution in each individual patient. A study using statistical parametric mapping compared hemispheric asymmetry on FDG-PET images in patients with mesial temporal lobe epilepsy with controls [41]. When the statistical parametric mapping program was used to detect temporal interhemispheric asymmetry, hypometabolism was identified on the side chosen for resection in most cases (sensitivity, 71%; specificity, 100%) and was predictive of favorable postsurgical outcome in 90% of the patients. After a correction for multiple comparisons, statistical parametric mapping also identified temporal lobe hypermetabolic areas and extratemporal cortical and subcortical hypometabolic areas on the side of resection, but also on the contralateral side. An analysis of interictal FDG-PET scans in 17 patients with surgically treated temporal lobe epilepsy showed that the mean z-scores were significantly more negative in anterolateral and mesial regions on the operated side than on the nonoperated side in those patients who were seizure free, but not in those with ongoing seizures postoperatively [42]. Statistical parametric imaging correctly lateralized 16 of 17 patients, but only the anterolateral region was significant in predicting surgical outcome.

PET studies have also shown changes in areas distant from the seizure focus in patients with temporal lobe epilepsy. One FDG-PET study showed ipsilateral hypometabolism of the seizure focus in the temporal pole, but relatively increased metabolism in the ipsilateral mesiobasal region [43]. Contralateral to the seizure focus, metabolism was increased in the lateral temporal cortex and mesiobasal regions. A study of patients with bilateral temporal lobe epilepsy demonstrated that approximately 10% of the PET scans from seizure patients had bilateral temporal lobe hypometabolism [44]. When compared with patients with unilateral temporal lobe hypometabolism, patients with bilateral temporal lobe hypometabolism had a higher percentage of generalized seizures; were more likely to have bilateral, diffuse, or extratemporal seizure onsets; and had bilateral or diffuse MR imaging findings. Medical treatment was less successful in patients with bilateral temporal lobe hypometabolism and these patients also had worse social and cognitive functioning. Finally, patients with bilateral temporal lobe hypometabolism had a worse prognosis for seizure remission after surgery. A more recent study showed that patients with bilateral temporal lobe hypometabolism had more frequent nonlateralized ictal EEG pattern, anterior temporal white matter changes, and less frequent aura and unilateral dystonic posturing [45]. This study showed no substantial difference in postoperative outcomes, however, between patients with bilateral or unilateral temporal lobe involvement on PET.

Another important aspect of seizure studies is how to distinguish those patients who will do well postoperatively from those who will be less likely to benefit from temporal lobectomy. In this regard, PET studies have yielded controversial results. One PET study did not find any correlation between the severity of abnormal temporal lobe blood flow and the frequency of postoperative seizures [46]. This study, however, had a limited number of patients and may not have been able to detect statistical differences. Other studies have shown that in those patients with hypometabolism only in the affected temporal lobe, there is a higher likelihood of a successful outcome [47–49]. It has also been shown that patients with a greater degree of hypometabolism in the temporal lobe (ie, a more distinct asymmetry) tended to have a better outcome than those with a lesser degree of asymmetry [48,50,51]. It may be that those patients without significant hypometabolism of the affected temporal lobe (ie, minimal asymmetry between the temporal lobes) might have extratemporal or bitemporal seizure foci. These patients may be less amenable to surgical resection. This is corroborated by other studies that have shown that patients with hypometabolism in the contralateral hemisphere to the epileptic focus on EEG may be more likely to have postoperative seizures [52,53] and those patients with extratemporal hypometabolism tend to have a higher likelihood of postoperative seizures (Fig. 6) [47,54].

Several studies have indicated that those patients with mesial temporal hypometabolism on PET imaging have a higher probability of being seizure free postoperatively than those patients with hypometabolism in other parts of the temporal lobe [51]. Other studies, however, have suggested that lateral temporal lobe hypometabolism is a good predictor of a seizure-free postoperative outcome [13,50]. Despite the findings regarding the association of temporal lobe hypometabolism with postoperative seizure outcome, several studies have not shown such a relationship [55,56]. Other investigators have explored the use of different statistical methods to show that using a discriminant and multivariate analysis, temporal lobe hypometabolism was a good predictor of postoperative seizure outcome [57]. Furthermore, a study comparing MR imaging with PET found that patients with white matter changes on MR imaging in the temporal lobes had greater reductions in glucose metabolism in the same regions [58]. These patients

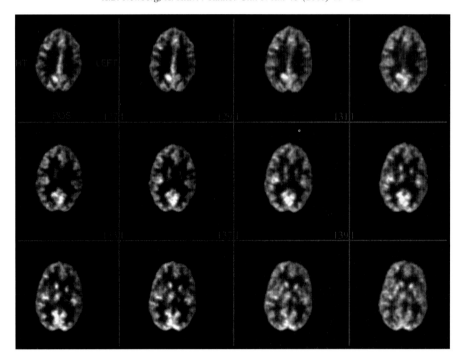

Fig. 6. Interictal FDG-PET study using a dedicated head PET of a subject demonstrating hypometabolism in the entire left hemisphere including the thalamus and basal ganglia. A specific seizure focus could not be identified.

also had better postsurgical outcomes suggesting that MR imaging and PET findings can be used in a complementary manner.

The thalamus may be an important structure to evaluate in patients with temporal lobe epilepsy with regard to postoperative seizure outcome. The findings from one study suggested that metabolic dysfunction of the thalamus ipsilateral to the seizure focus becomes more severe with long-standing temporal or frontal lobe epilepsy, and also with secondary generalization of seizures [59]. One research paper showed that of 64 patients who were seizure free postoperatively, all had either no thalamic metabolic asymmetry or asymmetry in the same direction as that of the temporal lobe removed (ie, the thalamus ipsilateral to the hypometabolic temporal lobe appeared to have reduced metabolism) [60]. No patients who were seizure free had thalamic asymmetry in the reverse direction as that of the temporal lobe removed (ie, the thalamus contralateral to the hypometabolic temporal lobe appeared to have reduced metabolism). In contrast, 5 (31%) of 16 patients with postoperative seizures of any degree had thalamic asymmetry in the reverse direction as that of the temporal lobe removed. Furthermore, all five patients with this reverse thalamic asymmetry were found to have some degree of postoperative seizures. Even patients with

ipsilateral thalamic hypometabolism had a slightly higher risk for having postoperative seizures in comparison with those patients with no asymmetry. Another study also demonstrated ipsilateral thalamic hypometabolism in patients with mesial temporal lobe epilepsy; however, the outcome associated with this finding was not described [61]. Contralateral thalamic hypometabolism as a predictor of poor postoperative seizure outcome may be taken to reflect a widespread pattern of seizure activity. Despite persistent seizures in patients with reverse thalamic asymmetry, however, there was still some degree of seizure activity improvement. Although the finding of reverse thalamic asymmetry may provide important prognostic information, surgery can still be an effective intervention in patients with medically refractory temporal lobe seizures.

PET imaging has also been used after surgical interventions to determine the metabolic landscape postsurgery. A study of eight patients undergoing temporal lobectomy had follow-up PET scans at least 6 months after surgery [62]. Half of the patients showed improved glucose metabolism in the formerly hypometabolic areas that were remote to the surgical site and ipsilateral to the epileptogenic foci. Patients who showed bilateral temporal hypometabolism preoperatively had contralateral temporal hypometabolism after surgery. Several areas, particularly the frontal lobes, actually showed increased glucose metabolism after surgery. The authors concluded that hypometabolism in remote areas ipsilateral to the seizure focus may demonstrate reversibility after surgery and may be caused by inhibition by the intercortical pathways. Contralateral temporal hypometabolic areas that persist after surgery may be caused by a different mechanism, and neither specifically indicates the presence of seizure foci nor affects the seizure outcome. PET imaging in a patient after entorhinoamygdalohippocampectomy performed with the newer surgical technique of gamma knife and low marginal doses showed relative improvement in metabolism in the lateral temporal lobe with persistently decreased metabolism in the mesial temporal lobe [63].

The other major site of the seizure focus in partial epilepsy is the frontal lobe (Fig. 7). Because many of these seizures begin in the medial or inferior aspects of the frontal lobe, scalp EEG readings do not provide adequate localization of foci [64–67]. Franck et al [68] used interictal FDG-PET to study 13 patients with presumed frontal lobe epilepsy and found PET to be the best modality for localizing seizure foci in this location. Further, the authors suggested that PET might help in determining the site of surgical excision or suggest a contraindication to surgical intervention in patients with multiple or bilateral foci. A study of 180 surgical specimens from patients with frontal lobe epilepsy found a high correlation between hypometabolic regions on interictal PET images and structural, histopathologic changes in the surgical specimens [69]. This study is supported by an earlier study in which FDG-PET images revealed decreased frontal lobe metabolism in 64% of patients with frontal lobe seizures as determined by electroclinical ictal localization [70]. A study of pediatric patients demonstrated a similar sensitivity of FDG-PET in detecting frontal lobe seizure foci [71]. PET scans, however, demonstrated hypometabolism restricted to

the frontal lobes in approximately 62%. The remaining patients demonstrated hypometabolism that exceeded the epileptogenic region indicated by ictal EEG. What this extrafrontal hypometabolism may actually represent is not clear, but may be caused by either additional epileptogenic areas, effects of diaschisis, seizure propagation sites, or secondary epileptogenic foci. Regardless, the findings from the studies on frontal lobe epilepsy suggest that FDG-PET scanning is a sensitive and specific technique for investigating patients with seizures of probable frontal lobe origins.

Seizure foci in other areas have also been detected using FDG-PET. A patient with seizures originating in the parietal lobe demonstrated hypermetabolism in the affected parietal lobe during an interictal PET scan [72]. The authors suggested that this hypermetabolism might have been related to the clustering of seizures in this patient so that the scan may have actually represented an ictal state. A more recent evaluation of parietal lobe seizures demonstrated that the sensitivity for detecting the seizure focus was comparable for MR imaging, PET, and SPECT, although MR imaging was the highest at approximately 64%, whereas PET had a sensitivity of only 50% [73]. The results indicate that parietal lobe seizures are much more difficult to localize than either temporal or frontal lobe seizures.

Ictal PET imaging

Performing ictal PET studies is more logistically impractical primarily because of the relatively short half-life of positron-emitting isotopes, such as [^{18}F] [74]. Several ictal PET studies have been reported, however, which have been successful in the determination of seizure foci in patients with partial seizures. In these studies, the seizure focus appears as a hypermetabolic area. In earlier studies, Chugani et al [75] have devised a classification system to describe

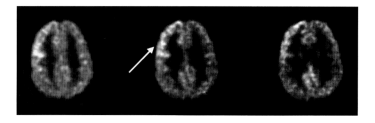

Fig. 7. Ictal FDG-PET study using a high-resolution GSO-dedicated head scanner of a subject demonstrating hypermetabolism in the right frontal lobe (*arrow*) compared with the rest of the cortical areas. This indicates a seizure focus in the right frontal lobe.

the metabolic patterns observed in children with partial complex seizures. Specifically, three major metabolic patterns were observed and were based on the degree and type of subcortical involvement. The type I pattern was defined as asymmetric glucose metabolism of the striatum and thalamus. Patients with this pattern often showed unilateral cortical and crossed cerebellar hypermetabolism. The type II pattern included symmetric hypermetabolism in the striatum and thalamus, which was associated with hypermetabolism of the hippocampal or insular cortex. Interestingly, the type II pattern also included diffuse neocortical hypometabolism and the absence of any cerebellar abnormalities. The type III pattern showed hypermetabolism that was restricted to the cerebral cortex with normal metabolism in the striatum and thalamus. Despite defining these three patterns of FDG-PET findings, this study could not correlate the PET findings with EEG or clinical features of the seizure disorders in these patients.

Another ictal PET study using oxygen-15–water ($[^{15}O]$-H_2O) showed that complex partial seizures are associated with bilaterally increased cerebral blood flow in a number of cortical areas, particularly the temporal and frontal lobes [76]. In addition, these patients also had increased blood flow to the subcortical areas, which are activated during ictus.

Surgical planning with PET

Several studies have used PET imaging for the purpose of planning surgical interventions. Duncan et al [77] used $[^{15}O]$-H_2O PET in conjunction with anatomic images from MR imaging, which helped to determine the brain regions involved with motor activity, visual perception, articulation, and receptive language tasks in pediatric patients before temporal, and even extratemporal, surgery. At follow-up, the patients who underwent both temporal lobectomy and extratemporal resection for a neoplastic or nonneoplastic seizure focus were seizure-free with minimal postoperative morbidity. The authors note that no child sustained a postoperative speech or language deficit. Interestingly, when patients had prenatal cortical injury, PET demonstrated reorganization of language areas to new adjacent areas or even to the contralateral hemisphere. One study used ictal PET overlaid onto the corresponding MR imaging to determine successfully the seizure focus and to help with neurosurgical planning [78]. Cognitive activation paradigms using PET imaging have been suggested as an alternative approach to the evaluation of functional and epileptogenic zones for presurgical

evaluation in patients with epilepsy [79]. More work is needed to determine the most clinically efficacious paradigms for different seizure types. The authors suggest that the strength of activation PET studies lies in the ability to study shifts in cognitive circuitry that accompany a fixed neuropathologic entity for both groups of similar subjects and individuals. These techniques may enhance the understanding of the fundamentals of brain plasticity and may be used in the future to predict precise surgical risks.

By combining PET and MR imaging data, these studies demonstrated an enhancement in surgical safety, definition of optimal surgical approach, delineation of the seizure focus, and facilitation of maximum resection and optimization of the timing of surgery. Noninvasive presurgical brain mapping with PET can reduce the risk and improve neurologic outcome in seizure patients undergoing surgical resection.

Receptor PET imaging

PET imaging to measure various neurotransmitter systems has been used to study patients with seizures. Initial studies of benzodiazepine receptor activity in temporal lobe epilepsy showed decreased benzodiazepine receptor activity in the medial temporal lobe [80]. This reduction in benzodiazepine receptor activity may correlate with the frequency of seizures [81]. A more recent study compared the results obtained from FDG with carbon-11–flumazenil ($[^{11}C]$-FMZ) [82]. FDG-PET images showed a large area of hypometabolism in the epileptogenic temporal lobe (as determined by other diagnostic studies including scalp EEG and MR imaging). Both FDG-PET and $[^{11}C]$-FMZ PET reliably revealed the epileptogenic temporal lobe and neither agent proved superior to the other. This study did not find any correlation between the degree of hypoactivity in either $[^{18}F]$-FDG or $[^{11}C]$-FMZ PET and the grading of mesial temporal sclerosis according to the Wyler criteria observed with MR imaging. Furthermore, this study compared the PET results with those obtained with interictal iodine-123–iomazenil ($[^{123}I]$-IMZ) SPECT and found that the later was highly inaccurate in localizing the affected temporal lobe. It has been suggested that in the pediatric population, $[^{11}C]$-FMZ PET may have a useful clinical role in patients with partial epilepsy who have normal or subtle changes on FDG-PET, in patients with bilateral FDG findings but unifocal seizure activity on EEG, and in patients after surgical resection who continue to have seizures [83]. This latter group often demonstrates large areas of hypometabolism on FDG-PET in the area of the resection that may also include remaining epileptogenic foci.

Another study compared changes in benzodiazepine receptors in the thalami of patients with temporal lobe epilepsy [84]. The dorsal medial nuclei showed significantly lower glucose metabolism and [^{11}C]-FMZ binding on the side of the epileptic focus. Interestingly, the lateral thalami showed bilateral hypermetabolism and increased [^{11}C]-FMZ binding. A significant correlation was found between the [^{11}C]-FMZ binding in the dorsal medial nuclei and that in the amygdala. These PET abnormalities were associated with a significant volume loss in the ipsilateral thalamus as determined by anatomic MR imaging. Decreased benzodiazepine receptor binding in the dorsal medial nucleus may be caused by neuronal loss, as suggested by volume loss on MR imaging, but this decrease also may indicate impaired γ-aminobutyric acid transmission in the dorsal medial nucleus, which has strong reciprocal connections with other parts of the limbic system. The increased glucose metabolism and [^{11}C]-FMZ binding in the lateral thalamus was hypothesized to represent an up-regulation of γ-aminobutyric acid–mediated inhibitory circuits. Frontal lobe epilepsy is associated with significantly reduced benzodiazepine receptor density in the anterior cerebellum contralateral to the seizure focus [85].

A study using the receptor ligand [^{11}C]-FMZ to evaluate six patients with frontal lobe seizures [86] reported that the seizure focus was correctly identified by [^{11}C]-FMZ PET as an area of decreased benzodiazepine receptor density in all patients studied. Furthermore, the area with reduced benzodiazepine receptor density was better delineated than the corresponding hypometabolic region observed with FDG-PET images. Several other studies of benzodiazepine receptors showed that the areas of abnormal benzodiazepine receptor binding were more extensive than anatomic abnormalities observed on MR imaging or even than the hypometabolic areas observed on interictal FDG-PET [87,88].

There are several studies that have demonstrated the involvement of the opioid neurotransmitter systems in seizure physiology. Several PET studies using the δ-receptor selective antagonist [^{11}C]-methylnaltrindole and [^{11}C]-carfentanil, which measures μ-receptor binding in patients with temporal lobe epilepsy, have shown increased receptor activity in the affected temporal lobe [89–91]. When compared with interictal FDG-PET, the binding of opiate receptors was increased and [^{18}F]-FDG uptake decreased in the temporal cortex ipsilateral to the seizure focus [91]. Furthermore, decreases in [^{18}F]-FDG uptake were more widespread than were the increases in opioid receptors. There were also different regional binding patterns for the δ- and μ-receptors. Increases in μ-receptor binding were localized to the middle aspect of the inferior temporal lobe and binding of δ receptors increased in the middle and superior temporal lobe. The fact that there are differences in the regional binding of the μ- and δ-opiate receptors suggests that they may play different roles in seizure physiology.

Other seizure disorders

There are many other types of seizure disorders that have been investigated using PET imaging. Absence seizures are a common form of epilepsy associated with brief spells of loss of consciousness and is associated with 3-Hz generalized spike-wave activity on EEG. The actual site of the seizure origin, however, has been difficult to detect and localize. An [^{15}O]-H$_2$O PET cerebral blood flow study was performed on eight patients with idiopathic generalized epilepsy in whom typical absence seizures were induced by voluntary hyperventilation [92]. This study showed that there was a global increase in blood flow during the typical absence seizures. There was also a focal increase in mean thalamic blood flow. This study, however, although indicating an important role of the thalamus in the pathogenesis of absence seizures, was unable to show that the thalamus was the origin of the seizure activity. An earlier ictal FDG-PET study of patients in absence status showed decreased metabolic rates throughout both cortical and subcortical structures compared with interictal scans [2]. A comparison with single absence attacks suggested that there is a pathophysiologic difference between the two states. A recent case study reported localizing absence seizures in one patient to the right frontal lobe using ictal PET [93]. No evidence was found for a change in [^{11}C]-FMZ binding with absence seizures. This result, together with those of a study showing no abnormality of [^{11}C]-FMZ binding interictally in patients with childhood and juvenile absence epilepsy, does not support a primary role for the benzodiazepine binding site of the γ-aminobutyric acid–A receptor in the pathogenesis of absence seizures [94].

Another unusual epileptic disorder consists of focal inhibitory motor seizures that result in ictal paralysis. A study of this type of seizure disorder showed that these patients had a centroparietal epileptogenic focus on SPECT that was also suggested by other neuroimaging studies [95]. In particular, MR imaging showed centroparietal structural lesions in most of the patients. In one patient with a normal MR imaging scan, there was right centroparietal hypometabolism on PET imaging. Given these findings, the authors suggest that it is important to distinguish such seizures from transient ischemic attacks and migraine, which may not have the same imaging findings.

There have been a few reports of imaging studies in patients with cortical heterotopia. A report of FDG-PET imaging in patients with diffuse band heterotopia revealed similar and even higher deoxyglucose uptake in the layer of cortical heterotopia compared with the normal cortex [96]. The authors suggested that the findings might represent persistent synaptic activity in the heterotopic neurons, which is unaffected by age or by the time-course of epilepsy. A hexamethylpropyleneamine oxime SPECT image has also been reported in an epileptic patient with a rare form of diffuse subcortical laminar heterotopia detected on MR imaging [97]. The interictal SPECT scan of this patient revealed identical or increased perfusion of the laminar heterotopia as compared with that of the overlying cortical mantle. The SPECT scan also showed decreased perfusion in the left temporal lobe that agreed with the type of complex partial seizures and the EEG finding of frequent generalized spike-wave complexes with a slight left-sided dominance.

Infantile spasms may occur either because of an underlying, identifiable cause (symptomatic group) or may be idiopathic (cryptogenic group). PET studies have found that cryptogenic spasms have focal cortical regions of hypometabolism in the interictal period [98,99]. Further, the focal areas found on PET correspond to areas of EEG abnormalities. A recent study suggested that there are multifocal areas of hypometabolism in such patients and that the structures involved are associated with specific disease characteristics [100]. For example, frontal hypometabolism correlated with the degree of mental retardation, hypotonia, and ataxia. Temporomesial hypometabolism correlated with the occurrence of obtunded states, and parietal changes were associated with the occurrence of myoclonic seizures and spike-wave discharges. Because of the poor prognosis of infants with infantile spasm, surgical removal of the abnormal foci identified by PET has been attempted. The results indicated that 75% of the patients remain seizure free, whereas others improved markedly after surgery [101].

Lennox-Gastaut syndrome, the triad of 1- to 2.5-Hz spike-wave pattern on EEG, intellectual im-pairment, and multiple seizure types, has been investigated with PET and four patterns have been described [102]. The four metabolic subtypes are (1) unilateral focal, (2) unilateral diffuse hypometabolism, (3) bilateral diffuse hypometabolism, and (4) normal metabolism [103,104]. Because this disorder is often refractory to anticonvulsant therapy, surgical intervention has been attempted with subsequent control of seizure activity [105]. PET imaging may provide useful information regarding the type of surgical intervention necessary in these patients. A more recent study of Lennox-Gastaut syndrome, in relation to other epileptic encephalopathies, demonstrated that PET scans were normal in all children with typical de novo Lennox-Gastaut syndrome but showed cortical metabolic abnormalities in three of four with atypical de novo Lennox-Gastaut syndrome, five of six with Lennox-Gastaut syndrome following infantile spasms, six of eight with severe myoclonic epilepsy in infancy, and four of six with an unclassified epileptic encephalopathy [106]. The findings from this study suggest that some children with epileptic encephalopathies previously thought to have primary generalized or multifocal seizures may have a unifocal origin for their seizures. If a focal origin is observed, then surgical intervention may be useful as a treatment modality in these cases.

Patients with Sturge-Weber syndrome, characterized by facial capillary nevus (port-wine stain) and ipsilateral leptomeningeal angiomatosis, often develop epileptic seizures because of the intracranial, extracerebral vascular malformation. Like infantile spasms and Lenox-Gastaut syndrome, Sturge-Weber syndrome is usually refractory to medications and requires surgical intervention. In conjunction with CT and MR imaging, PET has been useful in helping to determine the surgical technique (usually a hemispherectomy) necessary in these patients [107]. PET imaging usually shows widespread unilateral hypometabolism ipsilateral to the facial nevus [108]. Not unlike other seizure disorders, hypermetabolism is noted ipsilateral to the facial nevus during the ictal period.

Summary

PET imaging has been widely used in the evaluation and management of patients with seizure disorders. The ability of PET to measure cerebral function is ideal for studying the neurophysiologic correlates of seizure activity during both ictal and interictal states. PET imaging is also valuable for evaluating patients before surgical interventions to determine the best surgical method and maximize outcomes. PET will continue to play a major role, not only in the clinical arena, but also in investigating the pathogenesis and treatment of various seizure disorders.

References

[1] Duncan JS. Imaging and epilepsy. Brain 1997;120(Pt 2):339–77.

[2] Theodore WH, Brooks R, Margolin R, et al. Positron emission tomography in generalized seizures. Neurology 1985;35:684–90.

[3] Abou-Khalil BW, Siegel GJ, Sackellares JC, et al. Positron emission tomography studies of cerebral glucose metabolism in chronic partial epilepsy. Ann Neurol 1987;22:480–6.

[4] Engel Jr J, Brown WJ, Kuhl DE, et al. Pathologic findings underlying focal temporal lobe hypometabolism in partial epilepsy. Ann Neurol 1982;12:518–28.

[5] Engel Jr J, Kuhl DE, Phelps ME, et al. Comparative localization of the epileptic foci in partial epilepsy by PET and EEG. Ann Neurol 1982;12:529–37.

[6] Engel Jr J, Kuhl DE, Phelps ME, et al. Local cerebral metabolism during partial seizures. Neurology 1983; 33:400–13.

[7] Theodore WH, Brooks R, Sato S, et al. The role of positron emission tomography in the evaluation of seizure disorders. Ann Neurol 1984;15:S176–9.

[8] Theodore WH, Newmark ME, Sato S, et al. 18F fluorodeoxyglucose positron emission tomography in refractory complex partial seizures [abstract]. Ann Neurol 1983;13:537.

[9] Henry TR, Sutherling WW, Engel Jr J, et al. Interictal cerebral metabolism in partial epilepsies of neocortical origin. Epilepsy Res 1991;10:174–82.

[10] Engel Jr J. PET scanning inpartial epilepsy. Can J Neurol Sci 1991;18:588–92.

[11] Duncan R. Epilepsy, cerebral blood flow, and cerebral metabolic rate. Cerebrovasc Brain Metab Rev 1992; 4:105–21.

[12] Theodore WH, Holmes MD, Dorwart RH, et al. Complex partial seizures: cerebral structure and cerebral function. Epilepsia 1986;27:576–82.

[13] Theodore WH, Sato S, Kufta CV, et al. FDG-positron emission tomography and invasive EEG: seizure focus detection and surgical outcome. Epilepsia 1997; 38:81–6.

[14] Debets RM, van Veelen CW, Maquet P, et al. Quantitative analysis of 18/FDG-PET in the presurgical evaluation of patients suffering from refractory partial epilepsy: comparison with CT, MRI, and combined subdural and depth EEG. Acta Neurochir Suppl (Wien) 1990;50:88–94.

[15] Breier JI, Mullani NA, Thomas AB, et al. Effects of duration of epilepsy on the uncoupling of metabolism and blood flow in complex partial seizures. Neurology 1997;48:1047–53.

[16] Matheja P, Weckesser M, Debus O, et al. Drug-induced changes in cerebral glucose consumption in bifrontal epilepsy. Epilepsia 2000;41:588–93.

[17] Spanaki MV, Kopylev L, Liow K, et al. Relationship of seizure frequency to hippocampus volume and metabolism in temporal lobe epilepsy. Epilepsia 2000;41:1227–9.

[18] Savic I, Altshuler L, Baxter L, et al. Pattern of interictal hypometabolism in PET scans with fludeoxyglucose F 18 reflects prior seizure types in patients with mesial temporal lobe seizures. Arch Neurol 1997;54:129–36.

[19] Barrington SF, Koutroumanidis M, Agathonikou A, et al. Clinical value of "ictal" FDG-positron emission tomography and the routine use of simultaneous scalp EEG studies in patients with intractable partial epilepsies. Epilepsia 1998;39:753–66.

[20] Koutroumanidis M, Binnie CD, Elwes RD, et al. Interictal regional slow activity in temporal lobe epilepsy correlates with lateral temporal hypometabolism as imaged with 18FDG PET: neurophysiological and metabolic implications. J Neurol Neurosurg Psychiatry 1998;65:170–6.

[21] Gaillard WD, White S, Malow B, et al. FDG-PET in children and adolescents with partial seizures: role in epilepsy surgery evaluation. Epilepsy Res 1995; 20:77–84.

[22] Utsubo H, Chuang SH, Hwang PA, et al. Neuroimaging for investigation of seizures in children. Pediatr Neurosurg 1992;18:105–16.

[23] Verity CM, Strauss EH, Moyes PD, et al. Long-term follow-up after cerebral hemispherectomy: neurophysiologic, radiologic, and psychological findings. Neurology 1982;32:629.

[24] Juhasz C, Chugani DC, Muzik O, et al. Is epileptogenic cortex truly hypometabolic on interictal positron emission tomography? Ann Neurol 2000;48: 88–96.

[25] Engel Jr J, Kuhl DE, Phelps ME. Patterns of human local cerebral glucose metabolism during epileptic seizures. Science 1982;218:64–6.

[26] Markand ON, Salanova V, Worth R, et al. Comparative study of interictal PET and ictal SPECT in complex partial seizures. Acta Neurol Scand 1997;95: 129–36.

[27] Engel J, Kuhl DE, Phelps ME, et al. Patterns of ictal and interictal local cerebral metabolic rate studies in man with positron computed tomography. In: Akimoto H, Kazamatsure H, Setno M, et al, editors. Advances in epileptology. New York: Raven; 1982. p. 145.

[28] Theodore WH, Dorwart R, Holmes M, et al. Neuroimaging in refractory partial seizures. comparison of PET, CT, and MRI. Neurology 1986;36:750–9.

[29] Theodore WH, Fishbein D, Dubinsky R. Patterns of cerebral glucose metabolism in patients with partial seizures. Neurology 1988;38:1201–6.

[30] Kuhl DE, Engel J, Phelphs ME, et al. Epileptic pattern of local cerebral metabolism and perfusion in human determined by emission computed tomography of ^{18}FDG and ^{13}NH$_3$. Ann Neurol 1979;8: 348–60.

[31] Salanova V, Morris III HH, Rehm P, et al. Comparison of the intracarotid amobarbital procedure and interictal cerebral 18-fluorodeoxyglucose positron emission tomography scans in refractory temporal lobe epilepsy. Epilepsia 1992;33:635–8.

[32] Bernardi S, Trimble MR, Frackowiak RSJ, et al. An interictal study of partial epilepsy using positron emission tomography and oxygen 15 inhalation method. J Neurol Neurosurg Psychiatry 1983;46: 473–7.

[33] Franck G, Maquet P, Sadzot B, et al. Contribution of positron emission tomography to the investigation of epilepsies of frontal lobe origin. Adv Neurol 1992; 57:471–85.

[34] Och RF, Yamamoto Y, Gloor P. Correlations between the positron emission tomography measurement of glucose metabolism and oxygen utilization in focal epilepsy. Neurology 1984;34(Suppl 1):125.

[35] Yamamoto YL, Ochs R, Gloor P, et al. Pattern of rCBF and focal energy metabolism in relation to electroencephalographic abnormality in the interictal phase of partial epilepsy. In: Baldy-Moulinier M, Ingvar DH, Meldrum BS, editors. Cerebral blood flow, metabolism and epilepsy. Paris: John Libbey Eurotext; 1983.

[36] Salanova V, Markand O, Worth R, et al. FDG-PET and MRI in temporal lobe epilepsy: relationship to febrile seizures, hippocampal sclerosis and outcome. Acta Neurol Scand 1998;97:146–53.

[37] Knowlton RC, Laxer KD, Ende G, et al. Presurgical multimodality neuroimaging in electroencephalographic lateralized temporal lobe epilepsy. Ann Neurol 1997;42:829–37.

[38] Sperling M, Wilson G, Engel Jr J, et al. Magnetic resonance imaging in intractable partial epilepsy: correlative studies. Ann Neurol 1986;20:57–62.

[39] Nagarajan L, Schaul N, Eidelberg D, et al. Contralateral temporal hypometabolism on positron emission tomography in temporal lobe epilepsy. Acta Neurol Scand 1996;93:81–4.

[40] Salanova V, Markand O, Worth R, et al. Presurgical evaluation and surgical outcome of temporal lobe epilepsy. Pediatr Neurol 1999;20:179–84.

[41] Van Bogaert P, Massager N, Tugendhaft P, et al. Statistical parametric mapping of regional glucose metabolism in mesial temporal lobe epilepsy. Neuroimage 2000;12:129–38.

[42] Wong CY, Geller EB, Chen EQ, et al. Outcome of temporal lobe epilepsy surgery predicted by statistical parametric PET imaging. J Nucl Med 1996;37: 1094–100.

[43] Rubin E, Dhawan V, Moeller JR, et al. Cerebral metabolic topography in unilateral temporal lobe epilepsy. Neurology 1995;45:2212–23.

[44] Blum DE, Ehsan T, Dungan D, et al. Bilateral temporal hypometabolism in epilepsy. Epilepsia 1998;39:651–9.

[45] Joo EY, Lee EK, Tae WS, et al. Unitemporal vs bitemporal hypometabolism in mesial temporal lobe epilepsy. Arch Neurol 2004;61:1074–8.

[46] Theodore WH, Gaillard WD, Sato S, et al. Positron emission tomographic measurement of cerebral blood flow and temporal lobectomy. Ann Neurol 1994; 36:241–4.

[47] Manno EM, Sperling MR, Ding X, et al. Predictors of outcome after anterior temporal lobectomy: positron emission tomography. Neurology 1994;44:2331–6.

[48] Radtke RA, Hanson MW, Hoffman JM, et al. Temporal lobe hypometabolism on PET: predictor of seizure control after temporal lobectomy. Neurology 1993;43:1088–92.

[49] Wong C-Y, Geller EB, Chen EQ, et al. Outcome of temporal lobe epilepsy surgery predicted by statistical parametric PET imaging. J Nucl Med 1996;37: 1094–100.

[50] Theodore WH, Sato S, Kufta C, et al. Temporal lobectomy for uncontrolled seizures: the role of positron emission tomography. Ann Neurol 1992;32: 789–94.

[51] Delbeke D, Lawrence SK, Abou-Khalil BW, et al. Postsurgical outcome of patients with uncontrolled complex partial seizures and temporal lobe hypometabolism on 18FDG-positron emission tomography. Invest Radiol 1996;31:261–6.

[52] Benbadis SR, So NK, Antar MA, et al. The value of PET scan (and MRI and Wada test) in patients with bitemporal epileptiform abnormalities. Arch Neurol 1995;52:1062–8.

[53] Choi JY, Kim SJ, Hong SB, et al. Extratemporal hypometabolism on FDG PET in temporal lobe epilepsy as a predictor of seizure outcome after temporal lobectomy. Eur J Nucl Med Mol Imaging 2003; 30:581–7.

[54] Swartz BE, Tomiyasu U, Delgado-Escueta AV, et al. Neuroimaging in temporal lobe epilepsy: test sensitivity and relationships to pathology and postoperative outcome. Epilepsia 1992;33:624–34.

[55] Engel J, Babb TL, Phelps ME. Contributions of positron emission tomography to understanding mechanisms of epilepsy. In: Engel Jr J, Ojemann GA, Luders HO, et al, editors. Fundamental mechanisms of human brain function. New York: Raven Press; 1987. p. 209–18.

[56] Theodore WH, Katz D, Kufta C, et al. Pathology of temporal lobe foci: correlation with CT, MRI and PET. Neurology 1990;40:797–803.

[57] Dupont S, Semah F, Clemenceau S, et al. Accurate prediction of postoperative outcome in mesial temporal lobe epilepsy: a study using positron emission tomography with 18fluorodeoxyglucose. Arch Neurol 2000;57:1331–6.

[58] Choi D, Na DG, Byun HS, et al. White-matter change in mesial temporal sclerosis: correlation of MRI with

PET, pathology, and clinical features. Epilepsia 1999; 40:1634–41.

[59] Benedek K, Juhasz C, Muzik O, et al. Metabolic changes of subcortical structures in intractable focal epilepsy. Epilepsia 2004;45:1100–5.

[60] Newberg A, Alavi A, Sperling M, et al. Thalamic metabolic asymmetry on FDG-PET scans as a determinant of seizure outcome after temporal lobectomy. J Nucl Med 1997;38:92P.

[61] Khan N, Leenders KL, Hajek M, et al. Thalamic glucose metabolism in temporal lobe epilepsy measured with 18F-FDG positron emission tomography (PET). Epilepsy Res 1997;28:233–43.

[62] Akimura T, Yeh HS, Mantil JC, et al. Cerebral metabolism of the remote area after epilepsy surgery. Neurol Med Chir (Tokyo) 1999;39:16–25 [discussion: 25–7].

[63] Regis J, Semah F, Bryan RN, et al. Early and delayed MR and PET changes after selective temporomesial radiosurgery in mesial temporal lobe epilepsy. AJNR Am J Neuroradiol 1999;20:213–6.

[64] Quesney LF, Gloor P. Localization of epileptic foci. In: Gortman J, Ives JR, Gloor P, editors. Long term monitoring in epilepsy. EEG supplement 37. Amsterdam: Elsevier Science Publishers; 1985.

[65] Quesney LF, Olivier A, Andermann F, et al. Preoperative EEG investigation in patients with frontal lobe epilepsy. trends, results and pathophysiological considerations. J Clin Neurophysiol 1987; 4:208–9.

[66] Quesney LF. Extracranial EEG evaluations. In: Engel J, editor. Surgical treatment of the epilepsies. New York: Raven Press; 1987.

[67] Rasmussen T. Surgery of frontal lobe epilepsy. In: Purpura DP, Penry JK, Walter RD, editors. Advances in neurology, vol. 8. New York: Raven Press; 1975.

[68] Franck G, Maquet P, Sadzot B, et al. Contribution of positron emission tomography to the investigation of epilepsies of frontal lobe origin. Adv Neurol 1992; 57:471–85.

[69] Robitaille Y, Rasmussen T, Dubeau F, et al. Histopathology of nonneoplastic lesions in frontal lobe epilepsy: review of 180 cases with recent MRI and PET correlations. Adv Neurol 1992;57:499–511.

[70] Swartz BE, Halgren E, Delgado-Escueta AV, et al. Neuroimaging in patients with seizures of probable frontal lobe origin. Epilepsia 1989;30:547–58.

[71] da Silva EA, Chugani DC, Muzik O, et al. Identification of frontal lobe epileptic foci in children using positron emission tomography. Epilepsia 1997;38: 1198–208.

[72] Oka A, Kubota M, Sakakihara Y, et al. A case of parietal lobe epilepsy with distinctive clinical and neuroradiological features. Brain Dev 1998;20: 179–82.

[73] Kim DW, Lee SK, Yun CH, et al. Parietal lobe epilepsy: the semiology, yield of diagnostic workup, and surgical outcome. Epilepsia 2004;45:641–9.

[74] Alavi A, Hirsch LJ. Studies of central nervous system

disorders with single photon emission computed tomography and positron emission tomography: evolution over the past 2 decades. Semin Nucl Med 1991;21:58–81.

[75] Chugani HT, Rintahaka PJ, Shewmon DA. Ictal patterns of cerebral glucose utilization in children with epilepsy. Epilepsia 1994;35:813–22.

[76] Theodore WH, Balish M, Leiderman D, et al. Effect of seizures on cerebral blood flow measured with 15O–H2O and positron emission tomography. Epilepsia 1996;37:796–802.

[77] Duncan JD, Moss SD, Bandy DJ, et al. Use of positron emission tomography for presurgical localization of eloquent brain areas in children with seizures. Pediatr Neurosurg 1997;26:144–56.

[78] Meltzer CC, Adelson PD, Brenner RP, et al. Planned ictal FDG PET imaging for localization of extratemporal epileptic foci. Epilepsia 2000;41:193–200.

[79] Swartz BE, Mandelkern MA. Positron emission tomography: the contribution of cognitive activation paradigms to the understanding of the epilepsies. Adv Neurol 1999;79:901–15.

[80] Savic I, Persson A, Roland P, et al. In-vivo demonstration of reduced benzodiazepine receptor binding in human epileptic foci. Lancet 1988;2: 863–6.

[81] Savic I, Svanborg E, Thorell JO. Cortical benzodiazepine receptor changes are related to frequency of partial seizures: a positron emission tomography study. Epilepsia 1996;37:236–44.

[82] Debets RM, Sadzot B, van Isselt JW, et al. Is 11C-flumazenil PET superior to 18FDG PET and 123I-iomazenil SPECT in presurgical evaluation of temporal lobe epilepsy? J Neurol Neurosurg Psychiatry 1997;62:141–50.

[83] Chugani HT, Chugani DC. Basic mechanisms of childhood epilepsies: studies with positron emission tomography. Adv Neurol 1999;79:883–91.

[84] Juhasz C, Nagy F, Watson C, et al. Glucose and [11C]flumazenil positron emission tomography abnormalities of thalamic nuclei in temporal lobe epilepsy. Neurology 1999;53:2037–45.

[85] Savic I, Thorell JO. Localized cerebellar reductions in benzodiazepine receptor density in human partial epilepsy. Arch Neurol 1996;53:656–62.

[86] Savic I, Thorell JO, Roland P. [11C]flumazenil positron emission tomography visualizes frontal epileptogenic regions. Epilepsia 1995;36:1225–32.

[87] Arnold S, Berthele A, Drzezga A, et al. Reduction of benzodiazepine receptor binding is related to the seizure onset zone in extratemporal focal cortical dysplasia. Epilepsia 2000;41:818–24.

[88] Richardson MP, Koepp MJ, Brooks DJ, et al. Benzodiazepine receptors in focal epilepsy with cortical dysgenesis: an 11C-flumazenil PET study. Ann Neurol 1996;40:188–98.

[89] Fisher RS, Frost JJ. Epilepsy. J Nucl Med 1991;32: 651–9.

[90] Frost JJ, Mayhberg HS, Fisher RS, et al. Mu-opiate

receptors measured by positron emission tomography are increased in temporal lobe epilepsy. Ann Neurol 1988;23:231–7.

[91] Madar I, Lesser RP, Krauss G, et al. Imaging of delta- and mu-opioid receptors in temporal lobe epilepsy by positron emission tomography. Ann Neurol 1997;41: 358–67.

[92] Prevett MC, Duncan JS, Jones T, et al. Demonstration of thalamic activation during typical absence seizures using H2(15)O and PET. Neurology 1995;45: 1396–402.

[93] Millan E, Abou-Khalil B, Delbeke D, et al. Frontal localization of absence seizures demonstrated by ictal positron emission tomography. Epilepsy Behav 2001; 2:54–60.

[94] Prevett MC, Lammertsma AA, Brooks DJ, et al. Benzodiazepine-GABAA receptor binding during absence seizures. Epilepsia 1995;36:592–9.

[95] Abou-Khalil B, Fakhoury T, Jennings M, et al. Inhibitory motor seizures: correlation with centroparietal structural and functional abnormalities. Acta Neurol Scand 1995;91:103–8.

[96] De Volder AG, Gadisseux JF, Michel CJ, et al. Brain glucose utilization in band heterotopia: synaptic activity of double cortex. Pediatr Neurol 1994;11: 290–4.

[97] Matsuda H, Onuma T, Yagishita A. Brain SPECT imaging for laminar heterotopia. J Nucl Med 1995; 36:238–40.

[98] Chugani HT, Shields WD, Shewmon DA, et al. Infantile spasms. I. PET identifies focal cortical dysgenesis in cryptogenic cases for surgical treatment. Ann Neurol 1990;27:406–13.

[99] Chugani HT. The use of positron emission tomography in the clinical assessment of epilepsy. Semin Nucl Med 1992;22:247–53.

[100] Korinthenberg R, Bauer-Scheid C, Burkart P, et al. 18FDG-PET in epilepsies of infantile onset with pharmacoresistant generalized tonic-clonic seizures. Epilepsy Res 2004;60:53–61.

[101] Chugani HT, Shewmon DA, Sankar R, et al. Infantile spasms. II. Lenticular nuclei and brain stem activation on positron emission tomography. Ann Neurol 1992; 31:212–9.

[102] Iinuma K, Yanai K, Yanagisawa T, et al. Cerebral glucose metabolism in five patients with Lennox-Gastaut syndrome. Pediatr Neurol 1987;3:12–8.

[103] Chugani HT, Mazziotta JC, Engel Jr J, et al. Lennox Gastaut syndrome: metabolic subtypes determined by 18FDG positron emission tomography. Ann Neurol 1987;21:4–13.

[104] Theodore WH, Rose D, Patronas N, et al. Cerebral glucose metabolism in the Lennox-Gastaut syndrome. Ann Neurol 1987;21:14–21.

[105] Angelini L, Broggi G, Riva D, et al. A case of Lennox-Gastaut syndrome successfully treated by removal of a parietotemporal astrocytoma. Epilepsia 1979;20:665–9.

[106] Ferrie CD, Maisey M, Cox T, et al. Focal abnormalities detected by 18FDG PET in epileptic encephalopathies. Arch Dis Child 1996;75:102–7.

[107] Hoffman HJ, Hendrick EB, Dennis M, et al. Hemispherectomy for Sturge-Weber syndrome. Childs Brain 1979;5:233.

[108] Chugani HT, Mazziotta JC, Phelps ME. Sturge-Weber syndrome: a study of cerebral glucose utilization with positron emission tomography. J Pediatr 1989;114: 244–53.

ELSEVIER
SAUNDERS

RADIOLOGIC
CLINICS
of North America

Radiol Clin N Am 43 (2005) 93–106

Role of [18F]-dopa–PET imaging in assessing movement disorders

Alan J. Fischman, MD, PhD[a,b],*

[a]Division of Nuclear Medicine, Department of Radiology, Massachusetts General Hospital, 32 Fruit Street,
Boston, MA 02114, USA
[b]Department of Radiology, Harvard Medical School, Boston, MA, USA

Parkinson's disease (PD) is a chronic and progressive neurodegenerative condition that is characterized clinically by tremor at rest, rigidity, bradykinesia, and postural instability. The primary pathologic features of PD are degeneration of striatal dopamine neurons and their terminal fields in the caudate and putamen and 80% to 99% reductions in striatal concentrations of dopamine and its transporter (DAT) [1–4]. Currently, the most effective treatment for PD is dopamine replacement with levodopa (L-dopa) or receptor agonists. As the disease progresses, however, these therapies become less effective in relieving symptoms and drug-induced side effects become prominent. In recent years, research has been directed to the development of alternative medical and surgical approaches to treatment, such as neuroprotective agents [5], fetal cell transplants [6], and pallidotomy [7,8]. These therapies are designed to slow disease progression or permanently correct the deficit in striatal dopamine and there is a compelling need for an accurate, precise, and noninvasive procedure for monitoring disease activity.

Unfortunately, conventional imaging techniques, such as CT and MR imaging, are not useful for detecting early disease or monitoring subtle changes in disease activity. Furthermore, because dopamine neurons make a small contribution to overall striatal metabolism, PET tracers of glucose use and single-photon emission CT tracers of blood flow have not been effective for detecting decreases in striatal dopamine innervation before clinical symptoms are manifest [9,10]. In contrast, PET studies with L-fluorine-18 ([18F]) 6-FD have demonstrated that early asymptomatic disease can be detected at 50% to 60% loss [11].

General characteristics of L-[18F] 6-fluorodopa

FD is an analogue of L-dopa in which a proton at position-6 of the catechol ring is substituted with [18F] [12]. For nearly two decades this radiopharmaceutical has proved to be an extremely useful tracer for PET studies aimed at probing the integrity of the nigrostriatal dopaminergic system. It's most important application has been for diagnosis, evaluation of disease progression, and therapeutic monitoring of patients with movement disorders that may be attributed to PD and Parkinson-plus syndromes. Although other agents, such as tracers of DAT sites, have been used for these purposes, FD-PET remains the noninvasive gold standard for studying these patients.

The detailed kinetic model that has been used to describe the behavior of FD in plasma and striatal tissue is illustrated in Fig. 1. In this configuration, the tracer is accumulated and processed in four steps: (1) transport across the blood-brain barrier by the large neutral amino acid transporter; (2) decarboxylation in the brain by L-aromatic amino acid decarboxylase; (3) storage in synaptic vesicles; and (4) metabolism to [18F] dopamine, [18F] dopac, and [18F] HVA. For kinetic modeling, the tracer is considered to be in one

* Division of Nuclear Medicine, Department of Radiology, Massachusetts General Hospital, 32 Fruit Street, Boston, MA 02114.

E-mail address: fischman@pet.mgh.harvard.edu

0033-8389/05/$ – see front matter © 2004 Elsevier Inc. All rights reserved.
doi:10.1016/j.rcl.2004.08.002

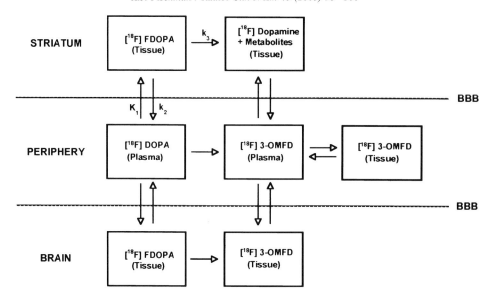

Fig. 1. Model for [^{18}F] dopa transport and metabolism. For kinetic modeling, the tracer is considered to be in one of three states: (1) a free pool, consisting of FD that is instantly available to other processes or reactions; (2) a slowly associating and dissociating reversible, nonsaturable, nonspecific binding pool; or (3) as [^{18}F] dopamine and metabolites. The transport rate of FD from plasma to brain tissue is K_1 (mL • min^{-1} • g^{-1}). FD in the free pool may return to plasma, according to the rate constant k_2 (min^{-1}); enter the nonspecific binding pool; or be converted to [^{18}F] dopamine and metabolites, according to the compound rate constant k_3. Fdopa, fluorodopa; 3-OMFD, 3-O-methyl-fluorodopa.

of three states: (1) a free pool, consisting of FD that is instantly available to other processes or reactions; (2) a slowly associating and dissociating reversible, nonsaturable, nonspecific binding pool; or (3) as [^{18}F] dopamine and metabolites. The transport rate of FD from plasma to brain tissue is K_1 (mL • min^{-1} • g^{-1}). FD in the free pool may return to plasma, according to the rate constant k_2 (min^{-1}); enter the nonspecific binding pool; or be converted to [^{18}F] dopamine and metabolites, according to the compound rate constant k_3. In brain regions that do not contain significant levels of L-aromatic amino acid decarboxylase (reference regions for kinetic modeling) FD remains unchanged.

Three general approaches have been developed for analyzing the results of FD-PET studies (Table 1):

(1) compartmental modeling [13,14], (2) graphical analysis [15,16], and (3) simple ratio methods [17–21]. Compartmental modeling of arterial blood and tissue time activity curves acquired by dynamic PET studies is the most rigorous analytical method and can be used to calculate individual values for some of the rate constants defined in Fig. 1. This approach can also yield information about the release of FD metabolites from the striatum, which is useful for evaluating the effects of inhibitors of dopamine metabolism, such as catechol O-methyl-transferase inhibitors. In early studies, the accuracy of these measurements was limited by signal noise; however, with the introduction of three-dimensional acquisition methods this problem has become less important. Unfortunately, because of the peripheral and central

Table 1
Analytical methods for evaluating fluorodopa-PET data

	Compartmental modeling	Graphical (Patlak)	Graphical (ref. region)	Ratios (ie, SOR)
Individual rate constants	Yes	No	No	No
Washout	Yes	Yes	Yes	No
Arterial blood sampling	Yes	Yes	No	No
Metabolite analysis	Yes	Yes	No	No
Imaging time	~120 min	~90 min	~90 min	10 min
Patient compliance	Poor	Poor	Fair	Excellent
Tracer economy	Poor	Poor	Poor	Good

Abbreviation: SOR, striatal-occipital ratio.

nervous system metabolism of FD, unless several assumptions are incorporated, compartmental modeling yields rate constants with high standard errors [13,22].

The graphical method makes use of the fact that although FD is extensively metabolized in the striatum, the metabolic products are retained in the striatum during the period of imaging. [^{18}F] uptake can be considered to be irreversible and described in terms of a single influx rate constant, K_i. With the graphical method, the ratio of background subtracted striatal [^{18}F] radioactivity (corrected for intravascular tracer) to metabolite corrected plasma FD concentration [$C_p(t)$] from time zero to the end of the acquisition (ordinant) is plotted against the ratio of metabolite corrected integrated plasma time activity data to $C_p(t)$ (abscissa). This plot becomes linear when pseudoequilibrium is reached. By assuming that there is no tracer back-flux, the asymptotic slope for the striatal data equals K_i, which represents the rate constant for tracer transport from blood to brain and striatal trapping. K_i depends on tracer transport, decarboxylation, and vesicular storage, and factors that affect any of these processes can alter its value. Because these processes are not rate limiting in dopamine metabolism the results of FD-PET studies are an index of the structural integrity of the nigrostriatal dopaminergic system (ie, K_i is directly correlated with the number of intact nigral pigmented neurons) [23,24]. Compared with compartmental modeling, the graphical method provides a more reliable estimate of FD metabolism and intact tracer plus metabolite release from the striatum; however, imaging times of up to 4 hours are required for these measurements. With this method the monotonic decrease in striatal radioactivity is described by a single rate constant that reflects tracer metabolism and release. Although the graphical analysis is simpler to perform than compartmental modeling, it still requires arterial blood collection and metabolite analysis, which are not practical for routine clinical applications. To address this issue, graphical procedures in which the blood information is replaced by region-of-interest data for a reference area of the brain that is devoid of L-aromatic amino acid decarboxylase activity have been developed [17,20,21]. K_i derived by this method has been shown to be highly correlated with the results of blood-based graphical methods and is extremely useful for studying patients with parkinsonian syndromes [19–21,25,26].

Although the reference region based graphical method of analysis represents a major advance for the clinical application of FD-PET, it still requires a prolonged dynamic acquisition. For debilitated patients, this prolonged imaging procedure is associated with both compliance issues and data bias introduced by motion. A ratio-based method, such as the striatal-occipital ratio (SOR), which uses FD-PET data acquired over a single short imaging period, could be of great value for quantifying nigrostriatal pathophysiology in PD and related conditions. Recently, the relative performance of SOR and K_i determined by the reference region method were compared in healthy volunteers and patients with PD of varying severity [21]. The results of this study demonstrated that both SOR and K_i were significantly reduced in the PD patients. SOR calculated for 10-minute images acquired between 65 and 95 minutes were statistically equivalent in group discrimination and were highly correlated ($P < .001$) with K_i (65–75 min, $r^2 = 0.85$; 75–85 min, $r^2 = 0.90$; 85–95 min, $r^2 = 0.92$). Both parameters were also significantly correlated with Parkinson's Disease Rating Scale (UPDRS) motor score. These results indicate that SOR is as accurate as K_i for distinguishing PD patients from healthy controls and for predicting clinical indices of disease severity. In another study it was demonstrated that SOR is superior to K_i for longitudinally monitoring fetal transplant viability in PD patients [27]. Based on these findings, it is clear that the SOR is the optimal analytical method for evaluating clinical FD-PET studies. Estimation of this parameter requires a single short image acquisition (<15 min including transmission imaging), which is less time consuming than a routine FDG brain scan. Also, tracer use is more efficient because multiple patients can be imaged with a single synthetic batch of FD.

FD has provided important information about nigrostriatal pathophysiology and the physical half-life of ^{18}F is well matched with the plasma half-life of L-dopa; however, it is far from an ideal tracer for several reasons. FD is difficult to produce and synthetic yields are relatively low compared with tracers like FDG. Modeling is complicated by peripheral metabolism of FD to 3-O-methyl-fluorodopa. FD-PET is almost always performed after pretreatment with carbidopa, which blocks peripheral decarboxylation and increases the amount of the dose that is delivered to the brain [28]. This blockade tends to be incomplete, however, and 3-O-methyl-fluorodopa accumulation in the brain reduces signal-to-background ratios to approximately 2:1 in healthy subjects and less in patients [29]. L-aromatic amino acid decarboxylase may be up-regulated in some disease states, which can reduce the difference between normal subjects and patients.

Normal brain distribution of L-[^{18}F] 6-fluorodopa

Until recently FD-PET was used exclusively to study the organization and pathophysiology of the striatal dopamine system in the human brain, particularly in PD. With the development of high-resolution three-dimensional PET cameras, however, it has become possible to study the pattern of extrastriatal tracer distribution. In a recent study [30], three-dimensional FD-PET studies were performed in 11 healthy volunteers. Regions of interest were constructed with individual coregistered volumetric MR images and K_is were calculated by the graphical method. The highest K_i values were measured in the neostriatum, with a rostrocaudal gradient of increasing K_i from the head of the caudate nucleus to rostral putamen to caudal putamen. Red nucleus and globus pallidus K_is were 81% and 40% of neostriatal values. In limbic areas, the highest K_i was detected in the amygdala (35% of neostriatal K_i). Compared with neostriatum, neocortical K_i values varied from 22% in temporal pole to 6% in occipital cortex. Hypothalamic K_i was high (45%) in comparison with thalamus (17%) and retina (17%). It was also demonstrated that FD is also taken up by serotonin (raphe, 51%) and noradrenaline (locus coeruleus, 37%) neurons.

Diagnosis of Parkinson's disease

The first clinical applications of FD-PET appeared in the mid-1980s and concerned patients with hemiparkinsonism [31,32]. These investigations demonstrated bilaterally reduced FD uptake in the putamen but normal uptake in the caudate nucleus. Putamen uptake was most reduced on the side contralateral to symptoms. The reduction in putamen uptake was of similar magnitude for PD patients with tremor and in

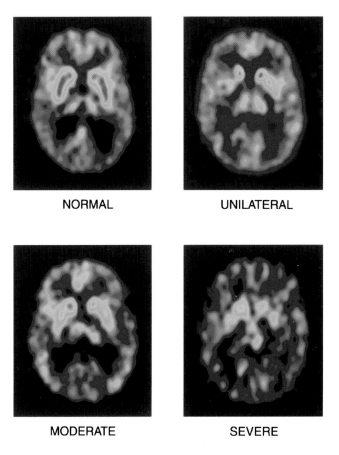

Fig. 2. Representative mid–striatal transaxial FD-PET images through the caudate and putamen of a healthy volunteer and patients with unilateral PD, moderate severity PD (left striatum worse than right), and severe PD.

akinetic rigid predominant disease. These studies were also the first to demonstrate subclinical involvement of the ipsilateral striatum. The findings of these studies were confirmed by later investigations that were extended to show that striatal uptake of FD decreases in proportion to disease severity (Fig. 2) [33–36]. PD patients with early disease and a continued response to L-dopa treatment retain FD in the striatum better than patients with long-standing PD and a fluctuating response to therapy. In general, average values for K_i in PD patients are reduced by 50% and 20% in putamen and caudate compared with controls [34]. The 50% reduction of K_i in the putamen is similar to the 60% reduction in striatal decarboxylase activity and 50% to 80% reduction in nigral compacta cell number reported in postmortem studies of PD patients [37,38]. It is considerably less than 90% reduction in dopamine content [39], indicating that FD-PET does not measure endogenous dopamine levels but rather the capacity of the striatum to decarboxylate dopa.

Longitudinal studies

In addition to the initial diagnosis of PD, FD-PET also has considerable value for following disease progression and monitoring response to therapy. For these applications, it is necessary to have information about the reliability of K_i measurements (ie, test-retest reproducibility). An early study of test-retest reproducibility in healthy subjects and PD patients demonstrated an 8% to 10% within-subject standard deviation [40]. Because the major component of the variation was in the blood data, it was suggested that graphical methods that substitute a brain tissue input function for blood data or simple ratio methods, such as SOR measurements, might prove to be more useful for longitudinal studies. This was verified in a later study of PD patients (Hoehn and Yahr stage I–III) in which within-subject standard deviations were determined to be 11%, 7%, and 2% for graphical analysis using a plasma input, graphical analysis using a cortical input, and a ratio method, respectively [41]. Because PD is largely a disease of the elderly, the effect of normal aging on K_i is another factor that must be considered for interpreting single time-point and longitudinal studies. Fortunately, several studies have demonstrated that K_i is not correlated with normal aging [42–44]. Because the number of dopaminergic neurons does decrease with aging, these findings most probably reflect compensatory up-regulation of decarboxylase activity in the remaining cells. Although it has been established that clinical doses of L-dopa do not have a measurable effect on

striatal K_i values [45], the effects of newer dopaminergic medications on FD uptake by the striatum are still under investigation.

The first demonstration that decline in whole striatal FD uptake in PD patients is more rapid than in age-matched controls was reported in 1994 [44]. A later study reported an average 12% per year decrease in putamen K_i for 17 PD patients with a mean clinical duration of 40 months [46]. This study was extended to include 32 patients with early PD and an overall 9% per year decrease was reported [47]. The average UPDRS score increased from 29 to 37 and K_i in the putamen decreased by 0.74% for each point on the UPDRS scale. By assuming a linear relationship between decline in putamen Ki and disease duration (and no effect of treatment of PD progression), the preclinical window for PD was estimated to be 6 ± 3 years; clinical symptoms started after 30% loss of dopaminergic function. These results are in agreement with the findings of a more recent longitudinal FD-PET study of 21 PD patients, 10 with de novo disease [48]. Over the observation period of 5 years, these patients demonstrated on average 8.3% ± 6.3% and 10.3% ± 4.3% annual decreases in K_i in the anterior and posterior putamen, respectively. In the caudate nucleus, K_i decreased by 5.9% ± 5.1% per year. These findings are in agreement with another study that correlated postmortem cell count with disease duration [49]. This investigation showed an exponential relationship between nigral cell number and clinical disease duration and estimated an approximately 5-year preclinical phase. It was also shown that the rate of nigral cell loss in PD is approximately 10-fold higher than in normal aging and by the time of onset of symptoms there is approximately 48% loss of nigral cells. The discordance between 30% functional decline at symptom onset in PD as determined by longitudinal FD-PET studies and the 50% cell loss measured in postmortem studies likely reflects up-regulation of decarboxylase activity in remaining terminals to increase dopamine synthesis and compensate for cell loss in early disease.

Preclinical Parkinson's disease

Autopsy studies have demonstrated that approximately 5% to 6% of normal individuals aged greater than or equal to 40 years have incidental Lewy bodies in the nigra, whereas only 0.3% to 0.4% of this group have clinical symptoms of PD [50]. Because both incidental Lewy body disease and PD are associated with the less pigmented ventral tier of the substantia nigra, it has been suggested that incidental Lewy body disease represents preclinical PD; parkinsonian

Parkinson-plus syndromes

Pathologic studies have shown that approximately 20% of patients diagnosed with PD on the basis of clinical criteria have other movement disorders [75–77]. Of these alternative pathologic etiologies, the most common are multiple system atrophy (MSA), progressive supranuclear palsy (PSP), corticobasal degeneration, and Alzheimer's disease. Although the number of FD-PET studies of patients with these conditions is much lower than in PD, a considerable amount of data has been reported.

Multiple system atrophy

MSA is an akinetic rigid movement disorder associated with autonomic dysfunction, cerebellar ataxia, and poor response to L-dopa treatment. Pathologically, the condition is characterized by neuronal loss in the putamen, caudate nucleus, globus pallidus, pigmented brain stem nuclei, cerebellar Purkinje cells, olives, and intermediolateral columns of the spinal cord. The clinical spectrum of MSA includes striatonigral degeneration, olivopontocerebellar atrophy, and pure autonomic failure. Although ventrolateral nigral dopaminergic projections to the putamen are lost in both MSA and PD, there is greater involvement of dorsomedial nigral projections in MSA, which suggests that dopamine terminals in the caudate should be more affected in MSA (Fig. 4). This possibility was confirmed in an early FD-PET study [34]. In this investigation, FD uptake in the caudate and putamen were compared in 10 patients with MSA and 8 patients with probable PD. In the putamen, FD uptake was reduced by a similar amount in MSA and PD (41% versus 38%). In contrast, there was a greater reduction in FD uptake in the caudate nucleus in the MSA patients (56% versus 73%). In another study [36], striatal uptake of FD in six patients with parkinsonism that was poorly respon-

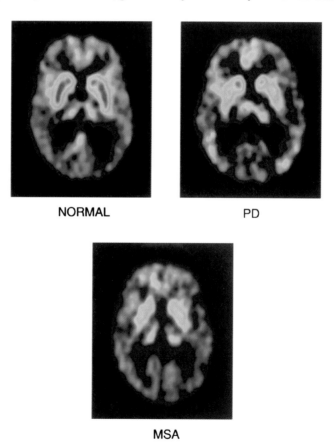

NORMAL   **PD**

MSA

Fig. 4. Representative mid-striatal transaxial FD-PET images through the caudate and putamen of a healthy volunteer and patients with PD of moderate severity and MSA. Note the relative sparing FD uptake in the caudate of the PD patient compared with the uniform reduction in the caudate and putamen of the MSA patient.

sive to L-dopa treatment (presumed diagnosis of striatonigral degeneration) was compared with eight PD patients. As in the earlier study, FD uptake in the putamen was equally reduced in both groups of patients but tracer uptake in the caudate was relatively spared in the PD patients. In a study of 28 patients with clinically probable PD and 25 with MSA that used discriminant analysis, clinical and PET categorization of MSA and PD agreed in only 60% of cases [78]. Although these findings establish that, on average, there is differential involvement of the caudate in MSA and PD, because of overlap of caudate uptake in the two conditions, FD-PET cannot reliably differentiate MSA from PD.

Several studies have indicated that FDG uptake is reduced in striatum, frontal cortex, and cerebellum in MSA [79] in contrast to normal or elevated striatal uptake that has been reported in PD [80,81,36]. This suggests that the combination of FDG and FD PET studies may be useful for differentiating the conditions. It has also been shown that striatal uptake of the nonselective opiate ligand ^{11}C diprenorphine is reduced in striatonigral degeneration but normal in PD [82].

Progressive supranuclear palsy

PSP (Steele-Richardson-Olszewski syndrome) is associated with rigidity, bradykinesia, axial dystonia, bulbar palsy, and frontal-type dementia. Pathologically, the condition is characterized by neuronal loss and neurofibrillar tangle inclusions in the basal ganglia, brainstem, and cerebellar nuclei. Usually, the cerebellar and cerebral cortices are spared; however, in some cases the frontal lobes are involved. Because all areas of the substantia nigra are involved in PSP, there are similar reductions in dopamine content in the caudate and putamen [83–86,49]. In an FD-PET study, FD uptake in the caudate and putamen were compared in 10 patients with PSP and 28 patients with probable PD. In the putamen, FD uptake was reduced by a similar amount in PSP and PD; however, as in the MSA, there was a greater reduction in FD uptake in the caudate nucleus in the PSP patients. As in the case of MSA, overlap of the ranges of K_i values in the PSP and PD groups was too great for effective differentiation of the conditions. Discriminant analysis was shown, however, to separate the conditions in 90% of cases [78]. In contrast to PD and MSA, striatal uptake in PSP is not correlated with disability [34]. It seems that PSP is primarily caused by degeneration of pallidal and brainstem neurons rather than nigrostriatal dopamine projections as in PD and MSA. FD-PET has also proved useful for identifying asymptomatic relatives of patients with PSP. In a recent study [87], two large kindreds with familial PSP were imaged to identify subclinical cases. In 4 of 15 first-degree asymptomatic relatives, caudate and putamen FD uptake was 2.5 standard deviations lower than the normal mean. A fifth asymptomatic relative with normal FD uptake showed a significant reduction of cortical and striatal glucose metabolism in a pattern similar to that of the affected relatives.

As with MSA, ^{18}F-fluorodeoxyglucose–PET has identified ^{18}F-fluorodeoxyglucose hypometabolism in striatum, frontal cortex, thalamus, and cerebellum in PSP [88–92] in contrast to normal or increased metabolism in PD. This suggests that the combination of ^{18}F-fluorodeoxyglucose– and FD-PET studies may be useful for differentiating the conditions. As in MSA, striatal uptake of ^{11}C diprenorphine is reduced in PSP [82].

Corticobasal degeneration

Corticobasal degeneration is associated with dyspraxic akinetic rigid limbs, myoclonus, supranuclear gaze problems, bulbar dysfunction, and rigidity. Dementia is uncommon but some patients are dysphasic. As with the other Parkinson-plus syndromes, response to L-dopa treatment is poor. Pathologically, the condition is characterized by collections of swollen achromatic Pick cells in the substantia nigra, cerebellar nuclei, and posterior frontal, parietal, and temporal cortices. Corticobasal degeneration should not be confused with Pick's disease, which affects the inferior frontal and temporal cortices and is associated with personality changes and dementia. In corticobasal degeneration, striatal uptake of FD is markedly reduced contralaterally to the most affected limbs. As in MSA and PSP the reductions are equal in caudate and putamen [93–95].

Other movement disorders

Dopa-responsive dystonia

Dopa-responsive dystonia is a familial disorder that usually presents in childhood with dystonic posturing of the legs and is extremely responsive to L-dopa therapy. Over time, the dystonia becomes more generalized and background parkinsonism becomes evident. In contrast to PD, however, FD uptake in the striatum is normal or only mildly reduced [96]. This suggests that dopa-responsive dystonia may be associated with a defect in the tyrosine hydroxylase complex that is effectively overcome by exogenous L-dopa that is decarboxylated normally to dopamine.

Drug-induced parkinsonism

The akinetic-rigid condition that can develop in patients taking clinical doses of dopamine receptor antagonists may be caused by the unmasking of subclinical nigral pathology by receptor blockade. In a study of 13 patients with drug-induced parkinsonism, striatal function was monitored by serial FD-PET studies for 2 years after discontinuing the drug. Four of the patients had reduced FD uptake in the putamen. One of these four patients improved after cessation of the drug, whereas three deteriorated. Eight of the nine patients with normal FD uptake improved clinically off dopamine antagonist. The ninth patient died before reassessment. These findings demonstrated that recovery from drug-induced parkinsonism can be associated with normal striatal uptake of FD but abnormal uptake did not necessarily indicate a poor prognosis.

Manganese-induced parkinsonism

It has been demonstrated that ingestion of manganese dioxide dust by manganese miners in Chile is associated with an akinetic-rigid syndrome that is poorly responsive to L-dopa. In contrast to PD and Parkinson-plus syndromes, however, striatal uptake of FD is normal [97], suggesting that the ore does not act as a direct nigral toxin.

Huntington's disease

Patients with the early onset variant of Huntington's disease can present with an akinetic-rigid syndrome that is poorly responsive to L-dopa. In contrast to PD patients, striatal FD uptake is preserved, whereas glucose metabolism and dopamine D2 receptor density are markedly reduced [98–101]. Pathologic analysis of the brains of these patients has revealed extensive striatal degeneration with loss of γ-aminobutyric acid projections to the internal and external pallidum [102]. This is in contrast to Huntington's disease patients with chorea in which there is minimal involvement of striatal projections to the internal pallidum, suggesting that loss of these may be the cause rigidity in early onset patients. In some cases, subclinical reductions in striatal glucose metabolism can be detected by [^{18}F]-fluorodeoxyglucose–PET in the same way that subclinical PD can be detected with FD-PET [103].

Summary

FD-PET has proved to be an extremely useful technique for the noninvasive evaluation of nigrostriatal pathophysiology in patients with PD and other movement disorders. The development of ratio methods for image analysis has greatly reduced the complexity of these PET studies and has facilitated data analysis. With the recent advances in cyclotron targetry and automated synthesis modules FD-PET will soon become an important component of the clinical armamentarium.

References

[1] Kish SJ, Shannak K, Hornykiewicz O. Uneven pattern of dopamine loss in the striatum of patients with idiopathic Parkinson's disease. N Engl J Med 1988; 318:876–80.

[2] Madras BK, Spealman RD, Fahey MA, Neumeyer JL, Saha JK, Milius RA. Cocaine receptors labeled by [^{3}H] 2 beta-carbomethoxy-3 beta-(4-fluorophenyl)tropane. Mol Pharmacol 1989;36:518–24.

[3] Madras BK, Fahey MA, Kaufman MJ. [^{3}H] CFT and [^{3}H] LU 19–005: markers for cocaine receptor/dopamine nerve terminals in Parkinson's disease [abstract]. Soc Neurosci Abstr 1990;16:14.

[4] Kaufman MJ, Madras BK. Severe depletion of cocaine recognition sites associated with the dopamine transporter in Parkinson's diseased striatum. Synapse 1991;9:43–9.

[5] Parkinson's Study Group. Effects of tocopherol and deprenyl on the progression of disability in early Parkinson's disease. N Engl J Med 1993;328:176–83.

[6] Freed CR, Breeze RE, Schneck SA. Transplantation of fetal mesencephalic tissue in Parkinson's disease. N Engl J Med 1995;333:730–1.

[7] Iacono RP, Shima F, Lonser RR, Kuniyoshi S, Maeda G, Yamada S. The results, indications, and physiology of posteroventral pallidotomy for patients with Parkinson's disease. Neurosurgery 1995;36:1118–25.

[8] Laitinen LV. Pallidotomy for Parkinson's disease. Neurosurg Clin N Am 1995;6:105–12.

[9] Kuhl DE, Metter EJ, Riege WH. Patterns of local cerebral glucose utilization determined in Parkinson's disease by the [^{18}F] fluorodeoxyglucose method. Ann Neurol 1984;15:419–24.

[10] Smith FW, Gemmell HG, Sharp PF, Besson JA. Technetium-99m HMPAO imaging in patients with basal ganglia disease. Br J Radiol 1988;61:914–20.

[11] Leenders KL, Salmon EP, Tyrrell P, Perani D, Brooks DJ, Sager H, et al. The nigrostriatal dopaminergic system assessed in vivo by positron emission tomography in healthy volunteer subjects and patients with Parkinson's disease. Arch Neurol 1990;47: 1290–8.

[12] Adam MJ, Jivan S. Synthesis and purification of

L-[^{18}F] 6-fluorodopa. Appl Radiat Isot 1988;39: 1203–6.

[13] Huang SC, Yu DC, Barrio JR, Grafton S, Melega WP, Hoffman JM, et al. Kinetics and modeling of L-6-[^{18}F]fluoro-dopa in human positron emission tomographic studies. J Cereb Blood Flow Metab 1991;11: 898–913.

[14] Wahl L, Nahmias C. Modeling of fluorine-18–6-fluoro-L-dopa in humans. J Nucl Med 1996;37: 432–7.

[15] Patlak CS, Blasberg RG. Graphical evaluation of blood-to-brain transfer constants from multiple-time uptake data: generalizations. J Cereb Blood Flow Metab 1985;5:584–90.

[16] Martin WRW, Palmer MR, Patlak CS, Calne DB. Nigrostriatal function in man studied with positron emission tomography. Ann Neurol 1989;26:535–42.

[17] Takikawa S, Dhawan V, Chaly T, Robeson W, Dahl R, Zanzi I, et al. Input functions for 6-[fluorine-18] fluorodopa quantitation in parkinsonism: comparative studies and clinical correlations. J Nucl Med 1994;35: 955–63.

[18] Vingerhoets FJ, Schulzer M, Ruth TJ, Holden JE, Snow BJ. Reproducibility and discriminating ability of fluorine-18–6-fluoro-L-dopa PET in Parkinson's disease. J Nucl Med 1996;37:421–6.

[19] Morrish PK, Rakshi JS, Bailey DL, Sawle GV, Brooks DJ. Measuring the rate of progression and estimating the preclinical period of Parkinson's disease with [^{18}F] dopa PET. J Neurol Neurosurg Psychiatry 1998;64: 314–9.

[20] Hoshi H, Kuwabara H, Leger G, Cumming P, Guttman M, Gjedde A. 6-[^{18}F] fluoro-L-dopa metabolism in living human brain: a comparison of six analytical methods. J Cereb Blood Flow Metab 1993; 13:57–69.

[21] Dhawan V, Ma Y, Pillai V, Spetsieris P, Chaly T, Belakhlkef A, et al. Comparative analysis of striatal Fdopa uptake in Parkinson's disease: ratio method versus graphical analysis. J Nucl Med 2002;43: 1324–30.

[22] Kuwabara H, Cumming P, Reith J, Leger G, Diksic M, Evans AC, et al. Human striatal L-dopa decarboxylase activity estimated in vivo using 6-[^{18}F]fluoro-dopa and positron emission tomography: error analysis and application to normal subjects. J Cereb Blood Flow Metab 1993;13:43–56.

[23] Pate BD, Kawamata T, Yamada T, McGeer EG, Hewitt KA, Snow BJ, et al. Correlation of striatal fluorodopa uptake in the MPTP-monkey with dopaminergic indices. Ann Neurol 1993;34:331–8.

[24] Snow BJ, Tooyama I, McGeer EG, Yamada T, Calne DB, Takahashi H, et al. Correlations in humans between premortem PET [^{18}F] fluorodopa uptake, postmortem cell counts and striatal dopamine levels. Ann Neurol 1993;34:324–30.

[25] Morrish PK, Sawle GV, Brooks DJ. Regional changes in [^{18}F]dopa metabolism in the striatum in Parkinson's disease. Brain 1996;119:2097–103.

[26] DeJesus OT, Endres CJ, Shelton SE, Nickles RJ, Holden JE. Evaluation of fluorinated m-tyrosine analogs as PET imaging agents of dopamine nerve terminals: comparison with 6-fluorodopa. J Nucl Med 1998;38:630–6.

[27] Nakamura T, Dhawan V, Chaly T, Fukuda M, Ma Y, Breeze R, et al. Blinded positron emission tomography study of dopamine cell implantation in Parkinson's disease. Ann Neurol 2001;50:181–7.

[28] Hoffman JM, Melaga WP, Hawk TC, Grafton SC, Luxen A, Mahoney DK, et al. The effect of carbidopa administration on 6-[^{18}F] fluoro-L-dopa kinetics in positron emission tomography. J Nucl Med 1992;33: 1472–7.

[29] Wahl L, Chirakal R, Firnau G, Garnett ES, Nahmias C. The distribution and kinetics of [^{18}F]6-fluoro-3-O-methyl-L-dopa in the human brain. J Cereb Blood Flow Metab 1994;14:664–70.

[30] Moore RY, Whone AL, McGowan S, Brooks DJ. Monoamine neuron innervation of the normal human brain: an ^{18}F-dopa PET study. Brain Res 2003;982: 137–45.

[31] Garnett ES, Nahmias C, Firnau G. Central dopaminergic pathways in hemiparkinsonism examined by positron emission tomography. Can J Neurol Sci 1984;11:174–9.

[32] Nahmias C, Garnett ES, Firnau G, Lang A. Striatal dopamine distribution in parkinsonian patients during life. J Neurol Sci 1985;69:223–30.

[33] Leenders KL, Palmer AJ, Quinn N, Clark JC, Firnau G, Garnett ES, et al. Brain dopamine metabolism in patients with Parkinson's disease measured with positron emission tomography. J Neurol Neurosurg Psychiatry 1986;49:853–60.

[34] Brooks DJ, Ibanez V, Sawle GV, Quinn N, Lees AJ, Mathias CJ, et al. Differing patterns of striatal ^{18}F-dopa uptake in Parkinson's disease, multiple system atrophy, and progressive supranuclear palsy. Ann Neurol 1990;28:547–55.

[35] Martin WRW, Adam MJ, Bergstrom M, Ammann W, Harrop R, Laihinen AO, et al. In vivo study of dopa metabolism in Parkinson's disease. In: Fajn S, Jenner P, Marsden CD, Teychenne PF, editors. Recent developments in Parkinson's disease. New York: Raven Press; 1986. p. 97–102.

[36] Otsuka M, Ichiya Y, Hosokawa S, Kuwabara Y, Tahara T, Fukumura T, et al. Striatal blood flow, glucose metabolism and ^{18}F-dopa uptake: difference in Parkinson's disease and atypical parkinsonism. J Neurol Neurosurg Psychiatry 1991;54:898–904.

[37] Goto S, Hirano A, Matsumoto S. Subdivisional involvement of nigrostriatal loop in idiopathic Parkinson's disease and striatonigral degeneration. Ann Neurol 1989;26:766–70.

[38] German DC, Manaye K, Smith WK, Woodward DJ, Saper CB. Midbrain dopaminergic cell loss in Parkinson's disease: computer visualization. Ann Neurol 1989;26:507–14.

[39] Bernheimer H, Birkmayer W, Hornykiewicz O,

Jellinger K, Seitelberger F. Brain dopamine and the syndromes of Parkinson and Huntington: clinical, morphological and neurochemical correlations. J Neurol Sci 1973;20:415–55.

[40] Vingerhoets FJ, Snow BJ, Schulzer M, Morrison S, Ruth TJ, Holden JE, et al. Reproducibility of fluorine-18–6-fluorodopa positron emission tomography in normal human subjects. J Nucl Med 1994;35:18–24.

[41] Vingerhoets FJ, Schulzer M, Ruth TJ, Holden JE, Snow BJ. Reproducibility and discriminating ability of fluorine-18–6-fluoro-L-dopa PET in Parkinson's disease. J Nucl Med 1996;37:421–6.

[42] Sawle GV, Colebatch JG, Shah A, Brooks DJ, Marsden CD, Frackowiak RS. Striatal function in normal aging: implications for Parkinson's disease. Ann Neurol 1990;28:799–804.

[43] Eidelberg D, Takikawa S, Dhawan V, Chaly T, Robeson W, Dahl R, et al. Striatal ^{18}F-dopa uptake: absence of an aging effect. J Cereb Blood Flow Metab 1993;13:881–8.

[44] Vingerhoets FJ, Snow BJ, Tetrud JW, Langston JW, Schulzer M, Calne DB. Positron emission tomographic evidence for progression of human MPTP-induced dopaminergic lesions. Ann Neurol 1994;36:765–70.

[45] Ceravolo R, Piccini P, Bailey DL, Jorga KM, Bryson H, Brooks DJ. ^{18}F-dopa PET evidence that tolcapone acts as a central COMT inhibitor in Parkinson's disease. Synapse 2002;43:201–7.

[46] Morrish PK, Sawle GV, Brooks DJ. An [^{18}F] dopa PET and clinical study of the rate of progression of Parkinson's disease. Brain 1996;119:585–91.

[47] Morrish PK, Rakshi JS, Sawle GV, Brooks DJ. Measuring the rate of progression and estimating the preclinical period of Parkinson's disease with [^{18}F] dopa PET. Neurol Neurosurg Psychiatry 1998;64:314–9.

[48] Nurmi E, Ruottinen HM, Bergman J, Haaparanta M, Solin O, Sonninen P, et al. Rate of progression in Parkinson's disease: a [^{18}F] fluoro-L-dopa pet study. mov disord 2001;16:608–15.

[49] Fearnley JM, Lees AJ. Ageing and Parkinson's disease: substantia nigra regional selectivity. Brain 1991;114:2283–301.

[50] Golbe LJ. The genetics of Parkinson's disease: a reconsideration. Neurology 1990;40:7–16.

[51] Calne DB, Langston JW, Martin WR, Stoessl AJ, Ruth TJ, Adam MJ, et al. Positron emission tomography after MPTP: observations relating to the cause of Parkinson's disease. Nature 1985;317:246–8.

[52] Sawle GV, Wroe SJ, Lees AJ, Brooks DJ, Frackowiak RS. The identification of presymptomatic parkinsonism: clinical and [^{18}F]dopa positron emission tomography studies in an Irish kindred. Ann Neurol 1992;32:609–17.

[53] Piccini P, Morrish PK, Turjanski N, Sawle GV, Burn DJ, Weeks RA, et al. Dopaminergic function in familial Parkinson's disease: a clinical and ^{18}F-dopa positron emission tomography study. Ann Neurol 1997;41:222–9.

[54] Khan NL, Brooks DJ, Pavese N, Sweeney MG, Wood NW, Lees AJ, et al. Progression of nigrostriatal dysfunction in a parkin kindred: an [18F]dopa PET and clinical study. Brain 2002;125:2248–56.

[55] Burn DJ, Mark MH, Playford ED, Maraganore DM, Zimmerman TR, Duvoisin RC, et al. Parkinson's disease in twins studied with 18F-dopa and positron emission tomography. Neurology 1992;42:1894–900.

[56] Alexander T, Sortwell CE, Sladek CD, Roth RH, Steece-Collier K. Comparison of neurotoxicity following repeated administration of L-dopa, D-dopa and dopamine to embryonic mesencephalic dopamine neurons in cultures derived from Fisher 344 and Sprague-Dawley donors. Cell Transplant 1997;6:309–15.

[57] Iida M, Miyazaki I, Tanaka K, Kabuto H, Iwata-Ichikawa E, Ogawa N. Dopamine D2 receptor-mediated antioxidant and neuroprotective effects of ropinirole, a dopamine agonist. Brain Res 1999;838:51–9.

[58] Olanow CW, Jenner P, Brooks D. Dopamine agonists and neuroprotection in Parkinson's disease. Ann Neurol 1998;44:167–74.

[59] Whone AL, Watts RL, Stoessl AJ, Davis M, Reske S, Nahmias C, et al. Slower progression of Parkinson's disease with ropinirole versus levodopa: the REAL-PET study. Ann Neurol 2003;54:93–101.

[60] Parkinson Study Group. Dopamine transporter brain imaging to assess the effects of pramipexole vs levodopas on Parkinson disease progression. JAMA 2002;287:1653–61.

[61] Lindvall O, Backlund EO, Farde L, Sedvall G, Freedman R, Hoffer B, et al. Transplantation in Parkinson's disease: two cases of adrenal medullary grafts to the putamen. Ann Neurol 1987;22:457–68.

[62] Lindvall O, Brundin P, Widner H, Rehncrona S, Gustavii B, Frackowiak R, et al. Grafts of fetal dopamine neurons survive and improve motor function in Parkinson's disease. Science 1990;247:574–7.

[63] Freed CR, Breeze RE, Rosenberg NL, Schneck SA, Kriek E, Qi JX, et al. Survival of implanted fetal dopamine cells and neurologic improvement 12 to 46 months after transplantation for Parkinson's disease. N Engl J Med 1992;327:1549–55.

[64] Peschanski M, Defer G, N'Guyen JP, Ricolfi F, Monfort JC, Remy P, et al. Bilateral motor improvement and alteration of L-dopa effect in two patients with parkinson's disease following intrastriatal transplantation of foetal ventral mesencephalon. brain 1994;117:487–99.

[65] Spencer DD, Robbins RJ, Naftolin F, Marek KL, Vollmer T, Leranth C, et al. Unilateral transplantation of human fetal mesencephalic tissue into the caudate nucleus of patients with Parkinson's disease. N Engl J Med 1992;327:1541–8.

[66] Widner H, Tetrud J, Rehncrona S, Snow B, Brundin P, Gustavii B, et al. Bilateral fetal mesencephalic grafting in two patients with parkinsonism induced

by 1-methyl-4-phenyl-1,2,3,6-tetrahydropyridine (MPTP). N Engl J Med 1992;327:1556–63.

[67] Freed CR, Greene PE, Breeze RE, Tsai WY, DuMouchel W, Kao R, et al. Transplantation of embryonic dopamine neurons for severe Parkinson's disease. N Engl J Med 2001;344:710–9.

[68] Nakamura T, Dhawan V, Chaly T, Fukuda M, Ma Y, Breeze R, et al. Blinded positron emission tomography study of dopamine cell implantation for Parkinson's disease. Ann Neurol 2001;50:181–7.

[69] Ding YS, Fowler JS, Volkow ND, Logan J, Gatley SJ, Sugano Y. Carbon-11-d-threo-methylphenidate binding to dopamine transporter in baboon brain. J Nucl Med 1995;36:2298–305.

[70] Kazumata K, Dhawan V, Chaly T, Antonini A, Margouleff C, Belakhlef A, et al. Dopamine transporter imaging with fluorine-18-FPCIT and PET. J Nucl Med 1998;39:1521–30.

[71] Fischman AJ, Bonab AA, Babich JW, Livni E, Alpert NM, Meltzer PC, et al. [(11)C, (127)I] Altropane: a highly selective ligand for PET imaging of dopamine transporter sites. Synapse 2001;39:332–42.

[72] Frey KA, Koeppe RA, Kilbourn MR, Vander Borght TM, Albin RL, Gilman S, et al. Presynaptic monoaminergic vesicles in Parkinson's disease and normal aging. Ann Neurol 1996;40:873–84.

[73] Gilman S, Frey KA, Koeppe RA, Junck L, Little R, Vander Borght TM, et al. Decreased striatal monoaminergic terminals in olivopontocerebellar atrophy and multiple system atrophy demonstrated with positron emission tomography. Ann Neurol 1996;40: 885–92.

[74] Lee CS, Samii A, Sossi V, Ruth TJ, Schulzer M, Holden JE, et al. In vivo positron emission tomographic evidence for compensatory changes in presynaptic dopaminergic nerve terminals in Parkinson's disease. Ann Neurol 2000;47:493–503.

[75] Fearnley JM, Lees AJ. Striatonigral degeneration: a clinicopathological study. Brain 1990;113:1823–42.

[76] Rajput AH, Rozdilsky B, Rajput A. Accuracy of clinical diagnosis in parkinsonism: a prospective study. Can J Neurol Sci 1991;18:275–8.

[77] Hughes AJ, Daniel SE, Kilford L, Lees AJ. Accuracy of clinical diagnosis of idiopathic Parkinson's disease: a clinico-pathological study of 100 cases. J Neurol Neurosurg Psychiatry 1992;55:181–4.

[78] Burn DJ, Sawle GV, Brooks DJ. Differential diagnosis of Parkinson's disease, multiple system atrophy, and Steele-Richardson-Olszewski syndrome: discriminant analysis of striatal ^{18}F-dopa PET data. J Neurol Neurosurg Psychiatry 1994;57:278–84.

[79] De Volder AG, Francart J, Laterre C, Dooms G, Bol A, Michel C, et al. Decreased glucose utilization in the striatum and frontal lobe in probable striatonigral degeneration. Ann Neurol 1989;26:239–47.

[80] Kuhl DE, Metter EJ, Riege WH. Patterns of local cerebral glucose utilization determined in Parkinson's disease by the [^{18}F]fluorodeoxyglucose method. Ann Neurol 1984;15:419–24.

[81] Wolfson LI, Leenders KL, Brown LL, Jones T. Alterations of regional cerebral blood flow and oxygen metabolism in Parkinson's disease. Neurology 1985;35:1399–405.

[82] Burn DJ, Rinne JO, Quinn NP, Lees AJ, Marsden CD, Brooks DJ. Striatal opioid receptor binding in Parkinson's disease, striatonigral degeneration and Steele-Richardson-Olszewski syndrome: a [^{11}C]diprenorphine PET study. Brain 1995;118:951–8.

[83] Jellinger K, Riederer P, Tomonaga M. Progressive supranuclear palsy: clinico-pathological and biochemical studies. J Neural Transm Suppl 1980;16: 111–28.

[84] Bokobza B, Ruberg M, Scatton B, Javoy-Agid F, Agid Y. [3H]spiperone binding, dopamine and HVA concentrations in Parkinson's disease and supranuclear palsy. Eur J Pharmacol 1984;99:167–75.

[85] Ruberg M, Bokobza B, Javoy-Agid F, Montfort JC, Agid Y. [^{3}H]spiperone binding in the nigrostriatal system in human brain. Eur J Pharmacol 1984;99: 159–65.

[86] Kish SJ, Chang LJ, Mirchandani L, Shannak K, Hornykiewicz O. Progressive supranuclear palsy: relationship between extrapyramidal disturbances, dementia, and brain neurotransmitter markers. Ann Neurol 1985;18:530–6.

[87] Piccini P, de Yebenez J, Lees AJ, Ceravolo R, Turjanski N, Pramstaller P, et al. Familial progressive supranuclear palsy: detection of subclinical cases using ^{18}F-dopa and 18fluorodeoxyglucose positron emission tomography. Arch Neurol 2001;58: 1846–51.

[88] D'Antona R, Baron JC, Samson Y, Serdaru M, Viader F, Agid Y, et al. Subcortical dementia: frontal cortex hypometabolism detected by positron tomography in patients with progressive supranuclear palsy. Brain 1985;108:785–99.

[89] Leenders KL, Frackowiak RS, Lees AJ. Steele-Richardson-Olszewski syndrome: brain energy metabolism, blood flow and fluorodopa uptake measured by positron emission tomography. Brain 1988;111: 615–30.

[90] Foster NL, Gilman S, Berent S, Morin EM, Brown MB, Koeppe RA. Cerebral hypometabolism in progressive supranuclear palsy studied with positron emission tomography. Ann Neurol 1988;24:399–406.

[91] Goffinet AM, De Volder AG, Gillain C, Rectem D, Bol A, Michel C, et al. Positron tomography demonstrates frontal lobe hypometabolism in progressive supranuclear palsy. Ann Neurol 1989;25: 131–9.

[92] Blin J, Baron JC, Dubois B, Pillon B, Cambon H, Cambier J, et al. Positron emission tomography study in progressive supranuclear palsy: brain hypometabolic pattern and clinicometabolic correlations. Arch Neurol 1990;47:747–52.

[93] Sawle GV, Brooks DJ, Marsden CD, Frackowiak RS. Corticobasal degeneration: a unique pattern of regional cortical oxygen hypometabolism and striatal

fluorodopa uptake demonstrated by positron emission tomography. Brain 1991;114:541–56.

[94] Eidelberg D, Dhawan V, Moeller JR, Sidtis JJ, Ginos JZ, Strother SC, et al. The metabolic landscape of cortico-basal ganglionic degeneration: regional asymmetries studied with positron emission tomography. J Neurol Neurosurg Psychiatry 1991;54:856–62.

[95] Nagasawa H, Tanji H, Nomura H, Saito H, Itoyama Y, Kimura I, et al. PET study of cerebral glucose metabolism and fluorodopa uptake in patients with corticobasal degeneration. J Neurol Sci 1996;139: 210–7.

[96] Sawle GV, Leenders KL, Brooks DJ, Harwood G, Lees AJ, Frackowiak RS, et al. Dopa-responsive dystonia: [^{18}F]dopa positron emission tomography. Ann Neurol 1991;30:24–30.

[97] Wolters SC, Huang CC, Clark C, Peppard RF, Okada J, Chu NS, et al. Positron emission tomography in manganese intoxication. Ann Neurol 1989;26: 647–51.

[98] Kuhl DE, Metter EJ, Riege WH, Markham CH. Patterns of local cerebral glucose utilization in Parkinson's disease and Huntington's disease. Ann Neurol 1984;15:119–25.

[99] Leenders KL, Frackowiak RS, Quinn N, Marsden CD. Brain energy metabolism and dopaminergic function in Huntington's disease measured in vivo using positron emission tomography. Mov Disord 1986;1:69–77.

[100] Young AB, Penney JB, Starosta-Rubinstein S, Markel DS, Berent S, Giordani B, et al. PET scan investigations of Huntington's disease: cerebral metabolic correlates of neurological features and functional decline. Ann Neurol 1986;20:296–303.

[101] Hagglund J, Aquilonius SM, Eckernas SA, Hartvig P, Lundquist H, Gullberg P, et al. Dopamine receptor properties in Parkinson's disease and Huntington's chorea evaluated by positron emission tomography using ^{11}C-N-methyl-spiperone. Acta Neurol Scand 1987;75:87–94.

[102] Albin RL, Reiner A, Anderson KD, Penney JB, Young AB. Striatal and nigral neuron subpopulations in rigid Huntington's disease: implications for the functional anatomy of chorea and rigidity-akinesia. Ann Neurol 1990;27:357–65.

[103] Grafton ST, Mazziotta JC, Pahl JJ, St. George-Hyslop P, Haines JL, Gusella J, et al. A comparison of neurological, metabolic, structural, and genetic evaluations in persons at risk for Huntington's disease. Ann Neurol 1990;28:614–21.

ELSEVIER
SAUNDERS

Radiol Clin N Am 43 (2005) 107–119

RADIOLOGIC
CLINICS
of North America

PET in cardiology

Amol Takalkar, MD, Ayse Mavi, MD, Abass Alavi, MD, Luis Araujo, MD*

Division of Nuclear Medicine, Department of Radiology, Hospital of the University of Pennsylvania, 110 Donner Building, 3400 Spruce Street, Philadelphia, PA 19104, USA

There has been considerable improvement in the morbidity and mortality from cardiovascular disease over the past few decades. Along with the advancements in interventional and therapeutic measures, the tremendous progress and innovations in diagnostic testing modalities have made a key contribution to this accomplishment. Nuclear cardiology techniques to assess cardiovascular diseases have evolved significantly to provide reliable and accurate assessment of the cardiac status of a patient to assist the physician in making beneficial management decisions. Historically, nuclear cardiology techniques primarily involved planar and single-photon emission CT (SPECT) myocardial imaging. The relative ease and the cost-effectiveness of cardiac SPECT made it immensely popular and successful. Myocardial SPECT imaging has been inherently limited, however, by suboptimal spatial and temporal resolution and attenuation correction. The development of PET has further improved the use of nuclear cardiology in evaluating cardiovascular diseases. PET offers several advantages over traditional SPECT imaging including better spatial and temporal resolution and absolute quantification of regional radiotracer uptake. PET has been extremely successful in evaluating myocardial viability. Combination of myocardial perfusion and metabolism imaging using PET is considered the gold standard for noninvasive assessment of myocardial viability. Recent advancements in PET instrumentation and technology along with the development of several new PET radiotracers for assessing an array of cardiovascular pathology may

place PET in the forefront for evaluation of cardiovascular disorders.

Cardiac PET radiotracers

Several radiopharmaceuticals labeled with positron-emitting radiotracers are currently available. These include tracers for assessing myocardial perfusion, myocardial metabolism, myocardial hypoxia, and the cardiac nervous system.

Myocardial perfusion tracers

Several PET tracers that can be used to evaluate myocardial blood flow have been developed. These include the cyclotron-produced nitrogen-13 (^{13}N)-labeled ammonia and oxygen-15–labed water ($[^{15}O]$-H_2O), and the generator produced rubidium-82 (^{82}Rb)-chloride and copper-62 (^{62}Cu)-labeled pyruvaldehyde bis (N4-methylthio-semicarbazone) or $[^{62}Cu]$-PTSM. Only ^{13}N and ^{82}Rb are approved by the Food and Drug Administration.

Rubidium-82–labeled chloride

^{82}Rb is obtained from a generator that uses strontium-82 (^{82}Sr) as the parent isotope. Because ^{82}Sr has a physical half-life of 25 days, the generator can be used for about 1 month. ^{82}Rb has a physical half-life of 75 seconds, positron energy of 3.15 MeV, and positron range of 2.8 mm. Its tissue uptake is similar to potassium and thallium-201 (^{201}Tl), and requires an active Na/K-ATPase pump for intracellular transport. Because of its very short half-life, the imaging studies can be accomplished within 30 minutes, but necessitate the administration of high doses to obtain

* Corresponding author.
E-mail address: AraujoL@uphs.upenn.edu (L. Araujo).

adequate counts. The usual protocol for [82]Rb myocardial perfusion imaging consists of administering 1110 to 2220 MBq (30–60 mCi) of [82]Rb intravenously over 30 to 60 seconds and obtaining a static image for 3 to 7 minutes after waiting 1 to 3 minutes for clearance of the tracer from arterial blood [1–3]. The characteristics of the positron emitted by [82]Rb (high positron energy and tissue range) mildly impair the spatial resolution of the images. The important advantage of this tracer, however, is that it is generator produced; no cyclotron is necessary to perform myocardial perfusion imaging. In addition, because of its very short half-life a repeat perfusion image can be obtained within few minutes without any background activity. A rest-stress study can be completed within 1 hour.

Nitrogen-13–labeled ammonia

[13]N is a cyclotron-produced radioisotope and has a physical half-life of 9.9 minutes. Its positron energy of 1.19 MeV and positron range of 0.4 mm results in excellent images. The actual mechanism for intracellular transport of ^{13}N-ammonia remains unclear, but it has a high extraction rate and prolonged myocardial retention because of metabolic trapping by the glutamine synthetase pathway. Protocols using ^{13}N-ammonia for myocardial perfusion imaging usually consist of 5 to 10 minutes of static imaging 5 to 10 minutes after the intravenous administration of 370 to 555 MBq (10–15 mCi) of N-13 ammonia. By virtue of its 10 minutes half-life, gated acquisition

is feasible. Dynamic imaging to obtain quantitative myocardial blood flow data is also possible and well validated [1–8]. The 10-minute half-life of this tracer makes it suitable to be imaged after treadmill exercise (Fig. 1) as opposed to [82]Rb, which has to be used in conjunction with pharmacologic stress only.

Oxygen-15–labeled water

[15]O is also cyclotron-produced with a physical half-life of 122 seconds, positron energy of 1.72 MeV, and positron range of 1.1 mm. Being freely diffusible and metabolically inert, ^{15}O-H_2O is the closest to an ideal perfusion tracer. Its accumulation in tissue is almost exclusively a function of blood flow. Typical protocols use 555 to 925 MBq (15–25 mCi) as an intravenous bolus followed by dynamic imaging for 5 minutes. Complex mathematical analysis is needed to obtain regional myocardial perfusion, however, and the images are too noisy to be visually interpretable. Moreover, it is not a Food and Drug Administration–approved tracer [1,3,9–11]. This technique is mostly used for clinical investigation.

Copper-62–labeled pyruvaldehyde bis (N4-methylthio-semicarbazone)

A novel agent, [62]Cu-PTSM, is also being evaluated for myocardial perfusion imaging. [62]Cu is obtained from a Zinc-62 ([62]Zn)–[62]Cu generator, has a half-life of 9.74 minutes, positron energy of 2.93 MeV, and a range of 2.7 mm. It exhibits a lipophilic nature with a high extraction ratio and pro-

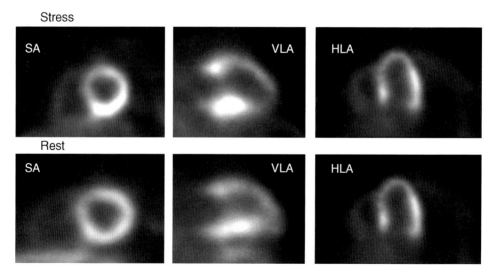

Fig. 1. Rest and stress myocardial perfusion imaging with PET using ^{13}N-ammonia in a 47-year-old man with history of essential hypertension complaining of exertional chest pain. The selected images of stress and rest myocardial perfusion in short axis (SA), vertical long axis (VLA), and horizontal long axis (HLA) demonstrate a large area of moderate reduction in tracer uptake in the mid and distal anterior wall and apex at peak exercise stress with normal myocardial perfusion at rest.

longed myocardial retention because of intracellular decoupling of Cu-62 and PTSM. The recommended dose is 4.44 to 7.4 MBq/kg (0.12–0.2 mCi/kg) as an intravenous bolus followed by dynamic imaging for 10 to 15 minutes. It has been proposed as an alternative myocardial perfusion agent using PET and is pending Food and Drug Administration approval [12,13].

Myocardial metabolic tracers

The human heart uses primarily free fatty acids (FFA) for oxidative metabolism under normal fasting conditions. In postprandial conditions after increased blood glucose and consequently insulin levels, however, it switches to glucose as the substrate for its oxidative metabolism and increases the intracellular glycogen pool. Moreover, ischemic and hypoxic myocardium predominantly uses glucose because of an increased anaerobic glycolytic rate. Under these conditions, the exogenous glucose use is independent of insulin. Accordingly, PET tracers have been developed to evaluate myocardial fatty acid and glucose metabolism to be able to image the ischemia-induced myocardial energy substrate use.

Fluorine-18–labeled fluorodeoxyglucose

Fluorine-18–labeled fluorodeoxyglucose ([^{18}F]-FDG) is the most established PET tracer. It has established itself as an important diagnostic agent in the work-up of several oncologic disorders and is making forays in the diagnosis of inflammatory diseases. In the myocardium, FDG is used to assess the glucose metabolism as a marker of myocardial metabolism. ^{18}F is cyclotron-produced and has a half-life of 110 minutes. Its positron energy is 0.63 MeV with a range of 0.3 mm. FDG is glucose analogue and is transported intracellularly by GLUT-1 and GLUT-4 transporters similar to glucose. After entering the myocytes, it undergoes phosphorylation to FDG-6-phosphate by the enzyme hexokinase. The enzyme isomerase has very poor affinity for FDG-6-phosphate and it does not proceed further along the glycolytic pathway, pentose shunt, or glycogenesis. The enzyme glucose-6-phosphatase also has relatively low affinity for FDG-6-phosphate and it undergoes negligible dephosphorylation. FDG remains metabolically trapped within the myocardium and provides a metabolic map of the myocardium [14–16].

The uptake of FDG in the myocardium has been shown to be heterogeneous and is dependent on myocardial substrate use. The hormonal milieu and the available substrate concentration considerably influence the myocardial substrate choice. High plasma FFA levels with low plasma glucose and insulin levels promote FFA as the primary myocardial substrate, whereas high plasma glucose and insulin levels promote glucose as the preferred myocardial substrate. FDG uptake in the myocardium is variable and frequently inadequate on PET studies performed under fasting conditions (as normal in oncologic PET studies). To overcome this variability, glucose loading is frequently practiced. The typical protocol consists of having the patient fast for 4 to 6 hours before the study and checking the blood sugar level. If the blood sugar level is less than 110 mg/dL and the patient is not a known diabetic, an oral glucose loading dose of 25 to 100 g is administered and 30 to 60 minutes later, 185 to 555 MBq (5–15 mCi) of FDG is administered intravenously. Images are typically obtained 60 to 90 minutes after the administration of FDG. If the patient is a diabetic or the blood sugar level is greater than 110 mg/dL, however, then oral glucose loading dose along with insulin supplementation is preferred to maintain a blood sugar level of 100 to 140 mg/dL at the time of FDG administration. There are alternative approaches to promote myocardial glucose uptake. Administration of intravenous glucose is useful in patients with altered gastrointestinal glucose absorption and in those who are unable to tolerate oral glucose. The hyperinsulinemic-euglycemic clamp technique provides controlled metabolic conditions for the study but is very cumbersome and difficult to implement. The drug Acipimox, a nicotinic acid derivative, indirectly promotes myocardial glucose uptake and has been successfully tried in Europe; however, it is not available in the United States [1].

Because the ischemic myocardium prefers glucose as its energy substrate, FDG may be used to image myocardial ischemia directly under stress conditions [17]. For imaging this exercise-induced ischemia, glucose loading is not necessary. FDG has also been evaluated to assess active atherosclerotic lesions by virtue of its ability to detect inflammatory lesions [18–22].

Carbon-11–labeled palmitate and acetate

Carbon-11 (^{11}C) is also a cyclotron-produced positron-emitter with a half-life of 20.4 minutes, positron energy of 0.96 MeV, and range of 0.4 mm. [^{11}C]-palmitate and [^{11}C]-acetate have been used as PET tracers to assess myocardial oxidative metabolism. [^{11}C]-palmitate was the introduced earlier than [^{11}C]-acetate; however, it has several metabolic pathways to enter after entering the cell, making the kinetics of [^{11}C]-palmitate very complicated. [^{11}C]-

acetate was later introduced as an alternative tracer to assess myocardial metabolism because it follows a straightforward metabolic course of entering the TCA cycle after getting converted to $[^{11}C]$-acetyl CoA within the myocytes. Although $[^{11}C]$-acetate can provide reliable assessment of myocardial metabolism, because of alterations in the myocardial substrate use, it could not provide an accurate representation of metabolism in the ischemic myocardium [14,16].

Other cardiac PET tracers

Several other cardiac PET tracers have been assessed for imaging various cardiac parameters. Radiopharmaceuticals, such as ^{18}F-labeled fluoromisonidazole (FMISO) and Cu-diacetyl-bis (N-4-methyl-thiosemicarbazone) or Cu-ATSM labeled with either ^{60}Cu, ^{62}Cu, or ^{64}Cu, have been used to assess myocardial hypoxia [23–27]. Several catecholamines or catecholamine-analogues have been radiolabeled with ^{18}F, ^{11}C, or bromine-76 (^{76}Br) to assess the cardiac sympathetic nervous system [28]. ^{11}C-labeled radiotracers have also been developed to assess the cardiac adrenoceptors and muscarinic receptors. These tracers are still in the investigational stage and have the potential to become clinically useful in the future.

Clinical applications of PET in cardiology

Management of patients with left ventricular dysfunction and coronary artery disease

Considerable advances have been made in understanding the natural progression of coronary artery disease (CAD) and aggressive treatment approaches along with various preventive measures have been established to decrease the morbidity and mortality from CAD. Despite this, ischemic heart disease poses a significant management dilemma to clinicians, especially in patients with severe left ventricular dysfunction and CAD. Clinical decisions regarding management range from cardiac transplantation to aggressive medical treatment to revascularization [14]. Cardiac transplantation suffers from the limited availability of donor hearts in addition to the associated periprocedure risks [14,15]. Despite the significant progress in medical therapy, long-term survival rates after revascularization remain superior to those of medical management mostly if myocardial ischemia is demonstrated [29–37]. Although the benefit of revascularization in patients with significant CAD and poor left ventricular function has been well documented in several studies, it has a signifi-

PET with Ammonia for perfusion

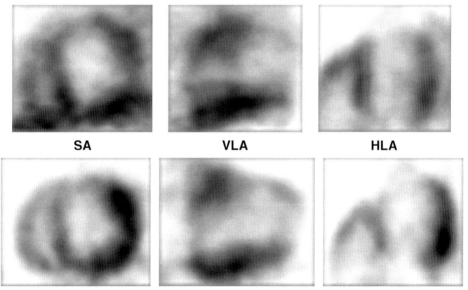

SA   VLA   HLA

PET with FDG for metabolism

Fig. 2. Myocardial viability assessment in an 82-year-old man with history of CAD and prior myocardial infarction. Images show selected short axis (SA), horizontal long axis (HLA), and vertical long axis (VLA) cardiac slices displaying decreased myocardial perfusion in the anterior wall, apex, and distal septum by PET using ^{13}N-ammonia with corresponding decreased FDG uptake in the same region indicating scar tissue.

cant periprocedure morbidity and mortality. Identification and selection of only those patients who will benefit maximally from revascularization has become crucial. The reversibility of contractile dysfunction contributes substantially to the improvement in the left ventricular function after revascularization. Identification of this viable myocardium (reversibly dysfunctional myocardium) and scar tissue (nonreversibly dysfunctional myocardium) is a critical component in the diagnostic work-up of these patients.

Myocardial viability can be assessed by several imaging modalities including stress echocardiography with low-dose dobutamine, ^{201}Tl rest-redistribution studies, SPECT with technetium-99m ([99m]T)-sestamibi, PET with myocardial perfusion and FDG [38], CT [39], and MR imaging [40]. PET with myocardial perfusion and [18F]-FDG can accurately assess myocardial viability and is regarded as the gold standard for assessing myocardial viability.

The cardiac applications of PET with myocardial perfusion and [18F]-FDG have been investigated considerably [14,15,41,42]. It has been used to assess a range of cardiovascular disorders including myocardial infarction [41,43], angina [41,44], cardiomyopathy [45], and CAD with left ventricular dysfunction [46]. Since the successful prediction of reversibility of wall motion abnormalities by Tillisch et al [47], PET has been used successfully by numerous investigators to assess myocardial viability in different clinical settings [48–56].

Diagnosis of myocardial viability

Ischemic insult to the myocardium may occur as a result of an acute occlusion of the coronary artery or because of more chronic hypoperfusion or repetitive ischemic processes. The myocardial response to the ischemic process depends on the severity and duration of ischemia and usually results in a dysfunctional myocardium if myocardial necrosis did not occur. The myocardium has several immediate and sustained mechanisms of adaptations to withstand acute or chronic ischemia. In patients with chronic CAD, these responses are in the form of hibernation, stunning, and ischemic preconditioning [16,57,58]. The myocardium in such patients may display an assortment of findings ranging from fully viable to partially viable to nonviable or scarred. The dysfunctional myocardium may represent necrosed and scarred myocardium that is nonviable, or stunned or hibernating but viable myocardium. Accurate identification of this viable myocardium in patients with decreased left ventricular function is crucial because

it has significant implications on therapy, functional recovery, remodeling, improvement in symptoms of congestive cardiac failure and quality of life, and long-term survival.

Identification of myocardial viability by PET

Assessment of regional blood flow alone is not adequate to determine the presence of viability in all cases of dysfunctional myocardium. Dysfunctional myocardial segments with a relatively normal blood flow most likely represent stunned myocardium, whereas those with significantly reduced blood flow are more likely to represent scarring. These extreme cases usually pose no significant assessment problems. A dysfunctional myocardium with an intermediate decline in blood flow, however, may represent either hibernating myocardium or necrosed subendocardial tissue mixed with relatively normal myocardium [15]. The assessment of myocardial viability requires the appraisal of myocardial blood flow in combination with evaluation of myocardial metabolism.

Myocardial metabolism is most commonly evaluated by assessing myocardial glucose uptake using [18F]-FDG and PET. During normal fasting conditions, FFAs are the preferred energy substrates for normal myocardium. Myocardial ischemia (either acute or chronic), however, alters the regional substrate use, resulting in increased myocardial glucose consumption in preference to FFA [59–68]. PET using [11C]-palmitate and [11C]-acetate can quantitatively assess myocardial oxidative metabolism [69,70], demonstrating decreased FFA use in ischemia; conversely, relatively increased myocardial glucose uptake can be shown with myocardial blood flow and [18F]-FDG [71,72]. The combination of these two physiologic parameters (myocardial blood flow and myocardial metabolism) has been extensively used to assess myocardial viability with PET. Three possible patterns have been described in the dysfunctional myocardium when myocardial blood flow is assessed in conjunction to myocardial glucose uptake: (1) normal myocardial blood flow and FDG activity; (2) decreased myocardial blood flow with normal or increased FDG activity (flow–metabolism mismatch); and (3) decreased myocardial blood flow and FDG activity [14,15]. Patterns 1 and 2 represent viable myocardial tissue, whereas pattern 3 represents necrosed or nonviable myocardium (Fig. 2). The flow-metabolism mismatch pattern (Fig. 3) is considered to be the hallmark of dysfunctional but viable myocardium with very important clinical implications.

Clinical implications of myocardial viability

Predicting functional recovery

Myocardial viability assessment can accurately predict the functional recovery in the form of improved global and regional left ventricular function after revascularization. Tillisch et al [47] found a positive predictive value and a negative predictive value of 85% and 92%, respectively. Several other investigators have demonstrated that PET can very accurately predict functional recovery by assessing myocardial viability before revascularization. Knuuti et al [73] reported a sensitivity of 85% and specificity of 84% to predict functional recovery with accuracy approaching 100% in patients with severely decreased flow, and Schoder et al [74] showed that the predictive accuracy of PET is maintained in patients with diabetes mellitus. Baer et al [75] reported 96% sensitivity and 69% specificity for the predictive value of [18F]-FDG–PET, and Bax et al [76] reported 87% sensitivity, 78% specificity, 72% positive predictive value and 90% negative predictive value with [18F]-FDG–SPECT. Factors that have an impact on the predictive accuracy of PET in investigations include timing to re-evaluate function after revascularization, revascularization technique and expertise, and patient selection. Additionally, the size of viable myocardial tissue before revascularization correlates well with the degree of functional recovery after revascularization. Pagano et al [77] found a linear correlation between the number of viable segments and the changes in left ventricular ejection fraction. Di Carli et al [78] reported a significantly higher functional improvement in patients with large mismatches (≥18%) on PET compared with those with minimal or no mismatch (<5%) on PET.

Predicting improvement in congestive heart failure symptoms, exercise capacity, and quality of life

Myocardial viability evaluation can also predict the degree of benefit in congestive heart failure symptoms after revascularization. The preoperative size of myocardial viability as determined by PET has a correlation to the magnitude of improvement in heart failure symptoms after coronary artery bypass grafting [78]. Marwick et al [79] reported a significantly higher improvement in the exercise capacity in patients with two or more viable regions on PET. Although there is significant improvement in the quality of life scores, it does not seem to correlate with the improvement in exercise capacity or extent of myocardial viability [80]. Assessing myocardial viability

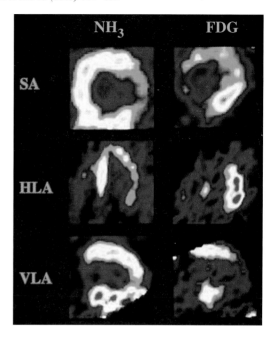

Fig. 3. Myocardial viability assessment in a 66-year-old man with history of prior coronary artery bypass grafting, presenting with recurrent angina and congestive heart failure. Recent cardiac catheterization had shown occlusion of the right coronary and left circumflex arterial grafts, patent left anterior descending artery graft, and anterolateral and apical akinesis with left ventricular ejection fraction of 30%. Images show selected short axis (SA), horizontal long axis (HLA), and vertical long axis (VLA) cardiac slices displaying decreased myocardial perfusion in the lateral wall by PET with 13N-ammonia and increased FDG uptake in the same region indicating myocardial viability. The left ventricular ejection fraction improved to 69% a month after repeat coronary artery bypass grafting.

with PET can help in predicting post-revascularization outcomes and provide significant information about the risk-benefit ratio for revascularization.

Predicting cardiac events, remodeling, and long-term survival

Patients with chronic ischemic heart disease with compromised left ventricular function are known to be prone for future cardiac events. Presence of viable myocardial tissue by PET seems to be risk factor for recurrent ischemic events and medical management of such patients does not minimize this risk. Eitzman et al [81] reported that patients with viable myocardium who do not undergo revascularization are more likely to have a cardiac event or death than those who did undergo revascularization. Based on their investigations to study the prognostic significance of viable myocardial tissue, Lee et al [82] concluded that the presence of viable myocardium and the lack of revascularization are independent predictors of ischemic events.

Left ventricular remodeling has an important bearing on the disease progression in heart failure patients and measures that halt or reverse ventricular remodeling favorably influence the natural history outcomes in such patients [83]. Senior et al [84] showed that revascularization had a significantly greater impact on reverse remodeling in patients with at least five myocardial viable segments. Although in this study myocardial viability was assessed by nitrate-enhanced ^{201}Tl- and nitrate-enhanced [^{99m}Tc]-sestamibi imaging, the results can easily be extrapolated to myocardial viability assessment by PET.

Di Carli et al [85] evaluated the long-term benefits of myocardial assessment before revascularization and found a significantly improved 4-year survival in patients with viable myocardium by PET receiving revascularization compared with those on medical therapy. In patients with minimal or no viable myocardium, revascularization improved survival and symptoms only in patients with severe angina. Several studies have confirmed that in chronic ischemic heart disease patients with left ventricular dysfunction, viable myocardium as determined by noninvasive imaging is independently associated with improved long-term survival after revascularization. Allman et al [86] pooled data from 24 viability studies using ^{201}Tl perfusion imaging, FDG PET metabolic imaging, or dobutamine echocardiography that reported patient survival after revascularization or medical therapy. This meta-analysis included 3088 patients and demonstrated a 79.6% reduction in annual mortality in patients with viable myocardium treated with revascularization compared with medical therapy (3.2% versus 16%, $P < .0001$). Patients without viability tended to have slightly higher mortality rates with revascularization, although the difference was not statistically significant. The failure to definitely identify significant myocardial viability should help the clinician to make the decision to treat these patients medically or by cardiac transplantation, if warranted.

Predicting perioperative complications and short-term survival

Presence of a viable myocardium before revascularization predicts a low perioperative morbidity and mortality. Haas et al [87] and Landoni et al [88] evaluated the effect of myocardial viability assessment before coronary artery bypass grafting surgery on predicting perioperative mortality and morbidity. Both studies confirmed that supplementation of PET viability data to the clinical and angiographic data in the decision-making process resulted in significantly less perioperative complications, less need for inotropic drugs, low early mortality, and promising short-term survival.

The adaptive responses in the ischemic myocardium do not last indefinitely and without restoration of blood flow, apoptosis and necrosis may ensue leading to irreversible myocardial damage. The hibernating myocytes are characterized by progressive loss of contractile proteins and replacement by perinuclear glycogen deposits, and changes in the extracellular matrix proteins with fibrosis. The process of myocardial hibernation has also been referred to as an incomplete adaptation to ischemia by Elsasser et al [89]. In the presence of sustained ischemia, there seems to be a transition from the adaptive mechanisms to apoptosis, but the cause of this transition remains unclear. This notion has further been strengthened by Beanlands et al [90], who examined the effect of prolonged waiting time in patients with left ventricular dysfunction directed to revascularization based on FDG-PET imaging. Patients who had delayed revascularization after the identification of viable myocardium by FDG-PET showed a significantly increased preoperative mortality and minimal functional improvement after successful but delayed revascularization. This suggests that the identification of viable myocardium in patients with chronic ischemic heart disease with decreased left ventricular function not only predicts good outcome after revascularization, but indicates a need for prompt revascularization in such patients, failure of which can lead to a suboptimal outcome and other more serious consequences including death.

Diagnosis of coronary artery disease

CAD is a complex syndrome resulting from decreased perfusion to the myocardium. It is highly prevalent in the United States with more than 650,000 deaths attributed to it per year. It is associated with significant morbidity and mortality evoking a huge burden in the form of health care costs. Coronary angiography is considered the gold standard for imaging coronary artery stenosis and myocardial perfusion imaging using gated SPECT has remained the primary investigation to assess inducible ischemia. PET has the ability to assess myocardial perfusion and is believed to provide superior data compared with SPECT.

Myocardial perfusion imaging

There are several PET agents that accurately assess myocardial perfusion. These agents can be used in place of the SPECT agents to assess myocardial perfusion imaging under resting and stress conditions (Fig. 1). It is also possible easily to gate these studies with the electrocardiogram to have gated PET data of myocardial perfusion. Moreover, because it is possible to obtain quantitative perfusion data, PET has the potential to assess endothelial dysfunction and coronary flow reserve as a measure of coronary stenosis [15]. PET is considerably more expensive than SPECT, however, and cost effectiveness of PET needs to be thoroughly evaluated, limiting the applicability of PET as a modality to image myocardial perfusion only in situations where the results of other established imaging modalities are indeterminate or inconclusive. This could be applicable to obese patients where SPECT techniques could have significant limitations because of attenuation artifacts.

Other cardiac applications of PET

The assessment of myocardial viability and the diagnosis of CAD disease have been the main focus in cardiac PET imaging. With rapid advances in PET instrumentation and the introduction of novel PET radiopharmaceuticals, however, hypoxia, atherosclerosis, and neuronal imaging may become valid indications for cardiac PET studies in the future.

Hypoxia imaging

The established radiotracers for imaging myocardial ischemia accumulate in the myocardium in proportion to the myocardial perfusion. Another approach to detect myocardial ischemia directly is to image the resultant myocardial hypoxia. Cu-ATSM has been evaluated as a possible hypoxia imaging agent using PET and has shown promising results in animal experiments [25–27]. ^{60}Cu, ^{62}Cu, and ^{64}Cu are cyclotron-produced positron-emitters and show positron decay similar to ^{18}F decay to provide excellent images [25]. Cu-ATSM seems to be a very good hypoxia imaging agent and has been shown to determine hypoxia accurately in various settings in animal experiments and is poised for human trials.

Another PET agent, ^{18}F-FMISO, has been evaluated as a tracer for myocardial hypoxia in animal studies [23,24]. Hypoxic cells metabolically trap FMISO preferentially as compared with cells with normal oxygen tension, and FMISO could potentially be useful to identify viable but hypoxic tissues. Because of its low cellular uptake and slightly longer clearance time from the normal tissue compared with Cu-ATSM, however, it requires imaging at a prolonged interval after administration of the agent [25].

Direct imaging of myocardial ischemia using FDG-PET is also feasible as reported by He et al [17]. In a study involving 26 patients, they found that ^{99m}Tc–sestamibi myocardial perfusion imaging during exercise combined with exercise ^{18}F-FDG–PET is superior to stress-rest myocardial perfusion imaging in identifying exercise-induced myocardial ischemia. Similar results have been reported earlier by Camici et al [91] using ^{82}Rb and FDG. They found increased FDG accumulation in exercise-induced perfusion defects. More extensive prospective studies are needed, however, to assess this finding.

Atherosclerosis imaging

Atherosclerosis is widely prevalent in the United States and the accurate imaging of vulnerable plaques that are considered to be responsible for most major acute coronary events would be an important breakthrough. Although various modalities like ultrasound, MR imaging, and CT scan can identify atheromas by assessing structural parameters including degree of calcification, degree of stenosis, intimal to media thickness ratio, and lipid content, these approaches fail to address the key element of active plaques: inflammation. Contrast-enhanced ultrasound using microbubbles targeted to inflammatory markers is in an investigational stage to assess inflammatory lesions in blood vessels. FDG-PET has been established for inflammatory imaging and has been suggested to image active atherosclerotic lesions by identifying the increased metabolic activity in these lesions. Several investigators have reported increased FDG uptake in atherosclerotic plaques in the aorta, carotids, and other major vessels [18–20]. Ogawa et al [21] investigated FDG accumulation in heritable hyperlipidemic rabbits and found a strong correlation with the number of macrophages in the atherosclerotic lesions. Future research must be directed in evaluating whether FDG accumulates specifically in these active vulnerable plaques with minimal accumulation in other atheromatous lesions to detect these vulnerable plaques reliably [22].

Cardiac neuronal imaging

Sympathetic and parasympathetic nerves innervating the human heart regulate various aspects of the cardiac function, and dysfunction of the cardiac nervous system is believed to play an important role in the pathophysiology of various cardiac diseases. Iodine-123 (^{123}I)-labeled metaiodobenzylguanidine (MIBG) has been previously used to assess the distribution and function of the cardiac sympathetic nervous system. MIBG imaging does not allow quantification of myocardial MIBG uptake and because the spatial resolution of PET is superior allowing better assessment of the regional myocardium, various PET radiotracers to image cardiac neuronal innervation have been developed. Several of them are in an investigational stage with animal experiments. These include ^{18}F-labeled 4- or 6-fluorometaraminol, 6-fluoronorepinephrine, para-fluorobensylguanidine, and [76]Br-labeled–meta-bromobenzylguanidine. Others, like ^{18}F-labeled 6-fluorodopamine and ^{11}C-labeled epinephrine, meta-hydroxyephedrine, and phenylephrine, have been tested successfully in humans and have shown promising results in detecting moderate to severe neuronal damage. There is still a need, however, to identify agents with optimal tracer kinetics for cardiac neuronal imaging. There are ongoing efforts focusing on imaging the cardiac sympathetic nervous system and it is hoped that one of the agents will find clinical use in the near future. The myocardium displays a low-density and focal distribution pattern for parasympathetic neurons, limiting the use of vesamicol-based agents (^{18}F-labeled fluoroethoxybenzovesamicol) for imaging the cardiac parasympathetic nervous system [28]. The past decade has also seen the development of several PET radiotracers to image the adrenergic and muscarinic receptors in the heart. These include ^{11}C-CGP 12,177 for β1 and β2 adrenoceptors [92], ^{11}C-GB67 for α1 adrenoceptors [93], and ^{11}C-MQNB for M1 and M2 muscarinic receptors [94,95].

The future

There is a need to standardize cardiac PET imaging. Specifically, protocols need to be established to maintain uniformity in metabolic conditions, administration of PET radiotracers, imaging parameters, and data interpretation. Another important consideration while reviewing cardiac PET studies is the heterogeneity of distribution of PET tracers (especially FDG-PET) in the myocardium. Metabolic tracers like FDG can show altered distribution depending on the fasting state of the patient, blood glucose and insulin levels, and regional variations in the metabolic milieu of the myocardium. Unlike

SPECT, data about normal variations in the distribution of most PET tracers are not yet available on a large scale. As the use of PET for noncardiac indications grows (especially for oncologic indications), it is hoped that more data will be generated about the normal variations in the PET tracer distribution.

PET offers several advantages over conventional nuclear medicine techniques and other imaging modalities used to assess the heart. It has better spatial and temporal resolution than SPECT and excellent contrast resolution. PET also provides quantitative data. As PET centers become ubiquitous, such issues as the cost-effectiveness of the cardiac applications of PET are hoped to be resolved. Cardiac PET has generated considerable interest and research is focusing on standardizing metabolic conditions and imaging parameters. With the introduction of novel PET radiopharmaceuticals and innovations in PET instrumentation, PET may cease to remain an investigative tool reserved for special circumstances and research purposes, and become a routine study to assess the human heart. With the entry of PET in the arena of noninvasive assessment of cardiac gene therapy [96,97], the future for PET in cardiac imaging seems bright.

References

[1] Bacharach SL, Bax JJ, Case J, et al. PET myocardial glucose metabolism and perfusion imaging. Part 1: Guidelines for data acquisition and patient preparation. J Nucl Cardiol 2003;10:543–56.

[2] Schwaiger M, Ziegler SI, Bengel FM. Assessment of myocardial blood flow with positron emission tomography. In: Shah PM, editor. Imaging in cardiovascular disease. Philadelphia: Lippincott Williams and Wilkins; 2000. p. 195–212.

[3] Beller GA, Bergmann SR. Myocardial perfusion imaging agents: SPECT and PET. J Nucl Cardiol 2004;11:71–86.

[4] Beanlands RS, Muzik O, Melon P, et al. Noninvasive quantification of regional myocardial flow reserve in patients with coronary atherosclerosis using nitrogen-13 ammonia positron emission tomography: determination of extent of altered vascular reactivity. J Am Coll Cardiol 1995;26:1465–75.

[5] Choi Y, Huang SC, Hawkins RA, et al. Quantification of myocardial blood flow using 13N-ammonia and PET: comparison of tracer models. J Nucl Med 1999; 40:1045–55.

[6] Choi Y, Huang SC, Hawkins RA, et al. A simplified method for quantification of myocardial blood flow using nitrogen-13-ammonia and dynamic PET. J Nucl Med 1993;34:488–97.

[7] Hutchins GD, Schwaiger M, Rosenspire KC, et al. Noninvasive quantification of regional blood flow in the human heart using N-13 ammonia and dynamic positron emission tomographic imaging. J Am Coll Cardiol 1990;15:1032–42.

[8] Krivokapich J, Smith GT, Huang SC, et al. 13N ammonia myocardial imaging at rest and with exercise in normal volunteers: quantification of absolute myocardial perfusion with dynamic positron emission tomography. Circulation 1989;80:1328–37.

[9] Huang SC, Schwaiger M, Carson RE, et al. Quantitative measurement of myocardial blood flow with oxygen-15 water and positron computed tomography: an assessment of potential and problems. J Nucl Med 1985;26:616–25.

[10] Herrero P, Markham J, Bergmann SR. Quantitation of myocardial blood flow with H2 15O and positron emission tomography: assessment and error analysis of a mathematical approach. J Comput Assist Tomogr 1989;13:862–73.

[11] Bergmann SR, Herrero P, Markham J, et al. Non-invasive quantitation of myocardial blood flow in human subjects with oxygen-15-labeled water and positron emission tomography. J Am Coll Cardiol 1989;14:639–52.

[12] Herrero P, Markham J, Weinheimer CJ, et al. Quantification of regional myocardial perfusion with generator-produced 62Cu-PTSM and positron emission tomography. Circulation 1993;87:173–83.

[13] Herrero P, Hartman JJ, Green MA, et al. Regional myocardial perfusion assessed with generator-produced copper-62-PTSM and PET. J Nucl Med 1996; 37:1294–300.

[14] Schelbert HR. 18F-Deoxyglucose and the assessment of myocardial viability. Semin Nucl Med 2002; 32:60–9.

[15] Keng FYJ. Clinical applications of positron emission tomography in cardiology: a review. Ann Acad Med Singapore 2004;33:175–82.

[16] Bengel FM, Schwaiger M. Assessment of myocardial viability by PET. In: Valk P, editor. Positron emission tomography: principles and clinical practice. London: Springer Verlag; 2003. p. 447–63.

[17] He ZX, Shi RF, Wu YJ, et al. Direct imaging of exercise-induced myocardial ischemia with fluorine-18-labeled deoxyglucose and Tc-99m-sestamibi in coronary artery disease. Circulation 2003;108:1208–13.

[18] Tatsumi M, Cohade C, Nakamoto Y, et al. Fluoro-deoxyglucose uptake in the aortic wall at PET/CT: possible finding for active atherosclerosis. Radiology 2003;229:831–7.

[19] Yun M, Jang S, Cucchiara A, et al. 18F FDG uptake in the large arteries: a correlation study with the atherogenic risk factors. Semin Nucl Med 2002;32:70–6.

[20] Rudd JH, Warburton EA, Fryer TD, et al. Imaging atherosclerotic plaque inflammation with [18F]-fluorodeoxyglucose positron emission tomography. Circulation 2002;105:2708–11.

[21] Ogawa M, Ishino S, Mukai T, et al. (18)F-FDG accumulation in atherosclerotic plaques: immunohistochemical and PET imaging study. J Nucl Med 2004; 45:1245–50.

[22] Strauss W, Dunphy M, Tokita N. Imaging the vulnerable plaque: a scintillating light at the end of the tunnel? J Nucl Med 2004;45:1106–7.

[23] Martin GV, Caldwell JH, Graham MM, et al. Noninvasive detection of hypoxic myocardium using fluorine-18-fluoromisonidazole and positron emission tomography. J Nucl Med 1992;33:2202–8.

[24] Shelton ME, Dence CS, Hwang DR, et al. In vivo delineation of myocardial hypoxia during coronary occlusion using fluorine-18 fluoromisonidazole and positron emission tomography: a potential approach for identification of jeopardized myocardium. J Am Coll Cardiol 1990;16:477–85.

[25] Lewis JS, Herrero P, Sharp TL, et al. Delineation of hypoxia in canine myocardium using PET and copper(II)-diacetyl-bis(N(4)-methylthiosemicarbazone). J Nucl Med 2002;43:1557–69.

[26] Fujibayashi Y, Taniuchi H, Yonekura Y, et al. Copper-62-ATSM: a new hypoxia imaging agent with high membrane permeability and low redox potential. J Nucl Med 1997;38:1155–60.

[27] Fujibayashi Y, Cutler CS, Anderson CJ, et al. Comparative studies of Cu-64-ATSM and C-11-acetate in an acute myocardial infarction model: ex vivo imaging of hypoxia in rats. Nucl Med Biol 1999;26:117–21.

[28] Langer O, Halldin C. PET and SPET tracers for mapping the cardiac nervous system. Eur J Nucl Med Mol Imaging 2002;29:416–34.

[29] Alderman EL, Fisher LD, Litwin P, et al. Results of coronary artery surgery in patients with poor left ventricular function (CASS). Circulation 1983;68:785–95.

[30] Emond M, Mock MB, Davis KB, et al. Long-term survival of medically treated patients in the Coronary Artery Surgery Study (CASS) Registry. Circulation 1994;90:2645–57.

[31] Passamani E, Davis KB, Gillespie MJ, et al. A randomized trial of coronary artery bypass surgery: survival of patients with a low ejection fraction. N Engl J Med 1985;312:1665–71.

[32] Alderman EL, Corley SD, Fisher LD, et al. Five-year angiographic follow-up of factors associated with progression of coronary artery disease in the Coronary Artery Surgery Study (CASS). CASS Participating Investigators and Staff. J Am Coll Cardiol 1993;22: 1141–54.

[33] Mickleborough LL, Maruyama H, Takagi Y, et al. Results of revascularization in patients with severe left ventricular dysfunction. Circulation 1995;92(9 Suppl): II73–9.

[34] Kaul T, Agnohotri A, Fields B, et al. Coronary artery bypass grafting in patients with an ejection fraction of twenty percent or less. J Thorac Cardiovasc Surg 1996; 111:1001–12.

[35] Miller D, Stinson E, Alderman E. Surgical treatment of ischemic cardiomyopathy: is it ever too late? Am J Surg 1981;141:688–93.

[36] Luciani G, Faggian T, Razzolini R, et al. Severe ischemic left ventricular failure: coronary operation or heart transplantation. Ann Thorac Surg 1993;557: 719–23.

[37] Ellis SG, Fisher L, Dushman-Ellis S, et al. Comparison of coronary angioplasty with medical treatment for single- and double-vessel coronary disease with left anterior descending coronary involvement: long-term outcome based on an Emory-CASS registry study. Am Heart J 1989;118:208–20.

[38] Bax JJ, Wijns W, Cornel JH, et al. Accuracy of currently available techniques for prediction of functional recovery after revascularization in patients with left ventricular dysfunction due to chronic coronary artery disease: comparison of pooled data. J Am Coll Cardiol 1997;30:1451–60.

[39] Lipton MJ, Bogaert J, Boxt LM, et al. Imaging of ischemic heart disease. Eur Radiol 2002;12:1061–80.

[40] Shan K, Constantine G, Sivananthan M, et al. Role of cardiac magnetic resonance imaging in the assessment of myocardial viability. Circulation 2004;109: 1328–34.

[41] Camici P, Araujo L, Spinks T, et al. Myocardial glucose utilization in ischaemic heart disease: preliminary results with F18-fluorodeoxyglucose and positron emission tomography. Eur Heart J 1986;7(Suppl C): 19–23.

[42] Schwaiger M, Hicks R. The clinical role of metabolic imaging of the heart by positron emission tomography. J Nucl Med 1991;32:565–78.

[43] Schwaiger M, Brunken R, Grover-McKay M, et al. Regional myocardial metabolism in patients with acute myocardial infarction assessed by positron emission tomography. J Am Col Cardiol 1986;8:800–8.

[44] Araujo LI, Camici P, Spinks TJ, et al. Abnormalities in myocardial metabolism in patients with unstable angina as assessed by positron emission tomography. Cardiovasc Drugs Ther 1988;2:41–6.

[45] Grover-McKay M, Schwaiger M, Krivokapich J, et al. Regional myocardial blood flow and metabolism at rest in mildly symptomatic patients with hypertrophic cardiomyopathy. J Am Coll Cardiol 1989;13: 317–24.

[46] Maddahi J, Schelbert H, Brunken R, et al. Role of thallium-201 and PET imaging in evaluation of myocardial viability and management of patients with coronary artery disease and left ventricular dysfunction. J Nucl Med 1994;35:707–15.

[47] Tillisch J, Brunken R, Marshall R, et al. Reversibility of cardiac wall-motion abnormalities predicted by positron tomography. N Engl J Med 1986;314:884–8.

[48] Gropler RJ, Geltman EM, Sampathkumaran K, et al. Comparison of carbon-11-acetate with fluorine-18-fluorodeoxyglucose for delineating viable myocardium by positron emission tomography. J Am Coll Cardiol 1993;22:1587–97.

[49] Lucignani G, Paolini G, Landoni C, et al. Presurgical identification of hibernating myocardium by combined use of technetium-99m hexakis 2-methoxyisobutylisonitrile single photon emission tomography and fluorine-18 fluoro-2-deoxy-D-glucose positron emission tomography in patients with coronary artery disease. Eur J Nucl Med 1992;19:874–81.

[50] Tamaki N, Ohtani H, Yamashita K, et al. Metabolic activity in the areas of new fill-in after thallium-201 reinjection: comparison with positron emission tomography using fluorine-18-deoxyglucose. J Nucl Med 1991;32:673–8.

[51] Marwick TH, MacIntyre WJ, Lafont A, et al. Metabolic responses of hibernating and infarcted myocardium to revascularization: a follow-up study of regional perfusion, function, and metabolism. Circulation 1992;85:1347–53.

[52] Tamaki N, Yonekura Y, Yamashita K, et al. Prediction of reversible ischemia after coronary artery bypass grafting by positron emission tomography. J Cardiol 1991;21:193–201.

[53] Tamaki N, Yonekura Y, Yamashita K, et al. Relation of change in wall motion and glucose metabolism after coronary artery bypass grafting: assessment with positron emission tomography. Jap Circulation J 1991;55: 923–9.

[54] Tamaki N, Yonekura Y, Yamashita K, et al. Positron emission tomography using fluorine-18 deoxyglucose in evaluation of coronary artery bypass grafting. Am J Cardiol 1989;64:860–5.

[55] Tamaki N, Yonekura Y, Yamashita K, et al. Value of rest-stress myocardial positron tomography using nitrogen-13 ammonia for the preoperative prediction of reversible asynergy. J Nucl Med 1989;30:1302–10.

[56] vom Dahl J, Eitzman DT, al-Aouar ZR, et al. Relation of regional function, perfusion, and metabolism in patients with advanced coronary artery disease undergoing surgical revascularization. Circulation 1994;90: 2356–66.

[57] Kloner R, Bolli R, Marban E, et al. Medical and cellular implications of stunning, hibernation and preconditioning: an NHLBI Workshop. Circulation 1998; 97:1848–67.

[58] Wijns W, Vatner SF, Camici PG. Hibernating myocardium. N Engl J Med 1998;339:173–81.

[59] Taegtmeyer H. Myocardial metabolism. In: Phelps M, Mazziotta J, Schelbert H, editors. Positron emission tomography and autoradiography: principles and applications for the brain and heart. New York: Raven Press; 1986. p. 149–95.

[60] Liedtke AJ. Alterations of carbohydrate and lipid metabolism in the acutely ischemic heart. Prog Cardiovasc Dis 1981;23:321–6.

[61] Liedtke AJ. The origins of myocardial substrate utilization from an evolutionary perspective: the enduring role of glucose in energy metabolism. J Mol Cell Cardiol 1997;29:1073–86.

[62] Liedtke AJ, Renstrom B, Hacker TA, et al. Effects of moderate repetitive ischemia on myocardial substrate utilization. Am J Physiol 1995;269(1 Pt 2):H246–53.

[63] Liedtke AJ, Renstrom B, Nellis SH, et al. Mechanical and metabolic functions in pig hearts after 4 days of

chronic coronary stenosis. J Am Coll Cardiol 1995;26:
815–25.

[64] Marwick TH, MacIntyre WJ, Lafont A, et al.
Metabolic responses of hibernating and infarcted
myocardium to revascularization: a follow-up study
of regional perfusion, function, and metabolism.
Circulation 1992;85:1347–53.

[65] Vanoverschelde JL, Wijns W, Depre C, et al. Mechanisms of chronic regional postischemic dysfunction
in humans: new insights from the study of noninfarcted
collateral-dependent myocardium. Circulation 1993;
87:1513–23.

[66] Schelbert HR, Henze E, Phelps ME, et al. Assessment
of regional myocardial ischemia by positron-emission
computed tomography. Am Heart J 1982;103(4 Pt 2):
588–97.

[67] Schwaiger M, Fishbein MC, Block M, et al. Metabolic
and ultrastructural abnormalities during ischemia in
canine myocardium: noninvasive assessment by positron emission tomography. J Mol Cell Cardiol 1987;
19:259–69.

[68] Kalff V, Schwaiger M, Nguyen N, et al. The relationship between myocardial blood flow and glucose
uptake in ischemic canine myocardium determined
with fluorine-18-deoxyglucose. J Nucl Med 1992;33:
1346–53.

[69] Bergmann SR, Weinheimer CJ, Markham J, et al.
Quantitation of myocardial fatty acid metabolism using
PET. J Nucl Med 1996;37:1723–30.

[70] Brown MA, Myears DW, Bergmann SR. Validity of
estimates of myocardial oxidative metabolism with
carbon-11 acetate and positron emission tomography
despite altered patterns of substrate utilization. J Nucl
Med 1989;30:187–93.

[71] Hicks RJ, Herman WH, Wolfe E, et al. Regional
variation in oxidative and glucose metabolism in the
normal heart: comparison of PET-derived C-11 acetate
and FDG kinetics. J Nucl Med 1990;31:774.

[72] Hicks RJ, Herman WH, Kalff V, et al. Quantitative
evaluation of regional substrate metabolism in the
human heart by positron emission tomography. J Am
Coll Cardiol 1991;18:101–11.

[73] Knuuti MJ, Saraste M, Nuutila P, et al. Myocardial
viability: fluorine-18-deoxyglucose positron emission
tomography in prediction of wall motion recovery
after revascularization. Am Heart J 1994;127(4 Pt 1):
785–96.

[74] Schoder H, Campisi R, Ohtake T, et al. Blood flow-
metabolism imaging with positron emission tomography in patients with diabetes mellitus for the assessment of reversible left ventricular contractile
dysfunction. J Am Coll Cardiol 1999;33:1328–37.

[75] Baer FM, Voth E, Deutsch HJ, et al. Predictive value of
low dose dobutamine transesophageal echocardiography and fluorine-18 fluorodeoxyglucose positron
emission tomography for recovery of regional left ventricular function after successful revascularization.
J Am Coll Cardiol 1996;28:60–9.

[76] Bax JJ, Cornel JH, Visser FC, et al. F18-fluorodeoxy-

glucose single-photon emission computed tomography
predicts functional outcome of dyssynergic myocardium after surgical revascularization. J Nucl Cardiol
1997;4:302–8.

[77] Pagano D, Townend JN, Littler WA, et al. Coronary
artery bypass surgery as treatment for ischemic heart
failure: the predictive value of viability assessment
with quantitative positron emission tomography for
symptomatic and functional outcome. J Thorac Cardiovasc Surg 1998;115:791–9.

[78] Di Carli MF, Asgarzadie F, Schelbert HR, et al.
Quantitative relation between myocardial viability
and improvement in heart failure symptoms after revascularization in patients with ischemic cardiomyopathy. Circulation 1995;92:3436–44.

[79] Marwick TH, Nemec JJ, Lafont A, et al. Prediction by
postexercise fluoro-18 deoxyglucose positron emission
tomography of improvement in exercise capacity after
revascularization. Am J Cardiol 1992;69:854–9.

[80] Marwick TH, Zuchowski C, Lauer MS, et al. Functional status and quality of life in patients with heart
failure undergoing coronary bypass surgery after
assessment of myocardial viability. J Am Coll Cardiol
1999;33:750–8.

[81] Eitzman D, al-Aouar Z, Kanter HL, et al. Clinical
outcome of patients with advanced coronary artery
disease after viability studies with positron emission
tomography. J Am Coll Cardiol 1992;20:559–65.

[82] Lee KS, Marwick TH, Cook SA, et al. Prognosis of
patients with left ventricular dysfunction, with and
without viable myocardium after myocardial infarction: relative efficacy of medical therapy and revascularization. Circulation 1994;90:2687–94.

[83] Udelson JE, Konstam MA. Relation between left
ventricular remodeling and clinical outcomes in heart
failure patients with left ventricular systolic dysfunction. J Card Fail 2002;8(6 Suppl):S465–71.

[84] Senior R, Kaul S, Raval U, et al. Impact of
revascularization and myocardial viability determined
by nitrate-enhanced Tc-99m sestamibi and Tl-201
imaging on mortality and functional outcome in
ischemic cardiomyopathy. J Nucl Cardiol 2002;9:
454–62.

[85] Di Carli MF, Maddahi J, Rokhsar S, et al. Long-term
survival of patients with coronary artery disease and
left ventricular dysfunction: implications for the role of
myocardial viability assessment in management decisions. J Thorac Cardiovasc Surg 1998;116:997–1004.

[86] Allman KC, Shaw LJ, Hachamovitch R, et al.
Myocardial viability testing and impact of revascularization on prognosis in patients with coronary artery
disease and left ventricular dysfunction: a meta-
analysis. J Am Coll Cardiol 2002;39:1151–8.

[87] Haas F, Haehnel CJ, Picker W, et al. Preoperative
positron emission tomographic viability assessment
and perioperative and postoperative risk in patients
with advanced ischemic heart disease. J Am Coll
Cardiol 1997;30:1693–700.

[88] Landoni C, Lucignani G, Paolini G, et al. Assessment

of CABG-related risk in patients with CAD and LVD: contribution of PET with [18F]FDG to the assessment of myocardial viability. J Cardiovasc Surg 1999;40: 363–72.

[89] Elsasser A, Schlepper M, Klovekorn WP, et al. Hibernating myocardium: an incomplete adaptation to ischemia. Circulation 1997;96:2920–31.

[90] Beanlands RS, Hendry PJ, Masters RG, et al. Delay in revascularization is associated with increased mortality rate in patients with severe left ventricular dysfunction and viable myocardium on fluorine 18-fluorodeoxy-glucose positron emission tomography imaging. Circulation 1998;98(19 Suppl):II51–6.

[91] Camici P, Araujo LI, Spinks T, et al. Increased uptake of 18F-fluorodeoxyglucose in postischemic myocardium of patients with exercise-induced angina. Circulation 1986;74:81–8.

[92] Delforge J, Syrota A, Lancon JP, et al. Cardiac beta-adrenergic receptor density measured in vivo using PET, CGP 12177, and a new graphical method. J Nucl Med 1991;32:739–48.

[93] Law MP, Osman S, Pike VW, et al. Evaluation of [11C]GB67, a novel radioligand for imaging myocardial alpha 1-adrenoceptors with positron emission tomography. Eur J Nucl Med 2000;27:7–17.

[94] Delforge J, Le Guludec D, Syrota A, et al. Quantification of myocardial muscarinic receptors with PET in humans. J Nucl Med 1993;34:981–91.

[95] Delforge J, Janier M, Syrota A, et al. Noninvasive quantification of muscarinic receptors in vivo with positron emission tomography in the dog heart. Circulation 1990;82:1494–504.

[96] Wu JC, Inubushi M, Sundaresan G, et al. Positron emission tomography imaging of cardiac reporter gene expression in living rats. Circulation 2002;106:180–3.

[97] Inubushi M, Wu JC, Gambhir SS, et al. Positron-emission tomography reporter gene expression imaging in rat myocardium. Circulation 2003;107:326–32.

RADIOLOGIC
CLINICS
of North America

Radiol Clin N Am 43 (2005) 121 – 134

Applications of fluorodeoxyglucose-PET imaging in the detection of infection and inflammation and other benign disorders

Hongming Zhuang, MD, PhD, Jian Q. Yu, MD, Abass Alavi, MD*

Division of Nuclear Medicine, Department of Radiology, Hospital of the University of Pennsylvania, 110 Donner Building, 3400 Spruce Street, Philadelphia, PA 19104, USA

Fluorodeoxyglucose-PET (FDG-PET) has evolved into one of the major imaging modalities commonly used in the management of a variety of malignancies [1,2]. This application stems from proved phenomenon of increased glucose metabolism in malignant cells [3]. Increased glucose metabolism, however, is not specific for tumor cells and in particular inflammatory cells using glucose as a main source of energy. Inflammatory cells usually demonstrate relatively low glucose uptake in the resting state, but increase significantly following in vivo or in vitro stimulation [4,5]. Inflammatory and infectious processes are frequently noted to have increased glucose metabolism and as a result cause false-positive interpretation of FDG-PET images when they are acquired for the evaluation of patients with various malignancies [6]. In fact, FDG uptake by the inflammatory cells is partly responsible for the overall increased FDG uptake by the malignant lesions. Kubota et al [7] have demonstrated that reactive inflammatory macrophages and leukocytes around the tumor are noted to have higher FDG uptake than the viable malignant cells in the same tissue sample. Animal experiments also have demonstrated that tumors in athymic nude mice that lack T lymphocytes are noted to have significantly less FDG uptake than that in the normal mice [8]. Initiating steroid hormone treatment, which is known to induce T cell apoptosis, has no effect on the tumor uptake in the athymic immunodeficient

mice, whereas it significantly reduces the tumor uptake in the immunocompetent mice [8,9]. These data suggest that the high tumor uptake of FDG observed in the immunologically intact subjects partially represents increased glucose metabolism in the infiltrating inflammatory cells within the tumor tissue, including T lymphocytes. Animal experiments also indicate that FDG uptake is higher in the infection site than that of any other radiotracers tested, including gallium, radiolabeled serum albumin, thymidine, and amino acid S-methionine [10].

Numerous reports have demonstrated increased FDG uptake at the sites of infection and inflammation. FDG is applicable to almost any type of infection or inflammation or any anatomic location, including the following: abscesses [11 – 17], pneumonia [18 – 20], tuberculosis [21 – 25], *Mycobacterium avium-intracellulare* infection [26 – 28], cryptococcosis [29], mastitis [30], enterocolitis [31 – 33], infectious mononucleosis [34], parasitic disease [35], *Clostridium perfringens* infection [36], osteomyelitis [37 – 42], infection or loosening following arthroplasty [43 – 45], fever of unknown origin (FUO) [46 – 48], thrombosis [49 – 51], amyloidosis [52], sarcoidosis [53,54], asthma [55], bronchitis [56], encephalitis [57], costochondritis [58], radiation pneumonitis [59], esophagitis [60,61], pancreatitis [62], thyroiditis [63 – 65], sinusitis [66], myositis [67], mediastinitis [68], gastritis [69], lobular panniculitis [70], dental cavity [71], and inflammation caused by foreign body [72 – 74]. Despite all of these findings, however, FDG-PET has not been fully accepted as an effective way to evaluate infection and inflammation. This

---

* Corresponding author.
E-mail address: abass.alavi@uphs.upenn.edu (A. Alavi).

article discusses the potentials of FDG-PET in this clinical setting.

Potential advantage of PET over conventional nuclear medicine modalities in the evaluation of infection and inflammation

Many imaging modalities are used for the management of patients with suspected infection and inflammation, including diagnosis, determining the extent, monitoring response to therapy, and detection of recurrence. Nuclear medicine modalities differ from anatomic imaging procedures, such as ultrasound, CT, and MR imaging, with regard to the type of formation that they can provide in such settings. Although radiologic techniques provide excellent structural spatial resolution, nuclear medicine procedures can assess the degree of disease activity based on physiologic and metabolic changes caused by the underlying pathologic states. Gallium 67 scintigraphy can detect infection and inflammation. Labeled autologous leukocyte scan has proved its value in the evaluation of a variety of infectious and inflammatory processes, especially in inflammatory bowel disease [75–77], abscess [78], arthroplasty-associated infection [79], and FUO [80]. Three-phase bone scan is commonly performed when osteomyelitis is suspected in the bony structure either in axial or in the appendicular skeleton. Some new techniques using radiolabeled antibodies [81,82], peptides [83], liposomes [84], and avidin-mediated compounds [85] are being investigated and seem to have promise for infection and inflammation imaging.

Almost all of these imaging methods have certain limitations, however, which may influence their routine use in the day-to-day procedure. Gallium 67 has unfavorable physical characteristics for gamma camera imaging and produces suboptimal images. In addition, gallium image is usually associated with significant bowel excretion, which renders it of a limited value in assessing abdominal inflammatory disorders. Radiolabeled white cell imaging to detect infection and inflammation is complex, time-consuming, and costly when it is combined with bone marrow and bone scintigraphy for a definitive answer in examining orthopedic complication.

In general, these techniques require waiting for an extended period of time before interpretable results can be obtained. This is a major deficiency and prevents timely use of appropriate therapeutic interventions.

FDG-PET imaging has several advantages over other conventional imaging modalities. PET generates tomographic scans with excellent spatial resolution, which can be interpreted with high levels of confidence in any anatomic site in the body. In addition, imaging is completed within 2 hours of the administration of the compounds. This substantially reduces the degree of inconvenience to the patient and allows generating results critical for timely management of these patients. Furthermore, PET is likely to produce highly accurate findings compared with other imaging modalities in many clinical settings, discussed in detail next.

HIV and AIDS

HIV–AIDS patients are prone to acquiring opportunistic infections and developing certain malignancies during the course of their disease. FDG-PET can be used effectively in the detection and differentiation of opportunistic infections and malignancies in patients with AIDS. In a study that included 57 patients, FDG-PET successfully localized sites of either infection or malignant transformation [86]. In this study, the overall sensitivity and specificity of FDG-PET imaging was 92% and 94%, respectively [86]. Recent reports indicate that FDG-PET can detect activated lymph nodes in asymptomatic HIV-positive patients and the metabolic activity in the involved nodes correlates well with the viral load [87]. It is also noted that there is a distinct pattern of lymphoid tissue FDG activity in the head and neck region during the acute stage of the disease, generalized peripheral lymph node activity at mid-stages, and involvement of the abdominal lymph nodes during late phase of the disease. Unexpectedly, HIV-1 progression was evident to follow a distinct anatomic sequence [87] similar to that noted in Hodgkin's disease and further suggests that lymphoid tissues are connected by a well-delineated connecting system.

FDG-PET can play an important role in the evaluation of the central nervous system of patients with AIDS. Approximately 50% of patients with AIDS have serious neurologic complications. Toxoplasmosis and central nervous system lymphomas have been noted to have high incidence in patients with AIDS. In these settings, it is difficult to distinguish between these two pathologies using conventional imaging modalities, such as CT or MR imaging, where both appear as ring-enhancing lesions. The therapy for these two pathologies and the prognoses are very different, and correct diagnosis is critical for the optimal management of these complications. Many reports have demonstrated that FDG-PET can successfully distinguish central nervous lymphoma from toxoplasmosis based on the degree of metabolic activity of these two distinct entities. Central nervous lymphomas show intense FDG activity, whereas the lesions' related toxoplasmosis appears with a mild degree of FDG uptake [86,88–90].

Orthopedic infections

Chronic osteomyelitis is a difficult infection to treat and is characterized by the progressive inflammatory destruction and new apposition of the surrounding bone. Diagnosis or exclusion of chronic osteomyelitis is frequently difficult with current noninvasive techniques, especially when the bone architecture has been compromised by previous surgery or trauma. Local pain combined with increased erythrocyte sedimentation rate, presence of elevated C-reactive protein levels, and other laboratory data can suggest acute osteomyelitis. In the case of chronic osteomyelitis, however, no laboratory tests are accurate enough and imaging studies are frequently required to help establish the accurate diagnosis. Plain radiographic studies of bone are inexpensive and are often the first imaging study requested in the work-up of osteomyelitis. Radiographic changes often occur relatively late, however, and are quite nonspecific because of the distorted anatomy and remodeling process in the evaluation for chronic osteomyelitis. In patients with prior trauma to the bones, radiologic signs suggestive of osteomyelitis in this setting on average appear 4.3 months after the assumed time of infection [91]. It is well established that CT and MR imaging provide excellent anatomic detail. CT can detect cortical destruction and periosteal new bone formation even when plain radiographs are normal. CT can accurately depict osseous changes, such as sequestration, intraosseous fistula tracts, and intramedullary gas collection. However, confirmation of active infection by CT is limited [92]. MR imaging has been used with excellent results in diagnosing osteomyelitis in several anatomic locations in the body [93]. Furthermore, its high spatial resolution provides the clinician with anatomic detail that can aid in planning surgery and other interventions. Criteria used to diagnose osteomyelitis by MR imaging include decreased signal intensity on T1-weighted images, increased intensity on T2-weighted or STIR scans, and marrow enhancement after the administration of gadolinium [94]. MR imaging in particular is quite useful in the evaluation of patients who have not had any surgical intervention [95]. There are a number of instances where MR imaging is less reliable, however, such as in posttraumatic and

postoperative states [96–98]. Three-phase bone scintigraphy has excellent sensitivity in the detection of osteomyelitis. Many other etiologies can produce similar findings on bone scan, however, and result in suboptimal specificity for the technique. In addition, positive bone scan can last for a considerably long period of time even after successful treatment [99], which further reduces its value in assessing response to the treatment and its overall specificity. Labeled leukocyte imaging is a reasonably accurate method when uncomplicated osteomyelitis is suspected in the peripheral skeleton [100]. It is well known, however, that leukocyte scintigraphy has only a limited sensitivity in the evaluation of central skeletal system where these cells are heavily taken up by the surrounding red marrow. In addition, previous fracture sites may result in false-positive results with this technique [101,102], but others dispute this observation.

Multiple reports indicate that FDG-PET is quite accurate in excluding or diagnosing chronic osteomyelitis. In contrast to bone scintigraphy, where degenerative changes [103] or history of fracture for a few months preceding the examination [104] are likely to cause false-positive results, FDG-PET imaging appears relatively negative in these clinical settings. The earliest evidence came from the study by Guhlmann et al [38]. They reported that the overall sensitivity and specificity of FDG-PET imaging were 100% and 92%, respectively, in assessing patients for chronic osteomyelitis. The same group also

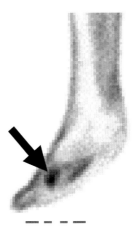

Fig. 1. A 70-year-old woman with diabetes. The patient had an Achilles tendon graft of the right ankle approximately 4 months ago with a nonhealing wound and wound infection. PET images increased FDG activity is also visualized in the soft tissues of the posterior aspect of the right lower leg and right foot and no bones were involved. The clinical follow-up excluded osteomyelitis.

noted that in the axial skeleton with high concentration of red marrow, FDG-PET is superior to labeled antibody imaging in the diagnosis of chronic osteomyelitis, where frequently the latter technique reveals a nonspecific photopenic defect and cannot differentiate between active and inactive tissues [37]. Several groups have reported that FDG-PET has a sensitivity of 100% in detecting bone infection (Fig. 1) [39,105,106]. Because of its high sensitivity, a negative PET scan essentially excludes osteomyelitis (Fig. 2). Unlike CT and MR imaging, FDG-PET is not affected by metal implants frequently inserted for fixing fracture sites [40]. FDG-PET may correctly identify chronic osteomyelitis when both MR imaging and labeled antibody imaging seem inconclusive [107]. In a study of 60 patients with suspected bone infection, De Winter et al [108] demonstrated that for the entire group the sensitivity, specificity, and accuracy of FDG-PET were 100%, 88%, and 93%, respectively. For the subgroup of patients with a suspected infection of the central skeleton, the rates were 100%, 90%, and 94%; for the subgroup of patients with a suspected infection of the peripheral skeleton the rates were 100%, 86%, and 93%. Unlike bone scintigraphy, fractures do not cause prolonged FDG accumulation in the fracture sites [104,109,110].

Increased FDG uptake at any sites with old fractures should raise the possibility of osteomyelitis or other pathology (Fig. 3). It has been proposed that FDG-PET as a single imaging modality is more accurate than the combination of bone scan and leukocyte scintigraphy in chronic bone infections [111].

Infectious spondylitis is a disease that results in osteomyelitis of two adjacent vertebrae, which spreads to intervening disk with destruction of the end plates. The diagnosis of this potentially debilitating disorder is difficult using conventional imaging techniques. Radiolabeled leukocyte scintigraphy is of limited value in this clinical setting because of its low sensitivity and specificity in detecting osteomyelitis of the vertebral bodies. Currently, a combination of bone scan, gallium 67 imaging, and MR imaging is used to evaluate this complex disorder. Gratz et al [112] assessed the role of FDG-PET in patients with suspected spondylitis. They demonstrated that FDG-PET was superior to MR imaging, gallium 67 citrate, and technetium 99m methylene diphosphonate, especially in patients with low-grade spondylitis (when compared with MR imaging), adjacent soft tissue infections (when compared with gallium 67 citrate), and advanced bone degeneration (when compared with technetium 99m methylene diphosphonate).

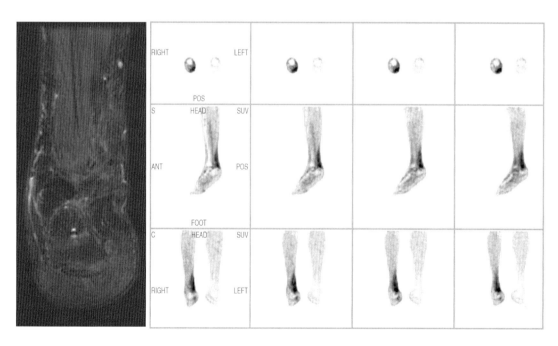

Fig. 2. The patient has a history peripheral vascular disease and cellulitis of left great toe. A three-phase bone scan rendered ambiguous diagnosis for osteomyelitis. A PET scan was performed for further evaluation. The images show intensely increased FDG activity in the left first phalanx, which is consistent with osteomyelitis. Subsequent surgery confirmed the diagnosis of osteomyelitis.

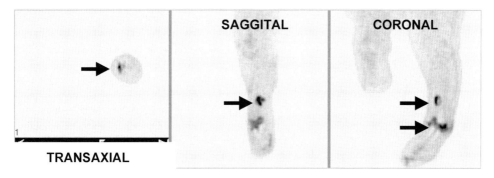

Fig. 3. A 58-year-old woman with history of diabetes, right below-knee amputation, and left lower extremity complex fracture. FDG-PET was acquired to evaluate possible osteomyelitis in the left lower leg. The PET images demonstrated intense FDG uptake at fracture site, indicating osteomyelitis. Osteomyelitis was confirmed by surgery.

Stumpe et al [103] performed FDG-PET prospectively in 30 consecutive patients with substantial end plate abnormalities of the lumbar spine, which were interpreted by MR imaging as being inconclusive for differentiating degenerative disease from an infectious process. They were able to demonstrate that PET did not show FDG uptake in the intervertebral spaces of patients with degenerative disease, whereas infected sites appeared positive on the scan. The sensitivity and specificity for MR imaging in detecting disk space infection were 50% and 96%, and for FDG-PET were 100% and 100%, respectively [103].

Considerable success of prosthetic joint replacement has greatly improved the quality of life for many individuals with disabling hip and knee joints. A fraction of patients experience persistent pain at the site of arthroplasty, however, which in most incidences is caused by mechanical loosening and infrequently by periprosthetic infection [113,114]. Distinguishing these two entities is important in the optimal management of patients with painful prostheses. Existing preoperative tests for the diagnosis of periprosthetic infection are not satisfactory, however, and the cause of a painful prosthesis often is unclear before a surgical procedure is planned for revision of prosthesis. Labeled leukocyte scintigraphy, when combined with sulfur colloid bone marrow imaging, provides a reasonable sensitivity and specificity in this clinical setting [79,115]. Because of the difficulties that are associated this technique, optimal results are not achievable in some centers [116].

Recently, favorable results have been demonstrated with FDG-PET imaging in the evaluation of possible periprosthetic infection of the lower-limb arthroplasty. PET has several theoretical advantages over other imaging modalities for this purpose. There is only a minimal degree of FDG accumulation in the remaining red bone marrow in these mostly elderly patients [105]. Although metal implants may cause artifacts on conventional nuclear medicine imaging and on CT and MR imaging, the accuracy of PET is not adversely affected by these devices [40,117]. Furthermore, FDG-PET images have superior spatial resolution compared with conventional nuclear medicine scans. Despite these advantages, the role of the FDG-PET technique in this clinical setting is unsettled at this time. Love et al [118] have reported an investigation involving 31 prostheses from 26 patients that showed sensitivity, specificity, and accuracy of FDG-PET of 100%, 55%, and 71%, respectively. The positive predictive value was 55% and the negative predictive value 100% [118]. The authors concluded that FDG-PET is very sensitive in detecting periprosthetic infection; however, it lacks optimal specificity for routine clinical application [118]. In contrast, in a study involving 17 prostheses, De Winter et al [111] demonstrated that FDG-PET had sensitivity of 100%, specificity of 89%, and an accuracy of 94%. Of the 53 hip prostheses studied in the authors' center, FDG-PET had an accuracy of 96.2%, sensitivity of 91.7%, and specificity of 97.6%. In the 36 knee prostheses examined with this technique, FDG-PET revealed an accuracy of 81%, a sensitivity of 92%, and a specificity of 75% [119]. It seems that FDG-PET is less successful in the evaluation of knee prostheses than in assessing the hip prostheses [43]. Vanquickenborne et al [120] compared the accuracy of a combined bone scan and technetium 99m–labeled leukocyte scintigraphy and FDG-PET in 24 subjects with hip prostheses. They reported that FDG-PET had a sensitivity of 88% and a specificity of 78% in detecting infected hip prostheses. In contrast, the combined bone scan and planar leukocyte scintigraphy had a sensitivity of

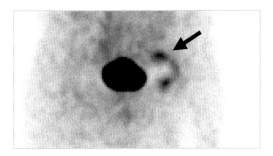

Fig. 4. A 73-year-old patient referred for oncology study, with asymptomatic hip prosthesis. Whole-body PET images demonstrate increased uptake in the head and neck region of the left hip prosthesis (*arrow*). This kind of uptake is typical for nonspecific uptake and cannot be interpreted as infection.

75% and a specificity of 78%, which further suggests superiority of FDG-PET imaging in this setting. In the same study, however, when single-photon emission CT (SPECT) images of labeled leukocytes were reconstructed, the sensitivity and specificity of this technique increased to 88% and 100%, respectively, which is comparable with PET results.

It is important to note that the diagnostic criteria for interpreting FDG-PET images in the assessment of painful hip prostheses have not been fully refined and some controversies remain with regard to the details that should be considered for optimal result. It is known that following hip arthroplasty, there is persistent nonspecific FDG activity in the neck and head region of prostheses in asymptomatic patients, which may last as long as 24 years (Fig. 4) [121]. Lack of awareness of this nonspecific uptake can

result in false-positive interpretations of these scans. It is becoming clear that the location of the abnormal FDG uptake is an important element in the diagnosis of infected prosthesis (Fig. 5) [122]. Using a dedicated PET camera, Manthey et al [123] has described a set of criteria for the diagnosis of loosening or infection of hip prosthesis. They propose that intense FDG uptake in the bone prostheses interface should be considered as positive for infection, mild uptake as suspect for loosening, and uptake only in the soft tissue as evidence of synovitis [123]. Recently, Cremerius et al [45] have reported that both loosening and infection can result in enhanced uptake in the proximal or middle segment of the lateral femoral interface and the proximal segment of the medial femoral interface. The degree of FDG uptake in infection is significantly higher, however, than in loosening. Based on these criteria, FDG-PET has an accuracy of 89% in the diagnosis of hip arthroplasty-related infection. Further investigation is warranted to establish the potential role of FDG-PET in this very difficult complication of a very common orthopedic procedure.

Fever of unknown origin

FUO is defined as a temperature of 101°F (38.3°C) or higher for 3 weeks or longer, the cause of which is not determined after 1 week of intensive in-hospital investigation [124]. More than 200 different pathologic entities can result in FUO [125]. Radionuclide agents that are currently available for investigating FUO are labeled leukocytes [80], gallium 67, and

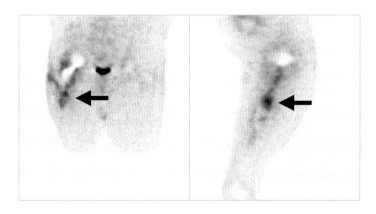

Fig. 5. A 47-year-old patient with history of right hip arthroplasty. The PET scan was ordered to exclude infection. The images demonstrate increased FDG uptake along the bone-prosthesis interface in the lower shaft portion of the prosthesis (*arrow*). This finding is consistent with arthroplasty-associated infection. Subsequent surgery confirmed periprosthetic infection.

radiolabeled immunoglobulin [126]. The lower specificity of gallium 67 is an advantage in this clinical setting because of the wide range of pathologic causes of FUO. In general, the labeled leukocyte scan is preferable in patients with suspected infection, whereas a gallium 67 scan should be considered in patients with possible tumor and autoimmune disease. The role of radiolabeled immunoglobulin in FUO is unsettled.

FDG-PET imaging can be a very useful tool in detecting the source of FUO. It is known that FDG can accumulate in many nonmalignant processes, which are considered a source of false-positive result when suspected or known cancer is examined with this technique. Searching for a source in patients with FUO, this nonspecificity is an advantage because high sensitivity of this method is more important than its low specificity in this setting. It has been shown that the major sources of FUO, including tumors, infections, and noninfectious inflammatory diseases (eg, arteritis and sarcoidosis), can be detected by FDG-PET. In addition, FDG-PET imaging can provide much higher resolution than gallium 67 and labeled leukocyte scintigraphy for surgical intervention if it is clinically indicated. It has been reported that FDG-PET has a very high negative predictive value and in no patient with a negative FDG-PET could a structural source be demonstrated in this population [48]. FDG-PET has the potential to become the single most effective imaging modality in the evaluation of FUO.

In a study involving 16 patients with FUO, pathologic sites of accumulations of FDG were determined, which led to the final diagnosis in 11 patients (69%) [48]. Meller et al [46] compared the efficacy of FDG-PET with gallium 67 SPECT in the evaluation of FUO in 18 patients. They found that the sensitivity of FDG-PET in detecting the focus of fever was 81% and the specificity was 86%. Positive and negative predictive values were 90% and 75%, respectively. In contrast, the gallium SPECT yielded a sensitivity of 67% and a specificity of 78% in detecting the focus of fever. Positive and negative predictive values for gallium 67 SPECT were 75% and 70%, respectively. In a subsequent publication by the same group, it was found that in a subgroup of patients with postoperative fever, the sensitivity of FDG-PET is also high [127]. The specificity is poor in this subgroup of patients, however, because of the uptake in granulative tissues at the sites of surgery [127]. Blockmans et al [47] also compared FDG-PET and gallium 67 scans in 40 patients with FUO. In this study, the authors demonstrated that FDG-PET scan and gallium scintigraphy were helpful in

detecting the source of the fever in 35% and 25%, respectively; both were noncontributory in 42% of the population examined. All lesions with abnormal gallium accumulation were also visible on FDG-PET scan. A recent study looked at 35 patients with FUO in whom a final diagnosis was established in 19 patients (54%) following FDG-PET imaging. The positive predictive value of FDG-PET in these patients was 87% and the negative predictive value 95% [128]. These results demonstrated that FDG-PET scan is superior to gallium scintigraphy in the evaluation for FUO [128]. The consistent high negative predictive value of FDG-PET in the evaluation of FUO indicates that in no patient with a negative FDG-PET can a morphologically significant source for the fever be determined [48], which further enhances the role of this technique in this population.

Soft tissue infection and inflammations

Sarcoidosis is a systemic disease that can affect any organ in the body, but the lungs and the associated lymph node are most frequently involved by this inflammatory disorder. Assessment of disease activity by conventional imaging methods is difficult and unreliable. Accurate determination of disease activity is essential, however, for timely administration of corticosteroids to control the disease.

Sarcoid lesions in the lungs and associated lymph nodes can have significantly increased FDG activity as described a decade ago [53,54,129]. It is believed that the levels of FDG uptake by the sarcoid lesions in the lungs reflect disease activity in the respective sites [53]. Subsequently, it was shown that FDG-PET can also detect sarcoid lesions in other organs [130–134]. If unsuspected, sarcoidosis easily can be confused with malignancies [131,133,135,136], such as lymphomas. Oriuchi et al [137] compared the uptake of [^{18}F]-fluoro-α-methyltyrosine with FDG in 10 patients with sarcoidosis and 10 patients with lung cancer to distinguish sarcoidosis from malignancy. Interestingly, they noted that in all 10 patients with sarcoidosis the mediastinal nodes were visualized with FDG with a relatively high intensity (SUV = 5), whereas [^{18}F]-fluoro-α-methyltyrosine PET demonstrated no significantly increased uptake (standard uptake value [SUV] = 0.8) at these sites. In contrast, in lung cancer, both [^{18}F]-fluoro-α-methyltyrosine and FDG demonstrated increased uptake [137]. This approach may be of value for distinguishing malignancy from sarcoidosis. PET may also provide some prognostic value in patients with sarcoidosis. Yamada et al [138] compared the uptake values of FDG and carbon-11–labeled methionine in the sarcoid lesions for this purpose [138]. They noted that response rate to treatment in patients with relatively high FDG uptake compared with methionine was significantly higher than those with relatively high methionine uptake (78% versus 33%).

Diagnoses of vasculitis, such as giant cell arteritis and Takayasu's arteritis, can be difficult because the symptoms related to these inflammatory disorders are frequently nonspecific and the management of these patients poses a challenge to clinicians. Several groups have demonstrated the use of FDG-PET in the evaluation of vasculitis [139–143]. In a study with 18 patients, Webb et al [144] demonstrated that FDG-PET achieved a sensitivity of 92%, a specificity of 100%, and negative and positive predictive values of 85% and 100%, respectively, in the initial assessment of active vasculitis in Takayasu's arteritis. The authors conclude that FDG-PET can be used to diagnose early disease; to detect active disease (even within chronic changes); and to monitor the effectiveness of treatment [144]. Meller et al [145] reported that the results from FDG-PET and MR imaging findings in the diagnosis of aortitis in this study were comparable, but FDG-PET identified more sites of vascular involvement than those visualized by MR imaging. In a study involving 27 patients with final diagnosis, Bleeker-Rovers et al [146] reported that FDG-PET has a positive predictive value of 100% and a negative predictive value of 82%. It has been reported that FDG-PET can detect Wegener's granulomatosis with negative labeled leukocyte imaging [142]. It should be pointed out that FDG-PET imaging is most successful in the detection of vasculitis of large blood vessels. Brodmann et al [147] compared findings from FDG-PET and duplex sonography in 22 patients with giant cell arteritis and noted that all patients with positive signs of giant cell arteritis in duplex sonography in the large arteries were also shown to have elevated FDG uptake in the same vessels, with complete agreement in the anatomic distribution of the involved sites. When the positive sonographic findings were limited to the small temporal arteries, however, FDG-PET was unable to detect these lesions [147]. The authors conclude that FDG-PET is suited to the demonstration of giant cell arteritis in arteries exceeding 4 mm in diameter [147].

FDG-PET is also suitable in the evaluation of several other disorders involving blood vessels. For example, several reports have demonstrated the ability of FDG-PET in detecting thrombosis [49,50,148]. In addition, FDG-PET can also detect septic thrombophlebitis [51,149,150] and vascular graft infection [151–153]. These data suggest a very promising role for FDG-PET in the evaluation of inflammation and infection involving blood vessels.

Summary

FDG-PET has great potential in the evaluation of a variety of inflammatory and infectious disorders and possibly other benign disorders. FDG-PET is very helpful in the evaluation of chronic osteomyelitis, sarcoidosis, FUO, and differentiating toxoplasmosis from lymphoma in the central nervous system in HIV-positive patients. The assessment of efficacy of FDG-PET in the evaluation of arthroplasty-associated infection, large-vessel vasculitis, and other inflammatory and infectious disorders is ongoing but seems quite promising at this time.

References

[1] Delbeke D. Oncological applications of FDG-PET imaging. J Nucl Med 1999;40:1706–15.

[2] Bar-Shalom R, Valdivia AY, Blaufox MD. PET imaging in oncology. Semin Nucl Med 2000;30: 150–85.

[3] Som P, Atkins HL, Bandoypadhyay D, Fowler JS, MacGregor RR, Matsui K, et al. A fluorinated glucose analog, 2-fluoro-2-deoxy-D-glucose (F-18): nontoxic tracer for rapid tumor detection. J Nucl Med 1980;21:670–5.

[4] Ahmed N, Kansara M, Berridge MV. Acute regulation of glucose transport in a monocyte-macrophage cell line: Glut-3 affinity for glucose is enhanced during the respiratory burst. Biochem J 1997;327: 369–75.

[5] Lehmann K, Behe M, Meller J, Becker W. F-18-FDG uptake in granulocytes: basis of F-18-FDG scintigraphy for imaging infection [abstract]. J Nucl Med 2001;42:1384.

[6] Bakheet SM, Powe J. Benign causes of 18-FDG uptake on whole body imaging. Semin Nucl Med 1998;28:352–8.

[7] Kubota R, Yamada S, Kubota K, Ishiwata K, Tamahashi N, Ido T. Intratumoral distribution of fluorine-18-fluorodeoxyglucose in vivo: high accumulation in macrophages and granulation tissues studied by microautoradiograph. J Nucl Med 1992; 33:1972–80.

[8] Mamede M, Saga T, Ishimori T, Nakamoto Y, Kobayashi H, Sato N, et al. Differential uptake of F-18-FDG in experimental tumors xenografted into immunocompetent and immunodeficient mice and the effect of steroid pretreatment on tumor uptake [abstract]. J Nucl Med 2001;42:1172.

[9] Mamede M, Saga T, Ishimori T, Nakamoto Y, Sato N, Higashi T, et al. Differential uptake of F-18-fluorodeoxyglucose by experimental tumors xenografted into immunocompetent and immunodeficient mice and the effect of immunomodification. Neoplasia 2003;5:179–83.

[10] Sugawara Y, Gutowski TD, Fisher SJ, Brown RS, Wahl RL. Uptake of positron emission tomography tracers in experimental bacterial infections: a comparative biodistribution study of radiolabeled FDG, thymidine, L-methionine, Ga-67-citrate, and I-125-HSA. Eur J Nucl Med 1999;26:333–41.

[11] Tahara T, Ichiya Y, Kuwabara Y, Otsuka M, Miyake Y, Gunasekera R, et al. High [18]-fluorodeoxyglucose uptake in abdominal abscesses: a PET study. J Comput Assist Tomogr 1989;5:829–31.

[12] Meyer MA, Frey KA, Schwaiger M. Discordance between F-18 fluorodeoxyglucose uptake and contrast enhancement in a brain abscess. Clin Nucl Med 1993;18:682–4.

[13] Yen RF, Chen ML, Liu FY, Ko SC, Chang YL, Chieng PU, et al. False-positive 2-[F-18]-fluoro-2-deoxy-D-glucose positron emission tomography studies for evaluation of focal pulmonary abnormalities. J Formos Med Assoc 1998;97:642–5.

[14] Kaya Z, Kotzerke J, Keller F. FDG-PET diagnosis of septic kidney in a renal transplant patient. Transpl Int 1999;12:156.

[15] Schroder W, Zimny M, Rudlowski C, Bull U, Rath W. The role of F-18-fluoro-deoxyglucose positron emission tomography (F-18-FDG-PET) in diagnosis of ovarian cancer. Int J Gynecol Cancer 1999;9: 117–22.

[16] Park CH, Lee MH, Oh CG. F-18FDG positron emission tomographic imaging in bilateral iliopsoas abscesses. Clin Nucl Med 2002;27:680–1.

[17] Tsuyuguchi N, Sunada I, Ohata K, Takami T, Nishio A, Hara M, et al. Evaluation of treatment effects in brain abscess with positron emission tomography: comparison of fluorine-18- fluorodeoxyglucose and carbon-11-methionine. Ann Nucl Med 2003;17: 47–51.

[18] Jones HA, Sriskandan S, Peters AM, Pride NB, Krausz T, Boobis AR, et al. Dissociation of neutrophil emigration and metabolic activity in lobar pneumonia and bronchiectasis. Eur Respir J 1997; 10:795–803.

[19] Kapucu LO, Meltzer CC, Townsend DW, Keenan RJ, Luketich JD. Fluorine-18-fluorodeoxyglucose uptake in pneumonia. J Nucl Med 1998;39:1267–9.

[20] Bakheet SM, Saleem M, Powe J, Al Amro A, Larsson SG, Mahassin Z. F-18 fluorodeoxyglucose chest uptake in lung inflammation and infection. Clin Nucl Med 2000;25:273–8.

[21] Bakheet SMB, Powe J, Ezzat A, Rostom A. F-18-FDG uptake in tuberculosis. Clin Nucl Med 1998; 23:739.

[22] Goo JM, Im JG, Do KH, Yeo JS, Seo JB, Kim HY, et al. Pulmonary tuberculoma evaluated by means of FDG-PET: findings in 10 cases. Radiology 2000; 216:117–21.

[23] Hara T, Kosaka N, Suzuki T, Kudo K, Niino H. Uptake rates of F-18-fluorodeoxyglucose and C-11-choline in lung cancer and pulmonary tuberculosis: a positron emission tomography study. Chest 2003; 124:893–901.

[24] Jeffry L, Kerrou K, Camatte S, Lelievre L, Metzger U, Robin F, et al. Peritoneal tuberculosis revealed by carcinomatosis on CT scan and uptake at FDG-PET. BJOG 2003;110:1129–31.

[25] Yang CM, Hsu CH, Lee CM, Wang FC. Intense uptake of F-18 -fluoro-2 deoxy-D-glucose in active pulmonary tuberculosis. Ann Nucl Med 2003;17: 407–10.

[26] Zhuang H, Pourdehnad M, Yamamoto AJ, Rossman MD, Alavi A. Intense F-18 fluorodeoxyglucose uptake caused by Mycobacterium avium-intracellulare infection. Clin Nucl Med 2001;26:458.

[27] El-Zeftawy H, LaBombardi V, Dakhel M, Heiba S, Dayem HA. Evaluation of F-18 FDG-PET imaging in diagnosis of disseminated Mycobacterium avium complex (DMAC) in AIDS patients [abstract]. J Nucl Med 2002;43:460.

[28] Bandoh S, Fujita J, Ueda Y, Tojo Y, Ishii T, Kubo A, et al. Uptake of fluorine-18-fluorodeoxyglucose in pulmonary Mycobacterium avium complex infection. Intern Med 2003;42:726–9.

[29] Hsu CH, Lee CM, Wang FC, Lin YH. F-18 fluorodeoxyglucose positron emission tomography in pulmonary cryptococcoma. Clin Nucl Med 2003;28: 791–3.

[30] Bakheet SMB, Powe J, Kandil A, Ezzat A, Rostom A, Amartey J. F-18FDG uptake in breast infection and inflammation. Clin Nucl Med 2000;25:100–3.

[31] Meyer MA. Diffusely increased colonic F-18 FDG uptake in acute enterocolitis. Clin Nucl Med 1995; 20:434–5.

[32] Hannah A, Scott AM, Akhurst T, Berlangieri S, Bishop J, McKay WJ. Abnormal colonic accumulation of fluorine-18-FDG in pseudomembranous colitis. J Nucl Med 1996;37:1683–5.

[33] Jacobson K, Mernagh JR, Green T, Moss L, Radoja C, Issenmam RM, et al. Positron emission tomography in the investigation of pediatric inflammatory bowel disease. Gastroenterology 1999;116:A742.

[34] Tomas MB, Tronco GG, Karayalcin G, Palestro CJ. FDG uptake in infectious mononucleosis. Clinical Position Imaging 2000;3:176.

[35] Watanabe SI, Nakamura Y, Kariatsumari K, Nagata T, Sakata R, Zinnouchi S, et al. Pulmonary paragonimiasis mimicking lung cancer on FDG-PET imaging. Anticancer Res 2003;23:3437–40.

[36] Zhuang H, Duarte PS, Rebenstock A, Feng Q, Alavi A. Pulmonary Clostridium perfringens infection detected by FDG positron emission tomography. Clin Nucl Med 2003;28:517–8.

[37] Guhlmann A, Brecht-Krauss D, Suger G, Glatting G, Kotzerke J, Kinzl L, et al. Fluorine-18-FDG-PET and

technetium-99m antigranulocyte antibody scintigraphy in chronic osteomyelitis. J Nucl Med 1998;39: 2145–52.

[38] Guhlmann A, Brecht-Krauss D, Suger G, Glatting G, Kotzerke J, Kinzl L, et al. Chronic osteomyelitis: detection with FDG-PET and correlation with histopathologic findings. Radiology 1998;206:749–54.

[39] Zhuang H, Duarte PS, Pourdehand M, Shnier D, Alavi A. Exclusion of chronic osteomyelitis with F-18 fluorodeoxyglucose positron emission tomographic imaging. Clin Nucl Med 2000;25:281–4.

[40] Kalicke T, Schmitz A, Risse JH, Arens S, Keller E, Hansis M, et al. Fluorine-18 fluorodeoxyglucose PET in infectious bone diseases: results of histologically confirmed cases. Eur J Nucl Med 2000;27:524–8.

[41] De Winter F, Gemmel F, Van de Wiele C, Vogelaers D, Uyttendaele D, Poffijn B, et al. Prospective comparison of 99m Tc ciprofloxacin (infection) SPECT and FDG-PET for the diagnosis of chronic osteomyelitis in the central skeleton: preliminary results [abstract]. Eur J Nucl Med 2001;28:OS101.

[42] Meller J, Koster G, Liersch T, Siefker U, Lehmann K, Meyer I, et al. Chronic bacterial osteomyelitis: prospective comparison of F- 18-FDG imaging with a dual-head coincidence camera and In-111–labeled autologous leucocyte scintigraphy. Eur J Nucl Med 2002;29:53–60.

[43] Zhuang H, Duarte PS, Pourdehnad M, Maes A, Van Acker F, Shnier D, et al. The promising role of F-18-FDG-PET in detecting infected lower limb prosthesis implants. J Nucl Med 2001;42:44–8.

[44] Kisielinski K, Cremerius U, Reinartz P, Niethard FU. Fluorodeoxyglucose positron emission tomography detection of inflammatory reactions due to polyethylene wear in total hip arthroplasty. J Arthroplast 2003;18:528–32.

[45] Cremerius U, Mumme T, Reinartz P, Wirtz D, Niethard FU, Bull U. Analysis of F-18-FDG uptake patterns in PET for diagnosis of septic and aseptic loosening after total hip arthroplasty. Nuklearmedizin 2003;42:234–9.

[46] Meller J, Altenvoerde G, Munzel U, Jauho A, Behe M, Gratz S, et al. Fever of unknown origin: prospective comparison of [F-18]FDG imaging with a double-head coincidence camera and gallium-67 citrate SPECT. Eur J Nucl Med 2000;27:1617–25.

[47] Blockmans D, Knockaert D, Maes A, De Caestecker J, Stroobants S, Bobbaers H, et al. Clinical value of [F-18]fluoro-deoxyglucose positron emission tomography for patients with fever of unknown origin. Clin Infect Dis 2001;32:191–6.

[48] Lorenzen J, Buchert R, Bohuslavizki KH. Value of FDG-PET in patients with fever of unknown origin. Nucl Med Commun 2001;22:779–83.

[49] Chang KJ, Zhuang H, Alavi A. Detection of chronic recurrent lower extremity deep venous thrombosis on fluorine-18 fluorodeoxyglucose positron emission tomography. Clin Nucl Med 2000;25:838–9.

[50] Lin EC, Quaife RA. FDG uptake in chronic superior

vena cava thrombus on positron emission tomographic imaging. Clin Nucl Med 2001;26:241–2.

[51] Bleeker-Rovers CP, Jager G, Tack CJ, van der Meer JWM, Oyen WJG. F-18-fluorodeoxyglucose positron emission tomography leading to a diagnosis of septic thrombophlebitis of the portal vein: description of a case history and review of the literature. J Intern Med 2004;255:419–23.

[52] Kung J, Zhuang H, Yu JQ, Duarte PS, Alavi A. Intense fluorodeoxyglucose activity in pulmonary amyloid lesions on positron emission tomography. Clin Nucl Med 2003;28:975–6.

[53] Brudin LH, Valind SO, Rhodes CG, Pantin CF, Sweatman M, Jones T, et al. Fluorine-18 deoxyglucose uptake in sarcoidosis measured with positron emission tomography. Eur J Nucl Med 1994;21: 297–305.

[54] Lewis PJ, Salama A. Uptake of fluorine-18-fluorodeoxyglucose in sarcoidosis. J Nucl Med 1994;35: 1647–9.

[55] Taylor IK, Hill AA, Hayes M, Rhodes CG, O'Shaughnessy KM, O'Connor BJ, et al. Imaging allergen-invoked airway inflammation in atopic asthma with [18F]-fluorodeoxyglucose and positron emission tomography. Lancet 1996;347:937–40.

[56] Kicska G, Zhuang H, Alavi A. Acute bronchitis imaged with F-18FDG positron emission tomography. Clin Nucl Med 2003;28:511–2.

[57] Dadparvar S, Anderson GS, Bhargava P, Guan L, Reich P, Alavi A, et al. Paraneoplastic encephalitis associated with cystic teratoma is detected by fluorodeoxyglucose positron emission tomography with negative magnetic resonance image findings. Clin Nucl Med 2003;28:893–6.

[58] Lin EC. Costochondritis mimicking a pulmonary nodule on FDG positron emission tomographic imaging. Clin Nucl Med 2002;27:591–2.

[59] Lin P, Delaney G, Chu J, Kiat H, Pocock N. Fluorine-18 FDG dual-head gamma camera coincidence imaging of radiation pneumonitis. Clin Nucl Med 2000; 25:866–9.

[60] Neto C, Zhuang H, Ghesani N, Alavi A. Detection of Barrett's esophagus superimposed by esophageal cancer by FDG positron emission tomography. Clin Nucl Med 2001;26:1060.

[61] Bhargava P, Reich P, Alavi A, Zhuang H. Radiation-induced esophagitis on FDG-PET imaging. Clin Nucl Med 2003;28:849–50.

[62] Shreve PD. Focal fluorine-18 fluorodeoxyglucose accumulation in inflammatory pancreatic disease. Eur J Nucl Med 1998;25:259–64.

[63] Yasuda S, Shohtsu A, Ide M, Takagi S, Suzuki Y, Tajima T. Diffuse F-18 FDG uptake in chronic thyroiditis. Clin Nucl Med 1997;22:341.

[64] Drieskens O, Blockmans D, Van den Bruel A, Mortelmans L. Riedel's thyroiditis and retroperitoneal fibrosis in multifocal fibrosclerosis positron emission tomographic findings. Clin Nucl Med 2002;27:413–5.

[65] Schmid DT, Kneifel S, Stoeckli SJ, Padberg BC,

Merrill G, Goerres GW. Increased 18F-FDG uptake mimicking thyroid cancer in a patient with Hashimoto's thyroiditis. Eur Radiol 2003;13:2119–21.

[66] Yasuda S, Shohtsu A, Ide M, Takagi S, Kijima H, Horiuchi M. Elevated F-18 FDG uptake in plasmacyte-rich chronic maxillary sinusitis. Clin Nucl Med 1998;23:176–8.

[67] Gysen M, Stroobants S, Mortelmans L. Proliferative myositis: a case of a pseudomalignant process. Clin Nucl Med 1998;23:836–8.

[68] Imran MB, Kubota K, Yoshioka S, Yamada S, Sato T, Fukuda H, et al. Sclerosing mediastinitis: findings on fluorine-18 fluorodeoxyglucose positron emission tomography. Clin Nucl Med 1999;24:305–8.

[69] Nunez RF, Yeung HW, Macapinlac H. Increased F-18 FDG uptake in the stomach. Clin Nucl Med 1999; 24:281–2.

[70] Yen R-F, Shun C-T, Pan M-H, Tsai Y-C, Wu Y-W. FDG-PET manifestation of lobular panniculitis. Clin Nucl Med 2004;29:442–3.

[71] Kao CH. Incidental findings of FDG uptake in dental caries. Clin Nucl Med 2003;28:610.

[72] Zhuang H, Cunnane ME, Ghesani NV, Mozley PD, Alavi A. Chest tube insertion as a potential source of false-positive FDG-positron emission tomographic results. Clin Nucl Med 2002;27:285–6.

[73] Hsu CH, Lee CM, Lin SY. Inflammatory pseudotumor resulting from foreign body in abdominal cavity detected by FDG-PET. Clin Nucl Med 2003; 28:842–4.

[74] Hurwitz R. F-18 FDG positron emission tomographic imaging in a case of ruptured breast implant: inflammation or recurrent tumor? Clin Nucl Med 2003;28: 755–6.

[75] Saverymuttu SH, Camilleri M, Rees H, Lavender JP, Hodgson HJ, Chadwick VS. Indium 111-granulocyte scanning in the assessment of disease extent and disease activity in inflammatory bowel disease: a comparison with colonoscopy, histology, and fecal indium 111-granulocyte excretion. Gastroenterology 1986;90:1121–8.

[76] Charron M, del Rosario JF, Kocoshis S. Use of technetium-tagged white blood cells in patients with Crohn's disease and ulcerative colitis: is differential diagnosis possible? Pediatr Radiol 1998;28:871–7.

[77] Charron M, Del Rosario F, Kocoshis S. Assessment of terminal ileal and colonic inflammation in Crohn's disease with 99mTc-WBC. Acta Paediatr 1999;88: 193–8.

[78] Saverymuttu SH, Crofton ME, Peters AM, Lavender JP. Indium-111 tropolonate leucocyte scanning in the detection of intra-abdominal abscesses. Clin Radiol 1983;34:593–6.

[79] Palestro CJ, Kim CK, Swyer AJ, Capozzi JD, Solomon RW, Goldsmith SJ. Total-hip arthroplasty: periprosthetic indium-111 labeled leukocyte activity and complementary technetium-99m-sulfur colloid imaging in suspected infection. J Nucl Med 1990; 31:1950–4.

[80] MacSweeney JE, Peters AM, Lavender JP. Indium labeled leucocyte scanning in pyrexia of unknown origin. Clin Radiol 1990;42:414–7.

[81] Becker W, Goldenberg DM, Wolf F. The use of monoclonal-antibodies and antibody fragments in the imaging of infectious lesions. Semin Nucl Med 1994; 24:142–53.

[82] Almers S, Granerus G, Franzen L, Strom M. Technetium-99m scintigraphy: more accurate assessment of ulcerative colitis with exametazime-labeled leucocytes than with antigranulocyte antibodies. Eur J Nucl Med 1996;23:247–55.

[83] Fischman AJ, Carter EA, Coco-Graham WA, Babich JW. Comparison of a Tc-99m chemotactic peptide with (18)FDG for imaging infection and sterile inflammation in rabbits [abstract]. J Nucl Med 1999; 40:894.

[84] Boerman O, Oyen W, Corstens F, Storm G. Liposomes for scintigraphic imaging: optimization of in vivo behavior. Q J Nucl Med 1998;42:271–9.

[85] Rusckowski M, Paganelli G, Hnatowich DJ, Magnani P, Virzi F, Fogarasi M, et al. Imaging osteomyelitis with streptavidin and indium-111-labeled biotin. J Nucl Med 1996;37:1655–62.

[86] O'Doherty MJ, Barrington SF, Campbell M, Lowe J, Bradbeer CS. PET scanning and the human immunodeficiency virus-positive patient. J Nucl Med 1997; 38:1575–83.

[87] Scharko AM, Perlman SB, Pyzalski RW, Graziano FM, Sosman J, Pauza CD. Whole-body positron emission tomography in patients with HIV-1 infection. Lancet 2003;362:959–61.

[88] Hoffman JM, Waskin HA, Schifter T, Hanson MW, Gray L, Rosenfeld S, et al. FDG-PET in differentiating lymphoma from nonmalignant central nervous system lesions in patients with AIDS. J Nucl Med 1993;34:567–75.

[89] Villringer K, Jager H, Dichgans M, Ziegler S, Poppinger J, Herz M, et al. Differential diagnosis of CNS lesions in AIDS patients by FDG-PET. J Comput Assist Tomogr 1995;19:532–6.

[90] Heald AE, Hoffman JM, Bartlett JA, Waskin HA. Differentiation of central nervous system lesions in AIDS patients using positron emission tomography (PET). Int J STD AIDS 1996;7:337.

[91] Laasonen EM, Porras M. Post-traumatic osteomyelitis: delay in appearance after infection and prognostic value of radiological signs. Eur J Radiol 1983;3:95–6.

[92] Wing VW, Jeffrey RB, Federle MP, Helms CA, Trafton P. Chronic osteomyelitis examined by CT. Radiology 1985;154:171–4.

[93] Craig JG, Amin MB, Wu K, Eyler WR, vanHolsbeeck MT, Bouffard JA, et al. Osteomyelitis of the diabetic foot: MR imaging. Pathologic correlation. Radiology 1997;203:849–55.

[94] Marcus CD, LadamMarcus VJ, Leone J, Malgrange D, BonnetGausserand FM, Menanteau BP. MR imaging of osteomyelitis and neuropathic osteo-

arthropathy in the feet of diabetics. Radiographics 1996;16:1337–48.

[95] Ma LD, Frassica FJ, Bluemke DA, Fishman EK. CT and MRI evaluation of musculoskeletal infection. Crit Rev Diagn Imaging 1997;38:535–68.

[96] Kaim A, Ledermann HP, Bongartz G, Messmer P, Muller-Brand J, Steinbrich W. Chronic post-traumatic osteomyelitis of the lower extremity: comparison of magnetic resonance imaging and combined bone scintigraphy/immunoscintigraphy with radiolabelled monoclonal antigranulocyte antibodies. Skeletal Radiol 2000;29:378–86.

[97] Ledermann HP, Kaim A, Bongartz G, Steinbrich W. Pitfalls and limitations of magnetic resonance imaging in chronic posttraumatic osteomyelitis. Eur Radiol 2000;10:1815–23.

[98] Sanders TG, Medynski MA, Feller JF, Lawhorn KW. Bone contusion patterns of the knee at MR imaging: footprint of the mechanism of injury. Radiographics 2000;20:S135–51.

[99] Schauwecker DS. The scintigraphic diagnosis of osteomyelitis. AJR Am J Roentgenol 1992;1:9–18.

[100] Kolindou A, Liu Y, Ozker K, Krasnow AZ, Isitman AT, Hellman RS, et al. In-111 WBC imaging of osteomyelitis in patients with underlying bone scan abnormalities. Clin Nucl Med 1996;21:183–91.

[101] Kim EE, Pjura GA, Lowry PA, Gobuty AH, Traina JF. Osteomyelitis complicating fracture: pitfalls of 111In leukocyte scintigraphy. AJR Am J Roentgenol 1987;148:927–30.

[102] Solomon M, Macdessi S, Van der Wall H. Utility of leukocyte scanning in osteomyelitis complicating a complex fracture. Clin Nucl Med 2001;26:858–9.

[103] Stumpe KDM, Zanetti M, Weishaupt D, Hodler J, Boos N, von Schulthess GK. FDG positron emission tomography for differentiation of degenerative and infectious endplate abnormalities in the lumbar spine detected on MR imaging. AJR Am J Roentgenol 2002;179:1151–7.

[104] Zhuang H, Sam JW, Chacko TK, Duarte PS, Hickeson M, Feng Q, et al. Rapid normalization of osseous FDG uptake following traumatic or surgical fractures. Eur J Nucl Med Mol Imaging 2003;30: 1096–103.

[105] Stumpe KDM, Dazzi H, Schaffner A, von Schulthess GK. Infection imaging using whole-body FDG-PET. Eur J Nucl Med 2000;27:822–32.

[106] De Winter F, Van de Wiele C, Vogelaers D, Verdonk R, De Smet K, De Clercq D, et al. FDG-PET is highly accurate in the diagnosis of chronic osteomyelitis in the central skeleton [abstract]. J Nucl Med 2000; 41:57.

[107] Robiller FC, Stumpe KDM, Kossmann T, Weisshaupt D, Bruder E, von Schulthess GK. Chronic osteomyelitis of the femur: value of PET imaging. Eur Radiol 2000;10:855–8.

[108] De Winter F, Van de Wiele C, Vogelaers D, De Smet K, Verdonk R, Dierckx RA. Fluorine-18 fluorodeoxy-glucose-positron emission tomography: a highly

accurate imaging modality for the diagnosis of chronic musculoskeletal infections. J Bone Joint Surg Am 2001;83:651–60.

[109] Paul R, Ahonen A, Virtama P, Aho A, Ekfors T. F-18 Fluorodeoxyglucose: its potential in differentiating between stress-fracture and neoplasia. Clin Nucl Med 1989;14:906–8.

[110] Schmitz A, Risse JH, Textor J, Zander D, Biersack HJ, Palmedo H. FDG-PET findings of vertebral compression fractures in osteoporosis: preliminary results. Osteoporos Int 2002;13:755–61.

[111] De Winter F, Dierckx R, De Bondt P, Vogelaers D, Verdonk R, Van De Wiele C. FDG-PET as a single technique is more accurate than the combination bone scan/white blood cell scan in chronic orthopedic infections (COI) [abstract]. J Nucl Med 2001;41:59.

[112] Gratz S, Dorner J, Fischer U, Behr TM, Behe M, Altenvoerde G, et al. F-18-FDG hybrid PET in patients with suspected spondylitis. Eur J Nucl Med Mol Imaging 2002;29:516–24.

[113] Andrews HJ, Arden GP, Hart GM, Owen JW. Deep infection after total hip replacement. J Bone Joint Surg Br 1981;63:53–7.

[114] Maderazo EG, Judson S, Pasternak H. Late infections of total joint prostheses: a review and recommendation for prevention. Clin Orthop 1988;229:131–42.

[115] Palestro CJ, Roumanas P, Swyer AJ, Kim CK, Goldsmith SJ. Diagnosis of musculoskeletal infection using combined In-111 labeled leukocyte and Tc-99m SC marrow imaging. Clin Nucl Med 1992; 17:269–73.

[116] Scher DM, Pak K, Lonner JH, Finkel JE, Zuckerman JD, Di Cesare PE. The predictive value of indium-111 leukocyte scans in the diagnosis of infected total hip, knee, or resection arthroplasties. J Arthroplast 2000; 15:295–300.

[117] Schmitz A, Risse HJ, Kalicke T, Grunwald F, Schmitt O. FDG-PET for diagnosis and follow-up of inflammatory processes: first results from an orthopedic view. Z Orthop Ihre Grenzgeb 2000;138:407–12.

[118] Love C, Pugliese PV, Afriyie MO, Tomas MB, Marvin SE, Palestro CJ. Utility of F18 FDG imaging for diagnosing the infected joint replacement. Clinical Positron Imaging 2000;3:159.

[119] Chacko TK, Moussavian B, Zhuang HM, Woods K, Alavi A. Critical role of FDG-PET imaging in the management of patients with suspected infection in diverse settings [abstract]. J Nucl Med 2002;43:456.

[120] Vanquickenborne B, Maes A, Nuyts J, Van Acker F, Stuyck J, Mulier M, et al. The value of (18)FDG-PET for the detection of infected hip prosthesis. Eur J Nucl Med Mol Imaging 2003;30:705–15.

[121] Zhuang H, Chacko TK, Hickeson M, Stevenson K, Feng Q, Ponzo F, et al. Persistent non-specific FDG uptake on PET imaging following hip arthroplasty. Eur J Nucl Med Mol Imaging 2002;29:1328–33.

[122] Chacko TK, Zhuang H, Stevenson K, Moussavian B, Alavi A. The importance of the location of fluorodeoxyglucose uptake in periprosthetic infection in

painful hip prostheses. Nucl Med Commun 2002;23: 851–5.

[123] Manthey N, Reinhard P, Moog F, Knesewitsch P, Hahn K, Tatsch K. The use of F-18 fluorodeoxyglucose positron emission tomography to differentiate between synovitis, loosening and infection of hip and knee prostheses. Nucl Med Commun 2002;23: 645–53.

[124] Cunha BA. Fever of unknown origin. Infect Dis Clin North Am 1996;10:111.

[125] Knockaert DC, Vanderschueren S, Blockmans D. Fever of unknown origin in adults: 40 years on. J Intern Med 2003;253:263–75.

[126] Meller J, Ivancevic V, Conrad M, Gratz S, Munz DL, Becker W. Clinical value of immunoscintigraphy in patients with fever of unknown origin. J Nucl Med 1998;39:1248–53.

[127] Meller J, Sahlmann CO, Lehmann K, Siefker U, Meyer I, Schreiber K, et al. F-18-FDG-hybrid-camera-PET in patients with postoperative fever. Nuklearmedizin 2002;41:22–9.

[128] Bleeker-Rovers CP, de Kleijn E, Corstens FHM, van der Meer JWM, Oyen WJG. Clinical value of FDG-PET in patients with fever of unknown origin and patients suspected of focal infection or inflammation. Eur J Nucl Med Mol Imaging 2004;31:29–37.

[129] Knopp MV, Bischoff HG. Evaluation of intrapulmonary nodules by positron emission tomography. Radiologe 1994;34:588–91.

[130] Kobayashi A, Shinozaki T, Shinjyo Y, Kato K, Oriuchi N, Watanabe H, et al. FDG-PET in the clinical evaluation of sarcoidosis with bone lesions. Ann Nucl Med 2000;14:311–3.

[131] Joe A, Hoegerle S, Moser E. Cervical lymph node sarcoidosis as a pitfall in F-18FDG positron emission tomography. Clin Nucl Med 2001;26:542.

[132] Dubey N, Miletich RS, Wasay M, Mechtler LL, Bakshi R. Role of fluorodeoxyglucose positron emission tomography in the diagnosis of neurosarcoidosis. J Neurol Sci 2002;205:77–81.

[133] Ludwig V, Fordice S, Lamar R, Martin WH, Delbeke D. Unsuspected skeletal sarcoidosis mimicking metastatic disease on FDG positron emission tomography and bone scintigraphy. Clin Nucl Med 2003; 28:176–9.

[134] Yamagishi H, Shirai N, Takagi M, Yoshiyama M, Akioka K, Takeuchi K, et al. Identification of cardiac sarcoidosis with N-13–NH3/F-18-FDG-PET. J Nucl Med 2003;44:1030–6.

[135] Cook GJ, Fogelman I, Maisey MN. Normal physiological and benign pathological variants of 18-fluoro-2-deoxyglucose positron-emission tomography scanning: potential for error in interpretation. Semin Nucl Med 1996;26:308–14.

[136] Gotway MB, Storto ML, Golden JA, Reddy GP, Webb WR. Incidental detection of thoracic sarcoidosis on whole-body (18)fluorine-2-fluoro-2-deoxy-D-glucose positron emission tomography. J Thorac Imaging 2000;15:201–4.

[137] Oriuchi N, Inoue T, Tomiyoshi K, Sando Y, Tsukakoshi M, Aoyagi K, et al. F-18-fluoro-alpha-methyl-tyrosine (FMT) and F-18- fluorodeoxyglucose (FDG) PET in patients with sarcoidosis [abstract]. J Nucl Med 1999;40:196P.

[138] Yamada Y, Uchida Y, Tatsumi K, Yamaguchi T, Kimura H, Kitahara H, et al. Fluorine-18-fluorodeoxyglucose and carbon-11-methionine evaluation of lymphadenopathy in sarcoidosis. J Nucl Med 1998; 39:1160–6.

[139] Hara M, Goodman PC, Leder RA. FDG-PET finding in early-phase Takayasu arteritis. J Comput Assist Tomogr 1999;23:16–8.

[140] De Winter F, Petrovic M, Van de Wiele C, Vogelaers D, Afschrift M, Dierckx RA. Imaging of giant cell arteritis: evidence of splenic involvement using FDG positron emission tomography. Clin Nucl Med 2000; 25:633–4.

[141] Turlakow A, Yeung HWD, Pui J, Macapinlac H, Liebovitz E, Rusch V, et al. Fludeoxyglucose positron emission tomography in the diagnosis of giant cell arteritis. Arch Intern Med 2001;161:1003–7.

[142] Beggs AD, Hain SF. F-18FDG-positron emission tomographic scanning and Wegener's granulomatosis. Clin Nucl Med 2002;27:705–6.

[143] Hoogendoorn EH, Oyen WJG, van Dijk APJ, van der Meer JWM. Pneumococcal aortitis, report of a case with emphasis on the contribution to diagnosis of positron emission tomography using fluorinated deoxyglucose. Clin Microbiol Infect 2003;9:73–6.

[144] Webb M, Chambers A, Al-Nahhas A, Mason JC, Maudlin L, Rahman L, et al. The role of F-18-FDG-PET in characterising disease activity in Takayasu arteritis. Eur J Nucl Med Mol Imaging 2004;31: 627–34.

[145] Meller J, Strutz F, Siefker J, Schee A, Sahmann CO, Lehmann K, et al. Early diagnosis and follow-up of aortitis with F-18 FDG-PET and MRI. Eur J Nucl Med Mol Imaging 2003;30:730–6.

[146] Bleeker-Rovers CP, Bredie SJH, van der Meer JWM, Corstens FHM, Oyen WJG. F-18-fluorodeoxyglucose positron emission tomography in diagnosis and follow-up of patients with different types of vasculitis. Neth J Med 2003;61:323–9.

[147] Brodmann M, Lipp RW, Passath A, Seinost G, Pabst E, Pilger E. The role of 2-F-18-fluoro-2-deoxy-D-glucose positron emission tomography in the diagnosis of giant cell arteritis of the temporal arteries. Rheumatology 2004;43:241–2.

[148] Raman S, Nunez R, Wong CO, Dworkin HJ. F-18FDG positron emission tomographic image of an aortic aneurysmal thrombus. Clin Nucl Med 2002; 27:213–4.

[149] Hutchings M, Eigtved A. Uptake of FDG in Lemierre's syndrome with normal leucocyte scintigraphy. Eur J Nucl Med Mol Imaging 2003;30:489.

[150] Miceli M, Atoui R, Walker R, Mahfouz T, Mirza N, Diaz J, et al. Diagnosis of deep septic thrombophlebitis in cancer patients by fluorine-18 fluorodeoxy-

glucose positron emission tomography scanning: a preliminary report. J Clin Oncol 2004;22:1949–56.

[151] Krupnick A, Lombardi J, Engels F, Kreisel D, Zhuang H, Alavi A, et al. 18-fluorodeoxyglucose positron emission tomography as a novel imaging tool for the diagnosis of aortoenteric fistula and aortic graft infection: a case report. Vasc Endovascular Surg 2003;37: 363–8.

[152] Keidar Z, Engel A, Nitecki S, Bar Shalom R, Hoffman A, Israel O. PET/CT using 2-deoxy-2-[18F]fluoro-D-glucose for the evaluation of suspected infected vascular graft. Mol Imaging Biol 2003;5: 23–5.

[153] Rohde H, Horstkotte MA, Loeper S, Aberle J, Jenicke L, Lampidis R, et al. Recurrent *Listeria monocytogenes* aortic graft infection: confirmation of relapse by molecular subtyping. Diagn Microbiol Infect Dis 2004;48:63–7.

ELSEVIER
SAUNDERS

Radiol Clin N Am 43 (2005) 135–152

RADIOLOGIC
CLINICS
of North America

PET in pediatric diseases

Hossein Jadvar, MD, PhD[a,b],*, Abass Alavi, MD[c], Ayse Mavi, MD[d],
Barry L. Shulkin, MD, MBA[e]

[a]Division of Nuclear Medicine, Departments of Radiology and Biomedical Engineering, Keck School of Medicine,
University of Southern California, 1200 North State Street, GNH 5250, Los Angeles, CA 90033, USA
[b]Bioengineering Program, California Institute of Technology, Pasadena, CA, USA
[c]Department of Radiology, University of Pennsylvania, Philadelphia, PA, USA
[d]University of Pennsylvania, Philadelphia, PA, USA
[e]Department of Radiology, University of Michigan, Ann Arbor, MI, USA

PET is emerging as an important diagnostic tool in the imaging evaluation of pediatric disorders. The recent advent of the dual-modality PET/CT imaging systems has provided unprecedented additional diagnostic capability by providing precise anatomic localization of metabolic information. The use of CT transmission scanning for attenuation correction has shortened the total acquisition time, a desirable attribute in pediatric imaging. Moreover, expansion of the regional distribution of the most common PET radiotracer, fluorine-18 fluorodeoxyglucose ([18F]-FDG), and the introduction of mobile PET units have greatly enhanced the access to this powerful diagnostic imaging technology. This article reviews the clinical applications of PET and PET/CT in pediatrics with an emphasis on the more common applications in epilepsy and oncology. General considerations in patient preparation and radiation dosimetry are discussed.

Patient preparation

The preparation of children and parents for nuclear medicine imaging has been thoroughly reviewed elsewhere [1,2]. Sheets wrapped around the body, sandbags, or special holding devices are often sufficient for immobilization. Parents may accompany the child during the course of a study to provide emotional support. Establishing reliable intravenous access is critical in pediatric imaging because patients and parents do not tolerate multiple access attempts. The skills of more experienced personnel such as pediatric anesthesiologists are helpful in this regard. Bladder catheterization may also be needed to avoid the obscuring of lesions by reconstruction artifacts in the pelvis and the possibility of spontaneous voiding during image acquisition with the resultant contamination. A full bladder may also cause discomfort and lead to patient motion and image degradation [3]. Sedation is indicated when it is anticipated that simple methods will be inadequate to assure acceptable image quality. Sedation protocols vary from institution to institution. Guidelines, such as those advanced by the Society of Nuclear Medicine, the American Academy of Pediatrics, and the American Society of Anesthesiology, are useful in developing an institutional sedation program [4–6]. It is also important to consider the potential effects of sedatives on FDG tracer biodistribution. Many sedatives may affect cerebral metabolism but are not known to cause significant changes in tumoral metabolism [7].

With combined PET/CT devices, imaging protocols are kept simple to facilitate the patient's tolerance of the imaging procedure [8–12]. Oral contrast may be given to outline the bowel without significant

* Corresponding author. Division of Nuclear Medicine, Keck School of Medicine, University of Southern California, 1200 North State Street, GNH 5250, Los Angeles, CA 90033.

E-mail address: jadvar@usc.edu (H. Jadvar).

0033-8389/05/$ – see front matter © 2004 Elsevier Inc. All rights reserved.
doi:10.1016/j.rcl.2004.09.008

untoward effects on image quality, although semi-quantitative measures such as the standardized uptake value (SUV) may be affected [13–15]. The calculation of optimal SUV in pediatric patients may be different from that used in adult patients because of the body changes that occur during childhood. Specifically, in pediatric patients an SUV calculation based on body surface area seems to be a more uniform parameter than an SUV calculation based on body weight [16]. Currently, intravenous contrast is not administered routinely in PET/CT imaging studies because of different contrast protocols needed for optimal CT imaging of various anatomic regions and the potential induction of artifacts related to attenuation correction. With appropriate imaging protocols, which may include alternative contrast application schemes or variations to the attenuation correction procedure, PET/CT diagnostic capacity may be improved with little or no compromise in image quality.

Radiation dosimetry

Administered doses of FDG ranging from 5 to 10 MBq (0.15–0.30 mCi)/kg have been recommended for pediatric use [17]. A minimal dose of 37 MBq (1 mCi) may be used. The maximal dose is 750 Mbq (20 mCi).

The radiation dose from an intravenous injection of FDG has been studied in adults [18]. The radiation dose to infants has been reported in one study [19]. The target organ is bladder wall, which receives an absorbed dose of 1.03 ± 2.10 mGy/MBq (3.81 ± 7.77 rad/mCi), about fourfold higher than the absorbed dose per unit of administered activity in adults. Good hydration and early drainage of the urine reduces the dose absorbed by the bladder wall. Infants also receive a 10-fold higher absorbed dose to the brain per unit of administered dose (0.24 ± 0.05 mGy/MBq or 0.89 ± 0.18 rad/mCi) than that received by the adult brain because the percentage of FDG uptake is slightly higher in the infant brain (8.8%) than in the adult brain (6.9%). Also the distribution of cerebral tracer is different in infants and adults, with higher tracer accumulation in subcortical gray matter in infants and higher uptake by cortical gray matter in adults. Heart, liver, and pancreas also receive higher absorbed dose per unit of administered activity in infants than in adults. Because of the low administered FDG dose in infants, the total-body absorbed radiation dose is lower than or similar to that of adults and to that imposed by the other radiographic and scintigraphic procedures [7,19].

Applications in neurology

Normal brain development

Glucose metabolism is initially high in the sensorimotor cortex, thalamus, brainstem, and cerebellar vermis. Glucose metabolism gradually increases in the basal ganglia and in the parietal, temporal, calcarine, and cerebellar cortices during the first 3 months of life. Maturation of the frontal cortex and the dorsolateral cortex occur during the second 6 months of life. Cerebral FDG biodistribution in children after the age of 1 year resembles that of adults [20–22].

Epilepsy

Epilepsy is a relatively common childhood neurologic disorder. Accurate preoperative localization of the epileptogenic region is often difficult. Invasive procedures such as surgical placement of electrode grids on the brain surface or insertion of depth electrodes carry risk to the patient. Therefore, non-invasive imaging-based localization of the seizure focus is often preferred. Structural lesions, which may potentially but not necessarily be the source of seizure activity, may be detected by CT and MR imaging [23]. Ictal or interictal single photon emission CT (SPECT) evaluation of regional cerebral blood flow (rCBF) with tracers such as technitium-99m hexamethylpropylene ([99mTc]-HMPAO) and [99mTc]–ethyl cysteinate dimer ([99mTc]-ECD) can localize the epileptogenic region regardless of the presence or absence of structural abnormalities. An epileptogenic region demonstrates relative zonal hyperperfusion on ictal SPECT, whereas relative zonal hypoperfusion is seen on interictal SPECT. The sensitivity of ictal rCBF tracer SPECT may approach 90%; the sensitivity of interictal SPECT is about 50% [24].

FDG-PET has proven useful in localization of the epileptogenic region [25,26]. FDG-PET is generally performed following an interictal injection. The sensitivity of interictal FDG-PET, which is indicated by regional hypometabolism, approaches that of ictal rCBF SPECT in localizing the epileptogenic region (Fig. 1). Seizure activity may originate in cortical areas bordering the hypometabolic regions rather than in the hypometabolic zone itself [27]. For interictal PET, FDG should be administered in a quiet setting where environmental stimuli are minimal and the child remains awake with minimal parental interaction during the uptake period. Sedatives are best withheld during this period to avoid untoward effects

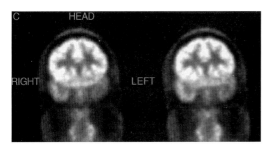

Fig. 1. Coronal images of the brain reveal significant hypometabolism in the left temporal lobe compared with the right side. This finding is typical in patients with temporal lobe epilepsy and correlates with other tests such as depth electrode recording. This pattern is seen in most patients with temporal lobe epilepsy, and imaging has replaced invasive procedures for definitive localization of seizure focus.

of sedation on cerebral metabolism. The relatively short half-life (110 minutes) of ^{18}F limits the window of opportunity during which it can be administered ictally. The approximately 30-minute uptake time of FDG may also depict a combination of the areas of seizure propagation and the actual seizure focus.

The use of FDG-PET in preoperative evaluation of epilepsy patients significantly reduces the need for intracranial electroencephalogram monitoring and the cost of preoperative evaluation [28,29]. The best results have been obtained in the localization of the epileptogenic focus within the temporal lobe origin [18,19]. Patients with bitemporal hypometabolism on FDG-PET have poor prognosis and are typically not candidates for resective surgery [30–33]. Use of FDG-PET in localizing extratemporal epileptogenic regions in children with intractable frontal lobe epilepsy and no structural abnormality has also been described [34].

FDG-PET is also helpful in the imaging evaluation of infantile spasms in which focal cortical areas of marked glucose hypometabolism are associated with malformative or dysplastic lesions not evident on anatomic imaging [35]. Incorporation of FDG-PET into the evaluation of children with infantile spasms has resulted in identification of a significant number of children who benefit from cortical resection.

PET radiotracers other than FDG that assess altered abundance or function of receptors, enzymes, and neurotransmitters have also been applied to localizing the epileptogenic region. Reduced uptake of carbon-11 ($[^{11}C]$)-flumazenil, a central benzodiazepine receptor antagonist, corresponds to the epileptogenic region, which may be smaller than the interictal hypometabolism on FDG-PET [36–39]. Decreased uptake of ^{11}C-labeled (S)-[*N*-methyl]ke-

tamine (which binds to the *N*-methyl-D-aspartate receptor-gated ion channel) and relative increases in uptake of $[^{11}C]$-carfentanil (a selective mu-opiate receptor agonist), and $[^{11}C]$-deprenyl (an irreversible inhibitor of monoamine oxidase type B) in epileptogenic areas have been described [40–42]. Other tracers such as α-$[^{11}C]$–methyl-L-tryptophan ($[^{11}C]$-AMT) may also differentiate between epileptogenic and nonepileptogenic tubers in patients with tuberous sclerosis [43].

Other neurologic applications

PET has been used to study the pathophysiology of many other childhood brain disorders such as Rasmussen's syndrome, hypoxic-ischemic encephalopathy, traumatic brain injury, autism, encephalitis, attention deficit hyperactivity disorder, schizophrenia, sickle cell encephalopathy, and anorexia and bulimia nervosa [44–55]. The exact role of PET in these clinical settings remains unclear, and further experience is needed.

Cardiac applications

Currently, PET plays a relatively minor role in pediatric cardiology. Cardiac applications of PET in children have been reviewed [56,57]. PET with nitrogen-13 ($[^{13}N]$)-ammonia has been employed to measure myocardial perfusion in infants after anatomic repair of congenital heart defects and after Norwood palliation for hypoplastic left heart syndrome [58]. Infants with repaired heart disease had higher resting blood flow and less coronary flow reserve than previously reported for adults. Infants with Norwood palliation had less perfusion and oxygen delivery to the systemic ventricle than infants with repaired congenital heart defect, which may explain in part the less favorable outcome for patients with Norwood palliation. Evaluation of myocardial perfusion with $[^{13}N]$-ammonia PET in infants following a neonatal arterial switch operation has demonstrated that patients with myocardial perfusion defects may have a more complicated postoperative course [59] (Fig. 2). PET can also assess the altered myocardial perfusion and impaired coronary flow reserve in patients with Fontan-like operations [60].

A major application of PET in adult cardiology is the assessment of myocardial viability with FDG. A recent study evaluated the regional glucose metabolism and contractile function by gated FDG-PET in infants and children after arterial switch operation and suspected myocardial infarction [61]. Gated FDG-

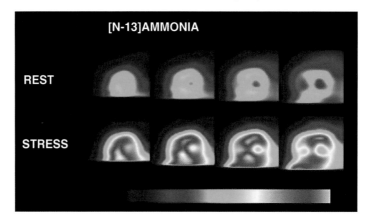

Fig. 2. A 27-day-old infant with D-transposition of the great vessels 13 days after repair. Images in the top row represent coronary perfusion at baseline. Images in the bottom row represent coronary perfusion following adenosine infusion. In this infant, the coronary flow reserve was approximately 1.5.

PET was found to contribute relevant information to guide additional therapy including a high-risk revascularization procedure. In another study, good agreement was documented between the findings on PET perfusion and metabolism imaging with those on coronary angiography, echocardiography, and histopathology in pediatric patients [62].

In children with Kawasaki disease, PET with [^{13}N]-ammonia and FDG showed abnormalities in about 60% of patients during the acute and subacute stages and in about 40% of patients during the convalescent stage of disease [63]. PET was specifically valuable in assessing the response to immunoglobulin therapy. PET has also been employed to study such fundamental functional abnormalities as mitochondrial dysfunction in children with hypertrophic and with dilated cardiomyopathy [64]. PET with [^{11}C]-acetate demonstrated reduced myocardial oxidative metabolism in children with cardiomyopathy despite normal myocardial perfusion. The diminished oxidative metabolism was associated with compensatory increased glycolysis activity as demonstrated on FDG-PET.

Although not yet studied extensively in children, PET scanning with tracers of the sympathetic nervous (eg, [^{11}C]-hydroxyephedrine) may be useful in helping identify which children with cardiomyopathies are at high risk for lethal dysrhythmias.

Applications in oncology

Cancer is second only to trauma as a cause of death in children [65]. The approximately 10% of deaths during childhood that are attributable to cancer

make it the leading cause of childhood disease-related death [66]. Of all the adult cancers to which FDG-PET has been most widely applied, only lymphomas and brain tumors occur with an appreciable incidence in children [3].

Before reviewing the applications of PET in pediatric oncology, it is important consider potential causes of misinterpretation of FDG-PET that relate to physiologic FDG distribution in children. The two important physiologic variations in FDG distribution encountered in children are the high FDG uptake in the thymus [67,68] and in the skeletal growth centers, particularly the long bone physes. Other potential pitfalls, similar to imaging in adults, include variable FDG uptake in working skeletal muscles, brown fat, myocardium, thyroid gland, and gastrointestinal tract, as well as accumulation of excreted FDG in the renal pelves, ureters, and bladder, and possible tracer accumulation in draining lymph nodes from extravasated tracer at the time of intravenous tracer administration [69–73]. Diffuse high FDG uptake in bone marrow and spleen following administration of hematopoietic stimulating factors may also resemble disseminated metastatic disease [74,75]. Elevated FDG uptake in bone marrow has been observed in patients as long as 4 weeks following completion of treatment with granulocyte colony-stimulating factor [74]. Thymic activity may also occasionally be elevated in a minority of young adults after chemotherapy because of reactive thymus hyperplasia [67,76]. Physiologic thymic hypermetabolism may also be seen in younger children before chemotherapy.

Some artifacts are unique to the relatively new combined PET/CT imaging systems. These artifacts may be caused by metallic objects, respiration, and oral and intravenous contrast agents. Overcorrection of dense metallic objects may result in hot-spot artifacts in the attenuation-corrected PET images [77]. Transient hot-spot artifacts may also be seen on PET as a result of the bolus passage of undiluted intravenous contrast material. The overestimation bias is modest (less than 15%) on the PET emission images of organs except for the kidneys, which may display higher bias [78]. Examination of the non–attenuation-corrected images can be helpful in distinguishing this technical artifact from physiologic/pathologic hypermetabolism. Attenuation correction of PET emission data using an artifactual CT map can yield false semiquantitative indices in the regions adjacent to metallic artifacts and probably in the presence of oral and intravenous contrasts [13].

Central nervous system tumors

Tumors of the central nervous system (CNS) account for about 20% of all pediatric cancers, second only to hematologic malignancies. The majority of pediatric brain tumors arise from neuro-epithelial tissue. CNS tumors are subclassified histopathologically by cell type and are graded for degree of malignancy using criteria that include mitotic activity, infiltration, and anaplasia [79,80].

The distribution of the most common CNS tumors may be categorized according to the major anatomic compartment involved. In the posterior fossa, medulloblastoma, cerebellar astrocytoma, ependymoma, and brain stem gliomas (Fig. 3) are most common. Tumors about the third ventricle include tumors that arise from suprasellar, pineal, and ventricular tissue. The most common neoplasms about the third ventricle are optic and hypothalamic gliomas, craniopharyngiomas, and germ cell tumors. Supratentorial tumors are most often astrocytomas, many of which are low grade [80]. MR imaging and CT are the principle imaging modalities used in staging and following children with CNS tumors. Their main limitation is distinguishing viable recurrent or residual tumor from posttherapy alterations. SPECT with thallium-201 ([^{201}Tl])- and [^{99m}Tc]-methoxyisobutylisonitrile (MIBI) have proven valuable for this determination in a number of pediatric brain tumors,

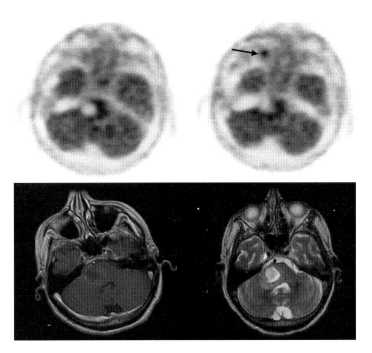

Fig. 3. (*Top row*) FDG-PET images of the brain at the cerebellar level reveal a large lesion in the pons that seems to have a central area of the hypometabolism surrounded by a rim of active tumor. This finding is suggestive of an aggressive tumor and generally predicts a poor prognosis. Because of the aggressive nature of this tumor, there is evidence of ocular muscle paralysis in the left orbit, but the ocular muscles in the right side seem to be within normal limits (*arrow*). (*Lower row*) Contrast-enhanced T1-weighted MR images of the brain show a hypointense lesion in the pons with a surrounding rim of mild enhancement. T2-weighted images show a hyperintense cystic area in the center of the enhanced lesion seen in the T1-weighted image.

generally demonstrating tracer uptake in the tumor and not in the scar tissue [81–84].

Use of FDG-PET in brain tumors has been widely reported in adult patients, and in these patients FDG-PET has helped distinguish viable tumor from post-therapeutic changes [85–87]. High FDG uptake relative to adjacent brain indicates residual or recurrent tumor, whereas low or absent FDG uptake is observed in areas of necrosis. This distinction is most readily made with high-grade tumors that show high uptake of FDG at diagnosis. FDG-PET does not, however, exclude microscopic tumor foci. FDG-PET results may also not accurately correlate with tumor progression after intensive radiation therapy [88]. Moreover, elevated FDG uptake may persist in the immediate posttherapy period [89]. The combined information from anatomic (MR) imaging and metabolic (PET) imaging has been shown to improve the diagnostic yield of stereotactic brain biopsy in children with infiltrative, ill-defined brain lesions while reducing tissue sampling in high-risk functional areas [90]. Moreover, FDG-PET has been applied to tumor grading and prognostication. Higher-grade aggressive tumors typically have higher FDG uptake than do lower-grade tumors, which may appear isometabolic or hypometabolic to the normal brain [91]. The development of hypermetabolism as evidenced by increased FDG uptake in a low-grade tumor that appeared hypometabolic at diagnosis indicates transformation to a higher grade [92]. The degree of FDG uptake seems to correlate with the biologic behavior of the tumor. Shorter survival times have been reported for patients whose tumors show the highest degree of FDG uptake [93]. Limited available data also suggest that FDG-PET findings correlate well with histopathology and clinical outcome in children [94–97]. A potential pediatric application entails a reported excellent correlation between FDG-PET findings and clinical outcome in children affected by neurofibromatosis who have low-grade astrocytomas [98].

Low-grade astrocytomas in patients with plexiform neurofibromatosis (NF$_1$) are often clinically silent, but some progress continuously, causing significant morbidity and even death. The objective of a prospective study designed as a collaborative effort between investigators at The Children's Hospital of Philadelphia and the Hospital of the University of Pennsylvania was to assess the diagnostic value of FDG uptake in NF$_1$-related low-grade astrocytomas and to compare tumor glucose uptake on PET imaging with clinical outcome. All patients had NF$_1$ and tumors of the optic pathways, thalamus, or brainstem. Patients were grouped initially into treatment versus no-treatment categories and then into stable-disease versus progressive-disease subgroups based on disease outcome. Tumor glucose uptake on FDG-PET was correlated with need for treatment, disease outcome, and histopathology.

Twenty-four patients were enrolled prospectively with a mean follow-up of 32.8 months. Thirteen of 14 patients (93%) in the no-treatment group had no increase in tumor glucose uptake on PET, a finding consistent with histologically proven benign tumors. Seven of 10 patients (70%) in the treatment group had increased tumor glucose uptake consistent with a malignant pathology. Sixteen of 17 patients (94%) with stable disease had no increased tumor glucose uptake, and seven patients (100%) with progressive disease had increased glucose uptake. Twenty-three of 24 patients (96%) had clinical outcomes (progressive disease versus stable disease) that correlated with tumor metabolic activity on FDG-PET ($P < 0.0005$). Three of four patients with pathologically proven low-grade astrocytomas had metabolically active tumors on PET despite benign histopathology. Based on these data, the authors believe that FDG-PET can accurately distinguish clinically stable astrocytomas from those with progressive growth. Tumor glucose uptake on [^{18}F]–FDG–PET correlated well with both need for treatment and clinical outcome and was not always supportive of histologic grade of tumor as determined by histologic examination. The latter finding also suggests that metabolic imaging may prove to be a reliable indicator of tumor activity (grade), and the information provided by FDG-PET should be taken into consideration in managing these patients (Fig. 4).

The role of FDG-PET imaging in the management of patients with NF$_1$ is unknown because of the limited level of experience that exists at this time. The authors have a relatively large sample of patients who underwent PET scans along with the standard techniques to assess the extent and the degree of disease activity in this population. Twenty-eight patients with clinical diagnosis of NF$_1$ were prospectively studied with a mean follow-up of 32.8 months. These patients were considered at high risk for progression; therefore the PET scan was ordered along with MR imaging to monitor disease activity over time. Based on clinical and radiologic examinations, the lesions were present in the face, neck, torso, and extremities. PET images in 24 of the 28 patients were correlated with MR scans which were performed within 3 months of the PET study. Index lesions were identified in 15 of the 28 patients. Correlation to MR scan results was made on a lesion-by-lesion basis when possible. In 4 of 28 patients,

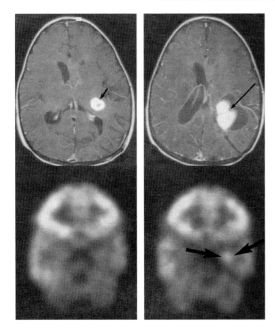

Fig. 4. The image on the left upper column represents a T1-weighted gadolinium-enhanced axial MR image that demonstrates a tumor in the left optic radiations. Based on clinical evaluation, this lesion was considered an inactive lesion. (*Right, upper column*) Follow-up MR imaging 1 year later demonstrates tumor progression at the same site. (*Left, lower column*) The initial FDG-PET image demonstrates no detectable area of increased glucose uptake corresponding to the lesion on MR imaging. This absence of increased uptake would indicate inactive disease. There is significant hypometabolism in the cerebellum, a common finding in patients with optic glioma. (*Right, lower column*) A follow-up FDG-PET image acquired 1 year later demonstrates increased glucose metabolism at the site of the tumor, indicating transformation of a low-grade tumor to a high-grade tumor during this interval.

there were no visible abnormal sites of focal uptake on PET images. In the remaining 24 patients, varying degrees of focal FDG uptake were noted and were correlated with the lesions seen on MR imaging. MR scans revealed all the known lesions but were unable to determine the disease activity based on the parameters established for this modality. Fewer lesions were detected by PET images than by MR scans. The SUV ranged from 1.0 to 4.0 on lesions identified on PET. The low sensitivity of PET was attributed to the varying degree of disease activity of the lesions noted on MR imaging. In other words, lesions that were not visualized on PET images were considered to be inactive and stable at the time of examination. A preliminary analysis of these data suggested that tumor FDG uptake on PET may

predict tumor growth better than histopathologic features. FDG-PET has the promise for following the course of the disease in patients with NF_1 (Fig. 5).

Another positron-emitting radiotracer that has been used to study pediatric brain tumors is the radiolabeled amino acid [^{11}C]-methionine ([^{11}C]-MET), which localizes to only a minimal degree in normal brain. Uptake of this radiotracer reflects transmethylation pathways that are present in some tumors. As with FDG, however, some low-grade gliomas may escape detection without clear limits of tumor-to-normal brain ratios that can accurately assess malignancy grade [99–101]. [^{11}C]-MET–PET has been reported to be useful in differentiating viable tumor from therapy-induced changes [99,102]. Like FDG, however, [^{11}C]-MET is not tumor specific because it has been shown to accumulate in some nontumoral CNS diseases, probably as a result of disruption of the blood–brain barrier [103]. Because of the relatively short 20-minute half-life of the ^{11}C label, [^{11}C]-MET must be produced locally for administration and is currently not commercially available.

Lymphoma

Non-Hodgkin's and Hodgkin's lymphomas account for between 10% and 15% of pediatric malignancies. Non-Hodgkin's lymphoma occurs throughout childhood. Lymphoblastic and small-cell tumors, including Burkitt's lymphoma, are the most common histologic types. The disease is usually widespread at diagnosis. Mediastinal and hilar involvement are common with lymphoblastic lymphoma. Burkitt's lymphoma most often occurs in the abdomen. Hodgkin's disease has a peak incidence during adolescence. Nodular sclerosing and mixed cellularity are the most common histologic types. The disease is rarely widespread at diagnosis, and the majority of cases have intrathoracic nodal involvement (Fig. 6) [65,104].

Gallium-67 ([^{67}Ga])-citrate scintigraphy has proven useful in staging and monitoring therapeutic response in patients with non-Hodgkin's and Hodgkin's lymphomas [105–109]. In numerous studies that predominantly included adult patients, FDG has been shown to accumulate in non-Hodgkin's and Hodgkin's lymphomas [69,110–134]. Similar to [^{67}Ga]-citrate, FDG uptake is generally greater in higher-grade lymphomas than in lower-grade lymphomas [117,119]. FDG-PET has been reported to reveal disease sites that are not detected by conventional staging methods, resulting in upstaging of disease with potential therapeutic ramifications

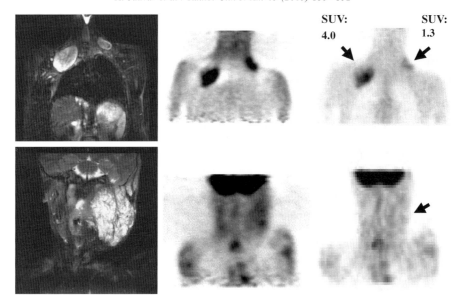

Fig. 5. (*Top row, left*) MR image of a 15-year-old male with neurofibromatosis demonstrates bilateral masses at the brachial plexi that are more prominent on the right side. The appearance of the abnormality cannot differentiate between active and inactive disease and therefore is nonspecific for assessing the state of the tumor at the time. (*Top row, middle and right*) FDG-PET scans of the same patient demonstrate increased uptake in both sides with more intense activity in the lesion on the right side than in the lesion on the left side (the middle image is not attenuation corrected, and the image on the right is attenuation corrected). The SUVs for the right and the left lesions are 4.0 and 1.3, respectively, which match the level of intensity seen on the scans. (*Lower row, left*) An MR image of an 8-year-old boy with neurofibromatosis reveals an extensive infiltrative mass in the left neck region that occupies most of the left neck. (*Lower row, middle and left*) Corresponding PET images demonstrate a mild degree of FDG uptake (*arrows*, SUV of 1.3) compared with the 15-year-old boy. These images demonstrate that the level of disease activity can be best assessed by combining structural and functional images.

[114,115,120–122]. Identification of areas of intense FDG uptake within the bone marrow can be particularly useful in directing the site of biopsy or even eliminating the need for biopsy at staging [115,128]. FDG-PET is also useful for assessing residual soft tissue masses shown by CT after therapy. Absence of FDG uptake in a residual mass is predictive of re-

mission, whereas high uptake indicates residual or recurrent tumor [122,130].

FDG-PET has been compared with [^{11}C]-MET–PET in a relatively small series of 14 patients with non-Hodgkin's lymphoma. [^{11}C]-MET–PET provided superior tumor-to-background contrast, whereas FDG-PET was superior in distinguishing between

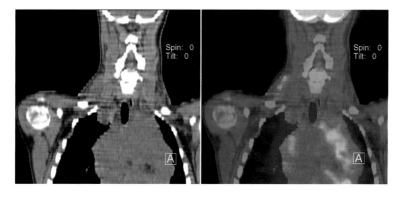

Fig. 6. A 14-year-old female with newly diagnosed Hodgkin's lymphoma confirmed by biopsy of a right cervical lymph node. PET/CT shows abnormal hypermetabolism involving the nodal basins of the right posterior cervical triangle and the anterior and superior mediastinum.

Before Therapy   **After Therapy**

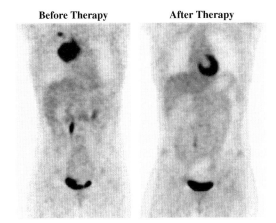

Fig. 7. An adolescent patient with non-Hodgkin's lymphoma. The image on the left demonstrates a large, round area of intense uptake that extends from mid-mediastinum to the right upper lung. In addition, there is a focal area of uptake in the right supraclavicular region that is also suggestive of an involved lymph node. The image on the right, which was obtained 3 months later following chemotherapy, reveals complete resolution of the involved sites. This finding is in general predictive of complete remission and therefore a good outcome in patients with lymphoma.

high- and low-grade lymphomas [113]. In summary, the existing relatively large body of evidence indicates that PET will play an increasingly important role in staging, evaluating tumor response, planning radiation treatment fields, and monitoring after completion of therapy in pediatric lymphoma (Fig. 7) [135–137].

Neuroblastoma

Neuroblastoma is the most common extracranial solid malignant tumor in children. The mean age of patients at presentation is 20 to 30 months, and it is rare after the age of 5 years [104]. The adrenal glands are the most common site of neuroblastoma. Other sites of origin include the paravertebral and presacral sympathetic chain, the organ of Zuckerkandl, posterior mediastinal sympathetic ganglia, and cervical sympathetic plexuses. Gross or microscopic calcification is often present in the tumor. Disseminated disease is present in up to 70% of neuroblastoma cases at diagnosis and most commonly involves cortical bone and bone marrow (Fig. 8). Less frequently, there is involvement of liver, skin, and lung. A primary tumor is not detected in up to 10% of children with disseminated neuroblastoma or in those who present with paraneoplastic syndromes [138].

Surgical excision is the preferred treatment of localized neuroblastoma. When local disease is ex-

tensive, intensive preoperative chemotherapy may be used. When distant metastases are present, prognosis is poor, but high-dose chemotherapy, total-body irradiation, and bone marrow reinfusion are beneficial for some children with this presentation.

Delineation of local disease extent is achieved with MR imaging, CT, and scintigraphy. These tests are also used in localizing the primary site in children who present with disseminated disease or with paraneoplastic syndrome. Metaiodobenzylguanidine (MIBG, an analogue of guanethidine and norepinephrine) and indium-111 ([^{111}In])-pentetreotide (somatostatin type 2 receptor agonist) scintigraphy have been employed in these settings with a sensitivity greater than 85% for detecting neuroblastoma. Uptake of MIBG into neuroblastoma is by a neuronal sodium- and energy-dependent transport mechanism. The localization of [^{111}In]-pentetreotide in neuroblastoma reflects the presence of somatostatin receptors on some neuroblastoma cells [139].

Bone scintigraphy has been most widely used to detect skeletal involvement for staging but is unable to distinguish active disease from bony repair on the basis of tracer uptake. Patients with residual unresected primary tumors are periodically evaluated with

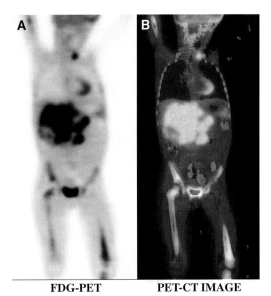

        FDG-PET   **PET-CT IMAGE**

Fig. 8. A 30-month-old girl who presented with leg pain and a limp. (*A*) A coronal image from an FDG-PET scan shows markedly increased uptake of FDG in the left lower neck, the right abdomen crossing the midline, the right ilium, both femurs, and the left proximal tibia. Normal myocardial and bladder activity are present. (*B*) A fusion image of the corresponding CT scan superimposed on the PET scan shown in A.

MR imaging or CT. These studies, however, cannot distinguish viable tumor from treatment-related scar. Specificity in establishing residual viable tumor can be improved with MIBG or [111In]-pentetreotide imaging when the primary tumor has been shown to accumulate one of these agents. These agents are also useful in assessing residual skeletal disease in patients with MIBG- or [111In]-pentetreotide–avid skeletal metastases. Neuroblastomas are metabolically active tumors. Neuroblastomas or their metastases avidly concentrated FDG before chemotherapy or radiation therapy in 16 of 17 patients studied with FDG-PET and MIBG imaging [140]. Uptake after therapy was variable but tended to be lower. FDG and MIBG results were concordant in most instances, but there were few discordant cases in which one tracer accumulated at a site of disease and the other did not. Overall, MIBG imaging was considered superior to FDG-PET, particularly in delineation of residual disease. An advantage of FDG-PET is the initiation of imaging 30 to 60 minutes after FDG administration. MIBG imaging is performed 1 or more days following tracer administration.

FDG-PET may be limited for the evaluation of the bone marrow involvement of neuroblastoma because of mild FDG accumulation by the normal bone marrow [140]. Pitfalls resulting from physiologic FDG uptake in the bowel and the thymus are additional factors that may limit the role for FDG-PET in neuroblastoma. Currently the primary role of FDG-PET in neuroblastoma is in the evaluation of known or suspected neuroblastomas that do not demonstrate MIBG uptake.

[11C]-hydroxyephedrine ([11C]-HED), an analogue of norepinephrine, and [11C]-epinephrine PET have also been used in evaluating neuroblastoma. All seven neuroblastomas studied showed uptake of [11C]-HED [141] and four of five neuroblastomas studied showed uptake of [11C]-epinephrine [142]. Uptake of these tracers is demonstrated within

minutes after tracer administration, an advantage over MIBG imaging. Practical current limitations regarding cost and the need for on-site synthesis of short-lived [11C] (half-life of 20 minutes) hinder their clinical utility, however. Compounds labeled with [18F], such as fluoronorepinephrine, fluorometaraminol, and fluorodopamine, may also be useful tracers. PET using 4-[18F]fluoro-3-iodobenzylguanidine [143] and iodine-124–labeled MIBG [144] has also been described.

Wilms' tumor

Wilms' tumor is the most common renal malignancy of childhood. Wilms' tumor is predominantly seen in younger children and is uncommonly encountered after the age of 5 years [65]. Bilateral renal involvement occurs in about 5% of all cases and can be identified synchronously or metachronously [104,145]. An asymptomatic abdominal mass is the typical mode of presentation. Nephrectomy with adjuvant chemotherapy is the treatment of choice. Radiation therapy is used in selected cases when resection is incomplete.

Radiography, ultrasonography, CT, and MR imaging are commonly employed in anatomic staging and detection of metastases, which predominantly involve lung, occasionally liver, and only rarely other sites (Fig. 9). Anatomic imaging, however, is limited in the assessment for residual or recurrent tumor [145]. Uptake of FDG by Wilms' tumor has been described [146], but a role for FDG-PET in Wilms' tumor has not been established. Normal excretion of FDG through the kidney is also a limiting factor, but careful correlation with anatomic cross-sectional imaging usually allows tumor uptake to be distinguished from normal renal FDG excretion. The authors have found FDG-PET most useful in identifying active tumor in residual masses that persist following radiation or chemotherapy.

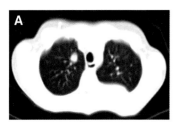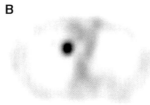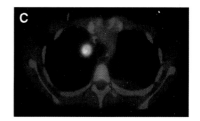

Fig. 9. A 12-year-old girl who presented with Wilms' tumor metastatic to the lungs 2 years previously. The tumor progressed despite chemotherapy. (*A*) Concurrent chest CT showing right lung nodule. (*B*) FDG-PET scan at same location showing markedly increased uptake of FDG within the right lung nodule. (*C*) Fusion of A and B.

Bone tumors

Osteosarcoma and Ewing's sarcoma are the two primary bone malignancies of childhood. Osteosarcoma is more common and predominantly affects adolescents and young adults with a second peak in older adults, principally individuals with a history of prior radiation to bone or Paget's disease. This tumor rarely affects children younger than 7 years of age. Osteosarcoma is typically a lesion of the long bones. The treatment of choice for osteosarcoma of an extremity is wide resection and limb-sparing surgery, which involves resection of tumor with a cuff of surrounding normal tissue at all margins and skeletal reconstruction. Limb-sparing procedures can be appropriately performed in 80% of patients by using the current chemotherapeutic regimens pre- and postoperatively and using imaging to define tumor extent and viability [147].

Almost all cases of Ewing's sarcoma occur between the ages of 5 and 30 years, with the highest incidence being in the second decade of life. In patients younger than 20 years, Ewing's sarcoma most often affects the appendicular skeleton (Fig. 10). Beyond that age, pelvic, rib, and vertebral lesions predominate. The tumor is believed to be of neuroectodermal origin and, along with the primitive neuroectodermal tumor, to be part of a spectrum of a single biologic entity [148]. Therapy for Ewing's sarcoma involves irradiation or surgery for control of the primary lesion and multiagent chemotherapy for eradication of metastatic disease [149].

MR imaging is used to define the local extent of osteosarcoma and Ewing's sarcoma in bone and soft tissue. Signal abnormalities caused by peritumoral edema can result in an overestimation of tumor extension, however [150]. Scintigraphy has been used primarily to detect osseous metastases of these tumors at diagnosis and during follow-up. With osteosarcoma, skeletal scintigraphy occasionally demonstrates extraosseous metastases, most often

pulmonary, resulting from osteoid production by the metastatic deposits. Because of the nonspecific appearance of viable tumor on MR imaging, variable results have been reported for assessing chemotherapeutic response in planning for limb-salvage surgery [151–156]. Scintigraphy with ^{201}Tl has been shown to be useful for assessing therapeutic response in osteosarcoma and Ewing's sarcoma [157–162]. Marked decrease in ^{201}Tl uptake by the tumor indicates a favorable response to chemotherapy. A change in therapy may be needed when tumor ^{201}Tl uptake does not decrease within weeks of chemotherapy. [^{99m}Tc]-MIBI may also be useful in osteosarcoma but seemingly not in Ewing's sarcoma [163,164].

The exact roles of FDG-PET in osteosarcoma and Ewing's sarcoma are unclear. Current experience, however, suggests that in patients with bone sarcomas, FDG-PET may play an important role in monitoring response to therapy (Fig. 11) [165–168]. Another diagnostic role may be in assessing patients with suspected metastatic disease; this assessment may have important therapeutic ramifications.

Soft tissue tumors

Rhabdomyosarcoma is the most common soft tissue malignancy of childhood. The peak incidence occurs between 3 and 6 years of age. Rhabdomyosarcomas can develop in any organ or tissue, and, contrary to what the name implies, do not usually arise in muscle. The most common anatomic locations are the head, particularly the orbit and paranasal sinuses, the neck, and the genitourinary tract. CT or MR imaging is important for establishing the extent of local disease. Radiography and CT are used to detect pulmonary metastases, and skeletal scintigraphy is used to identifyi osseous metastases. Radiation therapy and surgery are used to controllocal disease, and chemotherapy is used to treat metastatic disease. Rhabdomyosarcomas show varia-

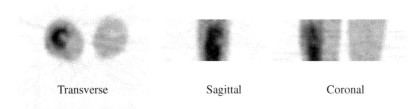

Transverse   Sagittal   Coronal

Fig. 10. This patient with Ewing's sarcoma in the right mid-femur demonstrates intense uptake that can be visualized in all three planes. The tumor seems to spare the medial aspect of the bone.

H. Jadvar et al / Radiol Clin N Am 43 (2005) 135–152

First PET   **Second PET**

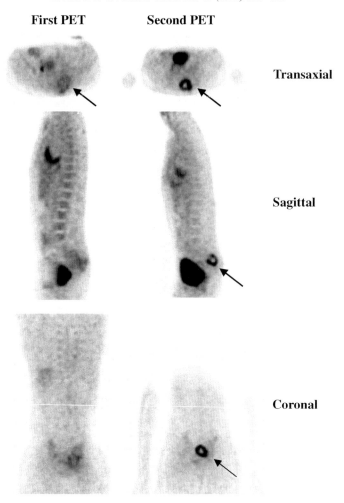

Fig. 11. (*Left*) The first set of images was obtained soon after the diagnosis of osteogenic sarcoma to the left sacrum adjacent to the sacroiliac joint. FDG-PET images reveal mild to moderately increased metabolic activity that is poorly defined on these initial images. (*Right*) The second set of images was acquired 3 months later and demonstrates intense uptake in the lesion with evidence of central necrosis (*arrows*). This intense uptake was interpreted as representing progression of the disease.

ble degrees of FDG accumulation. There are reports of diagnostic utility, but the exact clinical role of FDG-PET in rhabdomyosarcoma is currently not established [7,165,169].

Summary

FDG-PET is being increasingly applied to pediatric conditions, particularly in oncology. PET and PET/CT scanning in children are not currently supported by Centers for Medicare and Medicaid Services unless the disease condition coincides with a reimbursed adult condition. The recent merger of the Children's Cancer Group and the Pediatric Oncology Group to form the Children's Oncology Group creates an opportunity to examine the use of FDG-PET in the management of childhood tumors in multi-institutional, cooperative efforts. The interest in incorporating PET imaging technology in pediatric medicine has been evidenced by several recent review articles summarizing the ongoing progress in this area [170–172]. Future data will show that FDG-PET provides useful diagnostic information and can play a pivotal role in the clinical management and care of children with disease.

References

[1] Gordon I. Issues surrounding preparation, information, and handling the child and parent in nuclear medicine. J Nucl Med 1998;39:490–4.

[2] Treves ST. Introduction. In: Treves ST, editor. Pediatric nuclear medicine. 2nd edition. New York: Springer-Verlag; 1995. p. 1–11.

[3] Shulkin BL. PET imaging in pediatric oncology. Pediatr Radiol 2004;34:199–204.

[4] Mandell GA, Cooper JA, Majd M, et al. Procedure guidelines for pediatric sedation in nuclear medicine. J Nucl Med 1997;38:1640–3.

[5] American Academy of Pediatrics. Committee on Drugs. Guidelines for monitoring and management of pediatric patients during and after sedation for diagnostic and therapeutic procedures. Pediatrics 1992;89:1110–5.

[6] American Society of Anesthesiologists Task Force on Sedation and Analgesia by Non-anesthesiologists. Practice guidelines for sedation and analgesia by non-anesthesiologists. Anesthesiology 1996;84:459–71.

[7] Shulkin BL. PET applications in pediatrics. Q J Nucl Med 1997;41:281–91.

[8] Townsend DW, Beyer T. A combined PET-CT scanner: the path to true image fusion. Br J Radiol 2002; 75(Suppl):S24–30.

[9] Kaste SC. Issues specific to implementing PET-CT for pediatric oncology: what we have learned along the way. Pediatr Radiol 2004;34:205–13.

[10] Borgwardt L, Larsen HJ, Pedersen K, et al. Practical use and implementation of PET in children in a hospital PET center. Eur J Nucl Med Mol Imaging 2003;30(10):1389–97.

[11] Beyer T, Antoch G, Muller S, et al. Acquisition protocol considerations for combined PET/CT imaging. J Nucl Med 2004;45(Suppl 1):25S–35S.

[12] Cohade C, Wahl RL. Applications of positron emission tomography/computed tomography image fusion in clinical positron emission tomography—clinical use, interpretation methods, diagnostic improvements. Semin Nucl Med 2003;33(3):228–37.

[13] Visvikis D, Costa DC, Croasdale I, et al. CT-based attenuation correction in the calculation of semi-quantitative indices of [18F]FDG uptake in PET. Eur J Nucl Med Mol Imaging 2003;30(3):344–53.

[14] Nehmeh SA, Erdi YE, Kalaigian H, et al. Correction for oral contrast artifacts in CT attenuation-corrected PET images obtained by combined PET/CT. J Nucl Med 2003;44(12):1940–4.

[15] Dizendorf EV, Treyer V, von Schulthess GK, et al. Application of oral contrast media in coregistered positron emission tomography-CT. AJR Am J Roentgenol 2002;179(12):477–81.

[16] Yeung HW, Sanches A, Squire OD, et al. Standardized uptake value (SUV) in pediatric patients: an investigation to determine the optimum measurement parameter. Eur J Nucl Med Mol Imaging 2002;29(1): 61–6.

[17] Schelbert H, Hoh CK, Royal HD, et al. Procedure guideline for tumor imaging using Fluorine-18-FDG. J Nucl Med 1998;39:1302–5.

[18] Jones SC, Alavi A, Christman D, et al. The radiation dosimetry of 2-[18F]fluoro-2-deoxy-D-glucose in man. J Nucl Med 1982;23:613–7.

[19] Ruotsalainen U, Suhonen-Povli H, Eronen E, et al. Estimated radiation dose to the newborn in FDG-PET studies. J Nucl Med 1996;37:387–93.

[20] Chugani HT, Phelps ME. Maturational changes in cerebral function in infants determined by 18FDG positron emission tomography. Science 1986;231: 840–3.

[21] Chugani HT, Phelps ME, Mazziotta JC. Positron emission tomography study of human brain functional development. Ann Neurol 1987;22:487–97.

[22] Chugani HT. Positron emission tomography. In: Berg BO, editor. Principles of child neurology. New York: McGraw-Hill; 1996. p. 113–28.

[23] Kuzniecky R, Suggs S, Gaudier J, et al. Lateralization of epileptic foci by magnetic resonance imaging in temporal lobe epilepsy. J Neuroimaging 1991;1: 163–7.

[24] Treves ST, Connolly LP. Single photon emission computed tomography in pediatric epilepsy. Neurosurg Clin N Am 1995;6:473–80.

[25] Snead III OC, Chen LS, Mitchell WG, et al. Usefulness of [18F]fluorodeoxyglucose positron emission tomography in pediatric epilepsy surgery. Pediatr Neurol 1996;14:98–107.

[26] Meltzer CC, Adelson PD, Brenner RP, et al. Planned ictal FDG-PET imaging for localization of extratemporal epileptic foci. Epilepsia 2000;41(2):193–200.

[27] Juhasz C, Chugani DC, Muzik O, et al. Is epileptogenic cortex truly hypometabolic on interictal positron emission tomography? Ann Neurol 2000;48(1): 88–96.

[28] Cummings TJ, Chugani DC, Chugani HT. Positron emission tomography in pediatric epilepsy. Neurosurg Clin N Am 1995;6:465–72.

[29] Engel Jr J, Kuhl DE, Phelps ME. Patterns of human local cerebral glucose metabolism during epileptogenic seizures. Science 1982;218:64–6.

[30] Chugani HT, Shields WD, Shewmon DA, et al. Infantile spasms: I. PET identifies focal cortical dysgenesis in cryptogenic cases for surgical treatment. Ann Neurol 1990;27:406–13.

[31] Chuagni HT, Shewmon DA, Shields WD, et al. Surgery for intractable infantile spasms: neuroimaging perspectives. Epilepsia 1993;34:764–71.

[32] Chugani HT, Da Silva E, Chugani DC. Infantile spasms: III. Prognostic implications of bitemporal hypometabolism on positron emission tomography. Ann Neurol 1996;39:643–9.

[33] Chugani HT, Conti JR. Etiologic classification of infantile spasms in 140 cases: role of positron emission tomography. J Child Neurol 1996;11:44–8.

[34] da Silva EA, Chugani DC, Muzik O, et al. Identification of frontal lobe epileptic foci in children using

positron emission tomography. Epilepsia 1997;38: 1198–208.

[35] Hrachovy R, Frost J. Infantile spasms. Pediatr Clin North Am 1989;36:311–29.

[36] Savic I, Svanborg E, Thorell JO. Cortical benzodiazepine receptor changes are related to frequency of partial seizures: a positron emission tomography study. Epilepsia 1996;37:236–44.

[37] Arnold S, Berthele A, Drzezga A, et al. Reduction of benzodiazepine receptor binding is related to the seizure onset zone in extratemporal focal cortical dysplasia. Epilepsia 2000;41(7):818–24.

[38] Richardson MP, Koepp MJ, Brooks DJ, et al. 11C-flumanezil PET in neocortical epilepsy. Neurology 1998;51:485–92.

[39] Debets RM, Sadzot B, van Isselt JW, et al. Is 11C-flumazenil PET superior to 18FDG-PET and 123I-iomazenial SPECT in presurgical evaluation of temporal lobe epilepsy? J Neurol Neurosurg Psychiatry 1997;62:141–50.

[40] Kumlien E, Hartvig P, Valind S, et al. NMDA-receptor activity visualized with (S)-[N-methyl-11-C]ketamine and positron emission tomography in patients with medial temporal epilepsy. Epilepsia 1999;40:30–7.

[41] Mayberg HS, Sadzot B, Meltzer CC, et al. Quantification of mu and non-mu opiate receptors in temporal lobe epilepsy using positron emission tomography. Ann Neurol 1991;30:3–11.

[42] Kumlien E, Bergstrom M, Lilja A, et al. Positron emission tomography with [C-11]deuterium deprenyl in temporal lobe epilepsy. Epilepsia 1995;36:712–21.

[43] Chuagani DC, Chugani HT, Muzik O, et al. Imaging epileptogenic tubers in children with tuberous sclerosis complex using alpha-[C-11]methyl-L-tryptophan positron emission tomography. Ann Neurol 1998;44:858–66.

[44] Volpe JJ, Herscovitch P, Perlman JM, et al. Positron emission tomography in the newborn: extensive impairment of regional cerebral blood flow with intraventricular hemorrhage and hemorrhagic intracerebral involvement. Pediatrics 1983;72(5):589–601.

[45] Volpe JJ, Herscovitch P, Perlman JM, et al. Positron emission tomography in the asphyxiated term newborn: parasagittal impairment of cerebral blood flow. Ann Neurol 1985;17(3):287–96.

[46] Zilbovicius M, Boddaert N, Belin P, et al. Temporal lobe dysfunction in childhood autism: a PET study. Am J Psychiatry 2000;157(12):1988–93.

[47] Ernst M, Zametkin AJ, Matochik JA, et al. High midbrain [18F]DOPA accumulation in children with attention deficit hyperactivity disorder. Am J Psychiatry 1999;156(8):1209–15.

[48] Jacobson LK, Hamburger SD, Van Horn JD, et al. Cerebral glucose metabolism in childhood onset schizophrenia. Psychiatry Res 1997;75(3):131–44.

[49] Reed W, Jagust W, Al-Mateen M, et al. Role of positron emission tomography in determining the extent of CNS ischemia in patients with sickle cell disease. Am J Hematol 1999;60(4):268–72.

[50] Delvenne V, Lotstra F, Goldman S, et al. Brain hypometabolism of glucose in anorexia nervosa: a PET scan study. Biol Psychiatry 1995;37(3):161–9.

[51] Delvenne V, Goldman S, Simon Y, et al. Brain hypometabolism of glucose in bulimia nervosa. Int J Eat Disord 1997;21(4):313–20.

[52] Lee JS, Juhasz C, Kaddurah AK, et al. Patterns of cerebral glucose metabolism in early and late stages of Rasmussen's syndrome. J Child Neurol 2001; 16(11):798–805.

[53] Worley G, Hoffman JM, Paine SS, et al. 18-fluorodeoxyglucose positron emission tomography in children and adolescents with traumatic brain injury. Dev Med Child Neurol 1995;37(3):213–20.

[54] Yanai K, Iinuma K, Matsuzawa T, et al. Cerebral glucose utilization in pediatric neurological disorders determined by positron emission tomography. Eur J Nucl Med 1987;13(6):292–6.

[55] Mohan KK, Chugani DC, Chugani HT. Positron emission tomography in pediatric neurology. Semin Pediatr Neurol 1999;6(2):111–9.

[56] Schelbert HR, Schwaiger M, Phelps ME. Positron computed tomography and its applications in the young. J Am Coll Cardiol 1985;5(1 Suppl):140S–9S.

[57] Quinlivan RM, Robinson RO, Maisey MN. Positron emission tomography in pediatric cardiology. Arch Dis Child 1998;79(6):520–2.

[58] Donnelly JP, Raffel DM, Shulkin BL, et al. Resting coronary flow and coronary flow reserve in human infants after repair or palliation of congenital heart defects as measured by positron emission tomography. J Thorac Cardiovasc Surg 1998;115(1):103–10.

[59] Yates RW, Marsden PK, Badawi RD, et al. Evaluation of myocardial perfusion using positron emission tomography in infants following a neonatal arterial switch operation. Pediatr Cardiol 2000;21(2):111–8.

[60] Hauser M, Bengel FM, Kuhn A, et al. Myocardial perfusion and coronary flow reserve assessed by positron emission tomography in patients after Fontan-like operations. Pediatr Cardiol 2003;24(4): 386–92.

[61] Rickers C, Sasse K, Buchert R, et al. Myocardial viability assessed by positron emission tomography in infants and children after the arterial switch operation and suspected infarction. J Am Coll Cardiol 2000;36(5):1676–83.

[62] Hernandez-Pampaloni M, Allada V, Fishbein MC, et al. Myocardial perfusion and viability by positron emission tomography in infants and children with coronary abnormalities: correlation with echocardiography, coronary angiography, and histopathology. J Am Coll Cardiol 2003;41(4):618–26.

[63] Hwang B, Liu RS, Chu LS, et al. Positron emission tomography for the assessment of myocardial viability in Kawasaki disease using different therapies. Nucl Med Commun 2000;21(7):631–6.

[64] Litvinova I, Litvinov M, Loeonteva I, et al. PET for diagnosis of mitochondrial cardiomyopathy in children. Clin Positron Imaging 2000;3(4):172.

[65] Gurney JG, Severson RK, Davis S, et al. Incidence of cancer in children in the United States. Cancer 1995;75:2186–95.

[66] Robison L. General principles of the epidemiology of childhood cancer. In: Pizzo P, Poplack D, editors. Principles and practice of pediatric oncology. Philadelphia: Lippincott-Raven; 1997. p. 1–10.

[67] Weinblatt ME, Zanzi I, Belakhlef A, et al. False-positive FDG-PET imaging of the thymus of a child with Hodgkin's disease. J Nucl Med 1997;38: 888–90.

[68] Patel PM, Alibazoglu H, Ali A, et al. Normal thymic uptake of FDG on PET imaging. Clin Nucl Med 1996;21:772–5.

[69] Delbeke D. Oncological applications of FDG-PET imaging: colorectal cancer, lymphoma, and melanoma. J Nucl Med 1999;40:591–603.

[70] Yeung HW, Grewal RK, Gonen M, et al. Patterns of (18)F-FDG uptake in adipose tissue and muscle: a potential source of false-positives for PET. J Nucl Med 2003;44(11):1789–96.

[71] Minotti AJ, Shah L, Keller K. Positron emission tomography/computed tomography fusion imaging in brown adipose tissue. Clin Nucl Med 2004;29(1): 5–11.

[72] Hany TF, Gharehpapagh E, Kamel EM, et al. Brown adipose tissue: a factor to consider in symmetrical tracer uptake in the neck and upper chest region. Eur J Nucl Med Mol Imaging 2002;29:1393–8.

[73] Cohade C, Osman M, Pannu HK, et al. Uptake in supraclavicular area fat ("USA-Fat"): description on 18F-FDG-PET/CT. J Nucl Med 2003;44:170–6.

[74] Sugawara Y, Fisher SJ, Zasadny KR, et al. Preclinical and clinical studies of bone marrow uptake of fluorine-1-fluorodeoxyglucose with or without granulocyte colony-stimulating factor during chemotherapy. J Clin Oncol 1998;16:173–80.

[75] Hollinger EF, Alibazoglu H, Ali A, et al. Hematopoietic cytokine-mediated FDG uptake simulates the appearance of diffuse metastatic disease on whole-body PET imaging. Clin Nucl Med 1998;23:93–8.

[76] Brink I, Reinhardt MJ, Hoegerle S, et al. Increased metabolic activity in the thymus gland studied with 18F-FDG-PET: age dependency and frequency after chemotherapy. J Nucl Med 2001;42:591–5.

[77] Bujenovic S, Mannting F, Chakrabarti R, et al. Artifactual 2-deoxy-2-[(18)F]fluoro-D-deoxyglucose localization surrounding metallic objects in a PET/CT scanner using CT-based attenuation correction. Mol Imaging Biol 2003;5:20–2.

[78] Nakamoto Y, Chin RB, Kraitchman DL, et al. effects of nonionic intravenous contrast agents at PET/CT imaging: phantom and canine studies. Radiology 2003;227:817–24.

[79] Kleihues P, Burger P, Scheithauer B. The new WHO classification of brain tumors. Brain Pathol 1993;3: 255–68.

[80] Robertson R, Ball WJ, Barnes P. Skull and brain. In: Kirks D, editor. Practical pediatric imaging. Diagnostic radiology of infants and children. Philadelphia: Lippincott-Raven; 1997. p. 65–200.

[81] Maria B, Drane WB, Quisling RJ, et al. Correlation between gadolinium-diethylenetriaminepentaacetic acid contrast enhancement and thallium-201 chloride uptake in pediatric brainstem glioma. J Child Neurol 1997;12:341–8.

[82] O'Tuama L, Janicek M, Barnes P, et al. Tl-201/Tc-99m HMPAO SPECT imaging of treated childhood brain tumors. Pediatr Neurol 1991;7:249–57.

[83] O'Tuama L, Treves ST, Larar G, et al. Tl-201 versus Tc-99m MIBI SPECT in evaluation of childhood brain tumors. J Nucl Med 1993;34:1045–51.

[84] Rollins N, Lowry P, Shapiro K. Comparison of gadolinium-enhanced MR and thallium-201 single photon emission computed tomography in pediatric brain tumors. Pediatr Neurosurg 1995;22:8–14.

[85] Valk PE, Budinger TF, Levin VA, et al. PET of malignant cerebral tumors after interstitial brachytherapy. Demonstration of metabolic activity and correlation with clinical outcome. J Neurosurg 1988;69: 830–8.

[86] Di Chiro G, Oldfield E, Wright DC, et al. Cerebral necrosis after radiotherapy and/or intraarterial chemotherapy for brain tumors: PET and neuropathologic studies. AJR Am J Roentgenol 1988;150:189–97.

[87] Glantz MJ, Hoffman JM, Coleman RE, et al. Identification of early recurrence of primary central nervous system tumors by [18F]fluorodeoxyglucose positron emission tomograph. Ann Neurol 1991;29: 347–55.

[88] Janus T, Kim E, Tilbury R, et al. Use of [18F] fluorodeoxyglucose positron emission tomography in patients with primary malignant brain tumors. Ann Neurol 1993;33:540–8.

[89] Rozental JM, Levine RL, Nickles RJ. Changes in glucose uptake by malignant gliomas: preliminary study of prognostic significance. J Neurooncol 1991; 10:75–83.

[90] Pirotte B, Goldman S, Salzberg S, et al. Combined positron emission tomography and magnetic resonance imaging for the planning of stereotactic brain biopsies in children: experience in 9 cases. Pediatr Neurosurg 2003;38(3):146–55.

[91] Schifter T, Hoffman JM, Hanson MW, et al. Serial FDG-PET studies in the prediction of survival in patients with primary brain tumors. J Comput Assist Tomogr 1993;17:509–61.

[92] Francavilla TL, Miletich RS, Di Chiro G, et al. Positron emission tomography in the detection of malignant degeneration of low-grade gliomas. Neurosurgery 1989;24:1–5.

[93] Patronas NJ, Di Chiro G, Kufta C, et al. Prediction of survival in glioma patients by means of positron emission tomography. J Neurosurg 1985;62:816–22.

[94] Bruggers CS, Friedman HS, Fuller GN, et al. Comparison of serial PET and MRI scans in a pediatric patient with a brainstem glioma. Med Pediatr Oncol 1993;21(4):301–6.

[95] Molloy PT, Belasco J, Ngo K, et al. The role of FDG-PET imaging in the clinical management of pediatric brain tumors. J Nucl Med 1999;40:129P.

[96] Holthof VA, Herholz K, Berthold F, et al. In vivo metabolism of childhood posterior fossa tumors and primitive neuroectodermal tumors before and after treatment. Cancer 1993;1394–403.

[97] Hoffman JM, Hanson MW, Friedman HS, et al. FDG-PET in pediatric posterior fossa brain tumors. J Comput Assist Tomogr 1992;16:62–8.

[98] Molloy PT, Defeo R, Hunter J, et al. Excellent correlation of FDG-PET imaging with clinical outcome in patients with neurofibromatosis type I and low grade astrocytomas. J Nucl Med 1999;40:129P.

[99] O'Tuama LA, Phillips PC, Strauss LC, et al. Two-phase [11C]L-methionine PET in childhood brain tumors. Pediatr Neurol 1990;6:163–70.

[100] Mosskin M, von Holst H, Bergstrom M, et al. Positron emission tomography with 11C-methionine and computed tomography of intracranial tumors compared with histopathologic examination of multiple biopsies. Acta Radiol 1987;28:673–81.

[101] Utriainen M, Metsahonkala L, Salmi TT, et al. Metabolic characterization of childhood brain tumors: comparison of 18F-fluordeoxyglucose and 11C-methionine positron emission tomography. Cancer 2002; 95(6):1376–86.

[102] Lilja A, Lundqvist H, Olsson Y, et al. Positron emission tomography and computed tomography in differential diagnosis between recurrent or residual glioma and treatment-induced brain lesion. Acta Radiol 1989;38:121–8.

[103] Mineura K, Sasajima T, Kowada M, et al. Indications for differential diagnosis of nontumor central nervous system diseases from tumors. A positron emission tomography study. J Neuroimaging 1997;7:8–15.

[104] Cohen MD. Imaging of children with cancer. St. Louis (MO): Mosby Yearbook; 1992.

[105] Nadel HR, Rossleigh MA. Tumor imaging. In: Treves ST, editor. Pediatric nuclear medicine. 2nd edition. New York: Springer-Verlag; 1995. p. 496–527.

[106] Rossleigh MA, Murray IPC, Mackey DWJ. Pediatric solid tumors: evaluation by gallium-67 SPECT studies. J Nucl Med 1990;31:161–72.

[107] Howman-Giles R, Stevens M, Bergin M. Role of gallium-67 in management of pediatric solid tumors. Aust Pediatric J 1982;18:120–5.

[108] Yang SL, Alderson PO, Kaizer HA, et al. Serial Ga-67 citrate imaging in children with neoplastic disease: concise communication. J Nucl Med 1979;20: 210–4.

[109] Sty JR, Kun LE, Starshak RJ. Pediatric applications in nuclear oncology. Semin Nucl Med 1985;15: 171–200.

[110] Barrington SF, Carr R. Staging of Burkitt's lymphoma and response to treatment monitored by PET scanning. Clin Oncol 1995;7:334–5.

[111] Bangerter M, Moog F, Buchmann I, et al. Whole-body 2-[18F]-fluoro-2-deoxy-D-glucose positron emis-sion tomography (FDG-PET) for accurate staging of Hodgkin's disease. Ann Oncol 1998;9:1117–22.

[112] Jerusalem G, Warland V, Najjar F, et al. Whole-body 18F-FDG-PET for the evaluation of patients with Hodgkin's disease and non-Hodgkin's lymphoma. Nucl Med Commun 1999;20:13–20.

[113] Leskinen-Kallio S, Ruotsalainen U, Nagren K, et al. Uptake of carbon-11-methionine and fluorodeoxyglucose in non-Hodgkin's lymphoma: a PET study. J Nucl Med 1991;32:1211–8.

[114] Moog F, Bangerter M, Kotzerke J, et al. 18-F-fluorodeoxyglucose positron emission tomography as a new approach to detect lymphomatous bone marrow. J Clin Oncol 1998;16:603–9.

[115] Moog F, Bangerter M, Diederichs CG, et al. Extranodal malignant lymphoma: detection with FDG-PET versus CT. Radiology 1998;206:475–81.

[116] Moog F, Bangerter M, Diederichs CG, et al. Lymphoma: role of whole-body 2-deoxy-2-[F-18]fluoro-D-glucose (FDG) PET in nodal staging. Radiology 1997;203:795–800.

[117] Okada J, Yoshikawa K, Imazeki K, et al. The use of FDG-PET in the detection and management of malignant lymphoma: correlation of uptake with prognosis. J Nucl Med 1991;32:686–91.

[118] Okada J, Yoshikawa K, Itami M, et al. Positron emission tomography using fluorine-18-fluorodeoxyglucose in malignant lymphoma: a comparison with proliferative activity. J Nucl Med 1992;33:325–9.

[119] Rodriguez M, Rehn S, Ahlstrom H, et al. Predicting malignancy grade with PET in non-Hodgkin's lymphoma. J Nucl Med 1995;36:1790–6.

[120] Paul R. Comparison of fluorine-18–2-fluorodeoxyglucose and gallium-67 citrate imaging for detection of lymphoma. J Nucl Med 1987;28:288–92.

[121] Newman JS, Francis IR, Kaminski MS, et al. Imaging of lymphoma with PET with 2-[F-18]-fluoro-2-deoxy-D-glucose: correlation with CT. Radiology 1994;190:111–6.

[122] de Wit M, Bumann D, Beyer W, et al. Whole-body positron emission tomography (PET) for diagnosis of residual mass in patients with lymphoma. Ann Oncol 1997;8(Suppl 1):57–60.

[123] Cremerius U, Fabry U, Neuerburg J, et al. Positron emission tomography with 18-F-FDG to detect residual disease after therapy for malignant lymphoma. Nucl Med Commun 1998;19:1055–63.

[124] Hoh CK, Glaspy J, Rosen P, et al. Whole-body FDG-PET imaging for staging of Hodgkin's disease and lymphoma. J Nucl Med 1997;38:343–8.

[125] Romer W, Hanauske AR, Ziegler S, et al. Positron emission tomography in non-Hodgkin's lymphoma: assessment of chemotherapy with fluorodeoxyglucose. Blood 1998;91:4464–71.

[126] Stumpe KD, Urbinelli M, Steinert HC, et al. Whole-body positron emission tomography using fluorodeoxyglucose for staging of lymphoma: effectiveness and comparison with computed tomography. Eur J Nucl Med 1998;25:721–8.

[127] Lapela M, Leskinen S, Minn HR, et al. Increased glucose metabolism in untreated non-Hodgkin's lymphoma: a study with positron emission tomography and fluorine-18-fluorodeoxyglucose. Blood 1995;86:3522–7.

[128] Carr R, Barrington SF, Madan B, et al. Detection of lymphoma in bone marrow by whole-body positron emission tomography. Blood 1998;91:3340–6.

[129] Segall GM. FDG-PET imaging in patients with lymphoma: a clinical perspective. J Nucl Med 2001; 42(4):609–10.

[130] Moody R, Shulkin B, Yanik G, et al. PET FDG imaging in pediatric lymphomas. J Nucl Med 2001; 42(5 Suppl):39P.

[131] Kostakoglu L, Leonard JP, Coleman M, et al. Comparison of FDG-PET and Ga-67 SPECT in the staging of lymphoma. J Nucl Med 2000;41(5 Suppl):118P.

[132] Lin PC, Chu J, Pocock N. F-18 fluorodeoxyglucose imaging with coincidence dual-head gamma camera (hybrid FDG-PET) for staging of lymphoma: comparison with Ga-67 scintigraphy. J Nucl Med 2000; 41(5 Suppl):118P.

[133] Tomas MB, Manalili E, Leonidas JC, et al. F-18 FDG imaging of lymphoma in children using a hybrid pet system: comparison with Ga-67. J Nucl Med 2000;41(5 Suppl):96P.

[134] Tatsumi M, Kitayama H, Sugahara H, et al. Whole-body hybrid PET with 18F-FDG in the staging of non-Hodgkin's lymphoma. J Nucl Med 2001; 42(4):601–8.

[135] Hudson MM, Krasin MJ, Kaste SC. PET imaging in pediatric Hodgkin's lymphoma. Pediatr Radiol 2004;34:190–8.

[136] Krasin MJ, Hudson MM, Kaste SC. Positron emission tomography in pediatric radiation oncology: integration in the treatment-planning process. Pediatr Radiol 2004;34:214–21.

[137] Franzius C, Schober O. Assessment of therapy response by FDG-PET in pediatric patients. Q J Nucl Med 2003;47(1):41–5.

[138] Bousvaros A, Kirks DR, Grossman H. Imaging of neuroblastoma: an overview. Pediatr Radiol 1986; 16:89–106.

[139] Briganti V, Sestini R, Orlando C, et al. Imaging of somatostatin receptors by indium-111-pentetreotide correlates with quantitative determination of somatostatin receptor type 2 gene expression in neuroblastoma tumor. Clin Cancer Res 1997;3:2385–91.

[140] Shulkin BL, Hutchinson RJ, Castle VP, et al. Neuroblastoma: positron emission tomography with 2-[fluorine-18]-fluoro-2-deoxy-D-glucose compared with metaiodobenzylguanidine scintigraphy. Radiology 1996;199:743–50.

[141] Shulkin BL, Wieland DM, Baro ME, et al. PET hydroxyephedrine imaging of neuroblastoma. J Nucl Med 1996;37:16–21.

[142] Shulkin BL, Wieland DM, Castle VP, et al. Carbon-11 epinephrine PET imaging of neuroblastoma. J Nucl Med 1999;40:129P.

[143] Vaidyanathan G, Affleck DJ, Zalutsky MR. Validation of 4-[fluorine-18]fluoro-3-iodobenzylguanidine as a positron-emitting analog of MIBG. J Nucl Med 1995;36:644–50.

[144] Ott RJ, Tait D, Flower MA, et al. Treatment planning for 131I-mIBG radiotherapy of neural crest tumors using 124I-mIBG positron emission tomography. Br J Radiol 1992;65:787–91.

[145] Barnewolt CE, Paltiel HJ, Lebowitz RL, et al. Genitourinary system. In: Kirks DR, editor. Practical pediatric imaging. Diagnostic radiology of infants and children. 3rd edition. Philadelphia: Lippincott-Raven; 1997. p. 1009–170.

[146] Shulkin BL, Chang E, Strouse PJ, et al. PET FDG studies of Wilms' tumors. J Pediatr Hematol Oncol 1997;19:334–8.

[147] McDonald DJ. Limb salvage surgery for sarcomas of the extremities. AJR Am J Roentgenol 1994;163: 509–13.

[148] Triche TJ. Pathology of pediatric malignancies. In: Pizzo PA, Poplack DG, editors. Principles and practice of pediatric oncology. 2nd edition. Philadelphia: JB Lippincott; 1993. p. 115–52.

[149] O'Connor MI, Pritchard DJ. Ewing's sarcoma. Prognostic factors, disease control, and the reemerging role of surgical treatment. Clin Orthop 1991; 262:78–87.

[150] Jaramillo D, Laor T, Gebhardt M. Pediatric musculoskeletal neoplasms. Evaluation with MR imaging. MRI Clin North Am 1996;4:1–22.

[151] Frouge C, Vanel D, Coffre C, et al. The role of magnetic resonance imaging in the evaluation of Ewing sarcoma—a report of 27 cases. Skeletal Radiol 1988;17:387–92.

[152] MacVicar AD, Olliff JFC, Pringle J, et al. Ewing sarcoma: MR imaging of chemotherapy-induced changes with histologic correlation. Radiology 1992;184:859–64.

[153] Lemmi MA, Fletcher BD, Marina NM, et al. Use of MR imaging to assess results of chemotherapy for Ewing sarcoma. AJR Am J Roentgenol 1990; 155:343–6.

[154] Erlemann R, Sciuk J, Bosse A, et al. Response of osteosarcoma and Ewing sarcoma to preoperative chemotherapy: assessment with dynamic and static MR imaging and skeletal scintigraphy. Radiology 1990;175:791–6.

[155] Holscher HC, Bloem JL, Vanel D, et al. Osteosarcoma: chemotherapy-induced changes at MR imaging. Radiology 1992;182:839–44.

[156] Lawrence JA, Babyn PS, Chan HS, et al. Extremity osteosarcoma in childhood: prognostic value of radiologic imaging. Radiology 1993;189:43–7.

[157] Connolly LP, Laor T, Jaramillo D, et al. Prediction of chemotherapeutic response of osteosarcoma with quantitative thallium-201 scintigraphy and magnetic resonance imaging. Radiology 1996;201:349.

[158] Lin J, Leung WT. Quantitative evaluation of thallium-201 uptake in predicting chemotherapeutic

response of osteosarcoma. Eur J Nucl Med 1995;22: 553–5.

[159] Menendez LR, Fideler BM, Mirra J. Thallium-201 scanning for the evaluation of osteosarcoma and soft tissue sarcoma. J Bone Joint Surg [Am] 1993;75: 526–31.

[160] Ramanna L, Waxman A, Binney G, et al. Thallium-201 scintigraphy in bone sarcoma: comparison with gallium-67 and technetium-99m MDP in the evaluation of chemotherapeutic response. J Nucl Med 1990; 31:567–72.

[161] Rosen G, Loren GJ, Brien EW, et al. Serial thallium-201 scintigraphy in osteosarcoma. Correlation with tumor necrosis after preoperative chemotherapy. Clin Orthop 1993;293:302–6.

[162] Ohtomo K, Terui S, Yokoyama R, et al. Thallium-201 scintigraphy to assess effect of chemotherapy to osteosarcoma. J Nucl Med 1996;37:1444–8.

[163] Bar-Sever Z, Connolly LP, Treves ST, et al. Technetium-99m MIBI in the evaluation of children with Ewing's sarcoma. J Nucl Med 1997;38:13P.

[164] Caner B, Kitapel M, Unlu M, et al. Technetium-99m-MIBI uptake in benign and malignant bone lesions: a comparative study with technetium-99m-MDP. J Nucl Med 1992;33:319–24.

[165] Lenzo NP, Shulkin B, Castle VP, et al. FDG-PET in childhood soft tissue sarcoma. J Nucl Med 2000; 41(5 Suppl):96P.

[166] Abdel-Dayem HM. The role of nuclear medicine in primary bone and soft tissue tumors. Semin Nucl Med 1997;27:355–63.

[167] Shulkin BL, Mitchell DS, Ungar DR, et al. Neoplasms in a pediatric population: 2-[F-18]-fluoro-2-deoxy-D-glucose PET studies. Radiology 1995;194: 495–500.

[168] Hawkins DS, Rajendran JG, Conrad III EU, et al. Evaluation of chemotherapy response in pediatric bone sarcomas by [F-18]-fluorodeoxy-D-glucose positron emission tomography. Cancer 2002;94(12): 3277–84.

[169] Ben Arush MW, Israel O, Kedar Z, et al. Detection of isolated distant metastasis in soft tissue sarcoma by fluorodeoxyglucose positron emission tomography: case report. Pediatr Hematol Oncol 2001;18(4): 295–8.

[170] Jadvar H, Connolly LP, Shulkin BL, et al. Positron emission tomography in pediatrics. In: Freeman L.M., editors. Nuclear medicine annual. Philadelphia: Lippincott Williams & Wilkins; 2000. p. 53–83.

[171] Jadvar H, Connolly LP, Shulkin BL. Pediatrics. In: Wahl RL, editor. Principles and practice of positron emission tomography. Philadelphia: Lippincott Williams & Wilkins. p. 395–410.

[172] Jadvar H, Connolly LP, Shulkin BL. PET imaging in pediatric disorders. In: Valk PE, Bailey DL, Townsend DW, et al, editors. Positron emission tomography: basic science and clinical practice. London: Springer-Verlag; 2003. p. 755–74.

ELSEVIER
SAUNDERS

Radiol Clin N Am 43 (2005) 153–167

RADIOLOGIC
CLINICS
of North America

PET imaging of cellular proliferation

David A. Mankoff, MD, PhD[a],[*], Anthony F. Shields, MD, PhD[b],[c],
Kenneth A. Krohn, PhD[a],[d]

[a]Division of Nuclear Medicine, Department of Radiology, University of Washington, 1959 Northeast Pacific Street,
Room NN203, Box 356113, Seattle, WA 98195, USA
[b]Karmanos Cancer Institute, 4100 John R Street, 4 HWCRC, Detroit, MI 48201, USA
[c]Wayne State University, Detroit, MI, USA
[d]Department of Radiation Oncology, University of Washington, Seattle, WA, USA

Increased cellular proliferation is a hallmark of the cancer phenotype [1]. Measurements of tumor proliferation based on in vitro assays have played a key role in cancer research [2,3]. In patients, in vitro measures of cellular proliferation made on tumor biopsy specimens provide important prognostic information for most tumor types and have long been used to guide treatment selection [4]. Studies have also shown that a decrease in cellular proliferation is one of the earliest events in response to successful treatment. This was the basis of predictive assays using cultured cells and proliferation response to evaluate various cytotoxic agents, analogous to antibiotic sensitivity testing for bacteria [1,3,4]. These in vitro assays failed, however, to predict accurately the response to systemic therapy in the patient [4]. In vitro testing failed to account for host factors, including the delivery of the therapeutic agent and the in vivo biology of the tumor, which may mediate response. This spurred interest in an in vivo assay that can directly measure early tumor response in the patient and thereby provide timely guidance to allow individualized treatment selection.

Cellular proliferation imaging has a number of potential advantages over in vitro assay. Biopsy of large or multisite tumors is subject to sampling error; the portion of the tumor sampled may not be representative of the cancer as a whole and may lead to erroneous treatment choices. Imaging is well suited to serial studies, which are needed to assess the effect of a therapeutic intervention. Finally, PET imaging is uniquely quantitative; with knowledge of the specific activity of the radiopharmaceutical, PET images of metabolism can be expressed accurately in molar units. PET imaging tells how much the tumor is responding or progressing, not simply whether or not it is responding or progressing.

Cellular proliferation has a number of potential advantages over glucose metabolic imaging using fluorodeoxyglucose-PET (FDG-PET), which is the mainstay of current clinical PET imaging [5]. Cellular proliferation is specific to tumors, whereas a high level of energy metabolism is a feature of tumors, but also associated with a variety of other processes, including inflammation and tissue healing [1]. Cellular proliferation occurs early in response to treatment and is likely to provide earlier and more definitive evidence of response than changes in energy metabolism, which can be compounded by a variety of issues, including cellular repair. In the case of cytostatic agents, which stop cell division but not necessarily lead to cell death, tumor cellular proliferation drops, but tumor energy metabolism may not change. All these considerations provide an impetus for PET cellular proliferation imaging, especially as a tool for measuring early response. This article reviews the biology underlying proliferation imaging,

Supported by NIH Grants P01 CA42045, R01 CA72064, RO1 CA39566, K24 CA82645, and RO1 CA83131.

* Corresponding author.
E-mail address: dam@u.washington.edu
(D.A. Mankoff).

radiopharmaceuticals used for proliferation imaging, preclinical studies of proliferation imaging, and clinical results through 2003.

Biologic and quantitative considerations

DNA synthesis is required for cell growth and proliferation [1]. Nucleotides of the four bases (cytosine, guanine, adenine, and thymidine) are required for DNA synthesis, and measurements of the rate of their incorporation into DNA yield the DNA synthetic rate. Of the four nucleosides, thymidine is the only one incorporated exclusively into DNA, and not RNA, and provides a measure of DNA synthesis independent of RNA synthesis [2]. Thymidine exogenous to the cell can be incorporated into DNA by the salvage or exogenous pathway, illustrated in Fig. 1. Thymidine is also synthesized endogenously by the cell, as discussed later.

Early studies of cell proliferation used hydrogen-3 ([³H])-thymidine added to cell culture media or injected into animals [2,3]. The incorporation of labeled thymidine could be evaluated in one of two ways [2]. Histologic sections could be autoradiographed, and the fraction of labeled cells or labeling index estimated, a measure akin to the fraction of cells in S-phase. This had the advantage of counting label specifically associated with the cell, but could not identify how fast cells moved through the cell cycle. Alternatively, the measure of total thymidine uptake per unit cells or tissue provided an estimate of the thymidine flux into DNA directly proportional to the DNA synthetic rate. This had the ability to infer growth rates directly, but had the disadvantage that total uptake included label in the form of free thymidine, metabolites, phosphorylated precursors, and DNA. Both approaches have been used extensively in the cancer literature dating back to the 1950s [2].

The synthesis of carbon-11 ([¹¹C])-thymidine and the development of PET instrumentation led to the ability to image thymidine uptake and measure cell growth noninvasively [6–10]. The imaging approach is similar to in vitro measurements using [³H]-thymidine, using regional [¹¹C]-thymidine uptake as a measure of cellular proliferation. Unlike simple uptake measurements, however, dynamic PET imaging and kinetic modeling can estimate the rate at which thymidine is incorporated into DNA, overcoming the problem inherent in simple uptake measures (eg, standardized uptake value [SUV]), which include label present in species other than DNA [11].

The short half-life of [¹¹C] and the catabolism of thymidine make [¹¹C]-thymidine impractical for routine clinical use. This spurred the development of other compounds for cellular proliferation imaging [12], described later. Almost all cellular proliferation agents developed and tested to date are analogues of thymidine that also trace the exogenous pathway to DNA. Proper interpretation of images obtained using thymidine analogues requires a detailed knowledge of the biochemistry of the analogues, and an understanding of how their uptake into tissue reflects flux along the exogenous pathway as an estimate of the rate of thymidine incorporation into DNA [13,14].

Thymidine metabolism and consequences for imaging

PET with [¹¹C]-thymidine represents the standard for imaging proliferation, because it is the compound that is incorporated into DNA that is chemically identical to native thymidine, eliminating potential differences in uptake caused by differences in metabolism between thymidine and its analogues. The knowledge gained in the last 50 years of studying DNA synthesis using thymidine as a [³H]- or carbon-14 ([¹⁴C])-labeled pyrimidine can be applied directly to [¹¹C]-thymidine PET [2]. Cellular proliferation imaging with [¹¹C]-thymidine requires a consideration of in vivo factors in patients that are not present in historical in vitro or in vivo animal studies, however, where one can cut out, extract, and analyze pieces of tissues. For example, the role of blood delivery to the tumor site and other organs must be considered in thymidine imaging, because thymidine

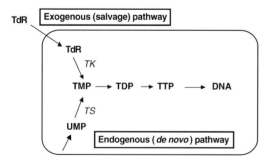

Fig. 1. Diagram of exogenous (*top*) pathway for thymidine incorporation into DNA versus endogenous (*bottom*) pathway. Flux through both pathways is ultimately controlled by the rate of DNA synthesis. Flux through the exogenous pathway is controlled by thymidine kinase, and flux through the endogenous is controlled by thymidylate synthase. TDP, thymidine diphosphate; TdR, thymidine; TK, *thymidine kinase*; TMP, thymidine monophosphate; TS, *thymidylate synthase*; TTP, thymidine triphosphate; UMP, uridine monophosphate.

is rapidly cleared from the circulation [15]. In the first minute after injection, the level of tracer in tissues reflects blood flow, but within a few minutes subsequent metabolism and incorporation into DNA become more important and determine thymidine retention. Thymidine is rapidly transported from the extracellular fluid into the cell using facilitated, non–energy-dependent nucleoside transporters and active, Na^+-dependent carriers [16–18]. This system provides rapid equilibration across the cell membrane. Once inside the cell, thymidine is phosphorylated by thymidine kinase (TK) to thymidine monophosphate, one of the rate-limiting steps in the pathway. It is subsequently phosphorylated twice more to yield thymidine triphosphate, which is incorporated into DNA. The rate of the DNA incorporation step ultimately controls flux of thymidine into the pathway; flux is directly proportional to the DNA synthetic rate [2].

Thymidine phosphorylation is accomplished by two different isoenzymes, TK1 and TK2. TK1 is the cytosolic form that is involved in the phosphorylation of thymidine involved in nuclear DNA synthesis. The level of TK1 in a cell increases several-fold as it goes from a resting state to the proliferative phase and is destroyed at the end of S-phase [19]. TK2 is a mitochondrial enzyme and a deficiency in TK2 results in a decline in mitochondrial DNA and is associated with a congenital myopathy [20]. It is not regulated by the cell cycle. Understanding the distribution of both forms of TK in the body is important for accurate interpretation of images obtained with thymidine and its analogues.

Once thymidine is taken up into the cytosol and phosphorylated by TK1, the exogenous thymidine monophosphate then mixes with the endogenously synthesized pool [2,21]. The exogenous pathway competes with endogenous (de novo) synthesis from uridylate. In the endogenous pathway, deoxyuridine monophosphate is methylated to form thymidine monophosphate by thymidylate synthase (TS), a rate-controlling step in the pathway. The thymidine monophosphate from the exogenous and endogenous synthesis pathways mixes in the phosphorylated thymidine precursor pool, which supplies thymidine triphosphate for DNA synthesis. If these two sources of thymidine varied greatly from tumor to tumor or over time, it would be difficult to infer the DNA synthetic rate from the flux of thymidine through the exogenous pathway. Previous studies, however, have shown that the relative use of these two sources of thymidine depends on the external concentration and is predictable across differing cell types and species [22]. The flux of thymidine through the exogenous pathway is a good measure of the DNA synthetic rate. Important enzymes in the DNA synthetic pathway, such as TK1 and TS, are typically all increased for highly proliferative cells. Nevertheless, the relative expression of TK1 and TS, and the relative use of the exogenous and endogenous pathway, are potentially confounding factors that must be considered in interpreting cellular proliferation imaging results [11,13,14].

Another factor that affects incorporation of a thymidine radiopharmaceutical into DNA is the

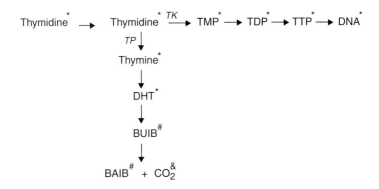

Fig. 2. Diagram of thymidine metabolism. In addition to incorporation into DNA through the exogenous pathway (*top*), thymidine can be catabolized by a series of enzymatic reactions, starting with thymidine phosphorylase, which controls flux through the catabolic pathway. This leads to labeled metabolites for [11C]-thymidine. Initially, the sugar is cleaved to form thymine, which is further metabolized to dihydrothymine. The nature of further labeled metabolites of [11C]-thymidine depends on the location of the [11C] label. For the methyl-labeled compound (#), small molecules, such as β-ureidoisobutyric acid and β-aminoisobutyric acid, are labeled with [11C]. These metabolites can become trapped in tissue like intact thymidine. For the ring-2 compound (&), the label is released as [11CO2], which forms a ubiquitous background, but is not trapped. BAIB, β-aminoisobutyric acid; BUIB, β-ureidoisobutyric acid; DHT, dihydrothymine; TP, thymidine phosphorylase.

in part because of image background from labeled TdR metabolites, both for the methyl compound [26] and the ring-2 compound [27,28]. Most patient series showed variability in tumor TdR uptake for different patients; in many cases, uptake correlated with tumor grade or other pathologic features indicative of tumor growth. In general, these studies were pilot-feasibility studies, limited by the difficulty of synthesizing [^{11}C]-thymidine and the need to analyze blood samples for metabolites or the requirement for a second scan with the major metabolite, [$^{11}CO_2$].

Brain tumor imaging has received considerable attention in pilot TdR-PET studies. These investigations were motivated in part by the difficulty encountered in FDG-PET brain tumor imaging, namely the high background of FDG uptake in normal brain tissue and the resulting difficulty in identifying tumor boundaries. Because normal brain cells do not proliferate, cell proliferation imaging offers a significant advantage over FDG in visualizing brain tumors and following their progression or response to treatment. Thymidine does not readily cross the normal blood-brain barrier, which also decreases background uptake [62]. Some early imaging trials met with limited success. De-Reuck et al [64] imaged patients with neoplastic and nonneoplastic brain lesions using methyl-labeled TdR and concluded that uptake was nonspecific, reflecting blood-brain barrier breakdown and trapping of labeled metabolites. Other studies using the ring-2 compound, where the major metabolite, [$^{11}CO_2$], is less likely to be trapped in brain, showed more

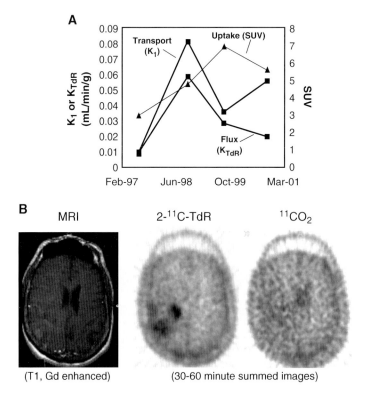

Fig. 7. Thymidine imaging of a brain tumor patient. A single patient was imaged four times using dual [$^{11}CO_2$]/2-[^{11}C]-thymidine imaging and compartmental analysis. The patient presented with a low-grade glioma (February, 1997) with clinical progression to a high-grade tumor, confirmed by biopsy (January, 1998). There was a good response after radiotherapy and chemotherapy (October, 1999). Subsequently, the MR imaging showed increased enhancement (March, 2001), which by clinical follow-up was necrosis rather than progressive tumor. (A) Estimates of thymidine transport (K_1) and flux (K_{TdR}) at each time point. The flux estimates correctly depict progression and response to treatment, including a progressive decline in thymidine flux with tumor necrosis. The increase in transport at the latest time point is the result of the progressive disruption of the blood-brain barrier associated with necrosis of the tumor and surrounding brain tissue. (B) Summed 2-[^{11}C]-thymidine and [$^{11}CO_2$] images at the point of tumor transformation to high-grade behavior (June, 1998). There is high uptake of thymidine, out of proportion to contrast enhancement on MR imaging. The $^{11}CO_2$ image shows relatively uniform uptake, indicating that the uptake in the tumor on the thymidine image is not caused by metabolite accumulation.

promising results. VanderBorght et al [65] imaged patients with brain tumors and found a good correlation between TdR uptake and tumor grade. Eary et al [66] studied a series of patients with TdR-PET, FDG-PET, and MR imaging and showed that TdR uptake correlated with the clinical and pathologic features of brain tumors. This study also found that the level and pattern of TdR uptake was distinct from tumor FDG uptake and from contrast enhancement on MR imaging. This qualitative analysis was later refined to provide a quantitative estimate of thymidine retention (flux) in brain tumors as an extension of a compartmental model developed for somatic tumors. The approach for brain tumors used dual CO_2-TdR scans [30]. In a pilot series of patients studied using the two-scan approach [61], the compartmental model showed promise in that it was able to separate the effects of enhanced TdR delivery versus increased thymidine retention because of incorporation into DNA. Estimates of thymidine flux into DNA agreed with clinical and pathologic features of the tumor, including grade and prior treatment.

In this series, a single patient was studied four times over the course of tumor progression and response to treatment [61], and TdR-PET with model analysis was able to distinguish increased proliferation associated with tumor transformation to a high-grade cancer, response to radiation and chemotherapy, and treatment-induced necrosis (Fig. 7). The transport parameter (K_1), uptake of FDG (SUV in the graph), and contrast-enhanced MR imaging all suggested worsening disease at the last time point. Only the thymidine flux parameter (K_{TdR}) accurately depicted the subsequent clinical course for this patient, who survived for several years after the last imaging study. This series showed the promise of cellular proliferation imaging for brain tumors but emphasized the need for rigorous quantitative analysis to interpret the results.

Other notable investigations studied novel applications of proliferation imaging. These studies indicate future clinical applications of cellular proliferation imaging that are likely to become important. Shields et al [32] studied a series of five patients with small cell lung cancer or high-grade sarcoma before and after a single cycle of chemotherapy with scans separated by 7 to 10 days. TdR-PET in these studies showed an early response to successful treatment, with a 100% decline in thymidine flux in the three patients who ultimately achieved a complete response, a 40% decline in a patient with a partial response, and no change in the patient with no response and ultimate disease progression. Changes in TdR flux were larger, and differentiated responders from nonresponders better than changes in FDG metabolism assessed at the same times (Fig. 8). This seminal study demonstrated the advantage of imaging cellular proliferation to assess early response and sets

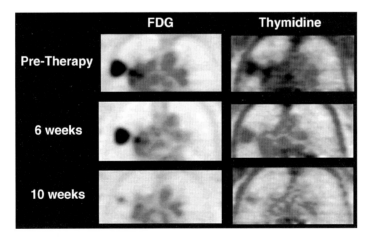

Fig. 8. Response to treatment. Coronal images through the mid-thorax are shown for a patient with non–small cell lung cancer with extensive hilar and mediastinal lymph node metastases. The pretherapy FDG and thymidine PET images show increased uptake at the tumor sites. Background is lower in the thymidine images because of labeled metabolites. The patient was treated with chemotherapy and radiation therapy. There is minimal changed by FDG-PET at 6 weeks, but by 10 weeks the FDG images show evidence of response. Thymidine images show an early decline in uptake, even for the raw images that have not been corrected for metabolites and unincorporated thymidine. This demonstrates the ability of cellular proliferation imaging to measure early response to treatment.

forth a paradigm for future clinical applications. Although glucose metabolism fuels the growth process, it supports much more than proliferation, and so FDG images are much less specific than proliferation images. Thymidine is either catabolized or it is phosphorylated and eventually incorporated into DNA; thymidine imaging provides a uniquely specific measure of proliferation.

A study by Wells et al [67] used TdR-PET to investigate the effect of drug therapy in vivo in the treated patient. In this novel study, the investigators performed TdR-PET in patients with gastrointestinal cancer before and after administration of a novel TS inhibitor, AG337. Given the competition between the endogenous pathway (modulated by TS activity) and the exogenous pathway (monitored by labeled TdR), one would expect successful inhibition of TS to show an early compensatory increase in flux through the exogenous pathway and an increase in TdR uptake. They found that TdR fractional retention of thymidine went up significantly at 1 hour after administration of AG337, a 5FU analogue, compared with controls imaged twice without therapeutic intervention. The authors also showed that the change in TdR fractional retention of thymidine in AG337-treated patients correlated with the exposure to AG337 estimated from drug clearance measurements. This imaginative study showed the value of cellular proliferation imaging in monitoring a specific drug effect and sets forth another paradigm for the use of PET imaging.

Patient imaging with fluorothymidine

Preclinical studies identified the potential of FLT as a PET imaging agent for cellular proliferation and examined the correlation between FLT uptake and TK enzyme activity as an assay of cellular proliferation in cell lines. Shields et al [41] published the first human studies using FLT-PET in a patient with non–small cell lung cancer, demonstrating the high image quality and low background afforded by FLT. Exquisite images are obtained from injection of 5 mCi or less of FLT, and imaging can be started as soon as 45 to 60 minutes after injection (Fig. 9). Recently, the radiation dosimetry has been published for FLT [68], showing that patient imaging is feasible with clinically acceptable radiation exposure for the subject. This is a critical issue for FLT because it is likely to be used in clinical applications that require repeated studies to measure response to therapy. These studies paved the way for a series of pilot studies examining FLT-PET imaging for a variety of tumors.

Most early series focused on testing the feasibility of FLT-PET imaging and comparing FLT uptake with in vitro measures of tumor proliferation, typically the Ki-67 (MIB-1) index [69]. Some studies also compared FLT-PET with FDG-PET, given the established clinical role of FDG for staging in the tumor types studied. Studies have shown good correlation between FLT uptake and the Ki-67 index for a variety of tumors, including lung cancer [70–72], lymphoma [73], and colorectal cancer [74]. In cases where FDG-

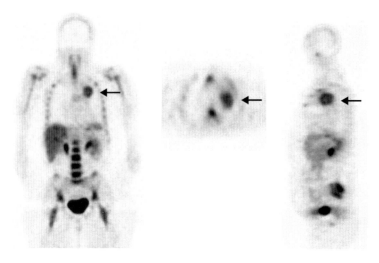

Fig. 9. FLT-PET images in a patient with lung cancer. A large centrally necrotic tumor is seen in the right upper lobe (*arrows*) seen on coronal (*left*), axial (*center*), and sagittal (*right*) slices. Prominent uptake is also seen in the marrow, a highly proliferative normal tissue.

Table 2
Summary of studies comparing 3′-fluorothymidine uptake and in vitro assay of cellular proliferation in patients

| | | | Correlation (P value) | |
Study	Tumor type	N	FLT vs Ki-67	FDG vs Ki-67
Vesselle et al [70]	Lung[a]	11	0.83 (.003)[b]	—
Buck et al [71]	Lung[c]	30	0.87 (<.0001)	—
Buck et al [72]	Lung[a]	26	0.92 (<.0001)	0.59 (<.001)
Wagner et al [73]	Lymphoma	10	0.95 (<.005)	—
Francis et al [74]	Colorectal	13[d]	0.80 (<0.01)	0.4 (NS)

Abbreviation: NS, not significant.
  [a] Benign and malignant lesions included.
  [b] Number of lesions; some patents had more than one lesion.
  [c] Solitary pulmonary nodule.
  [d] Spearman ρ value.

PET was also performed, the correlation for FLT uptake versus Ki-67 index was much better than the correlation for FDG uptake versus Ki-67. In some cases the correlation between FDG uptake and Ki-67 was not statistically significant, confirming the earlier comment that FDG is used to fuel much more than cellular growth. Results are summarized in Table 2.

Most studies evaluated FLT uptake by a simple uptake measure (ie, SUV) or by model-independent calculation of the flux of FLT trapping using graphical analysis. One exception was the study by Visvikis et al [75], which applied a compartmental model to dynamic FLT data obtained in patients with colorectal cancer and found that the data were fit well by a three-parameter model. Estimates of flux by compartmental analysis agreed with estimates from graphical analysis. This result was distinct from experience at the University of Washington [76]; preliminary studies suggested that many tumors exhibited release of label from the trapped compartment for tumors, necessitating a k_4 parameter. A late downward curvature to the graphical analysis function indicated a finite k_4, causing discrepancies between compartmental and graphical estimates of flux. This was also reported in other preliminary studies [77]. These early studies support the hypothesis that FLT uptake reflects tumor proliferation; however, more work is needed to understand the kinetics of FLT in a variety of tumors and clinical settings to choose the optimal approach to image analysis. At this time, the approximation of a simple uptake value, such as SUV, or simple graphical analysis has not been validated.

Some recent studies have examined the performance of FLT-PET as a cancer staging tool, although this is unlikely to be the most important role for FLT-PET. Preliminary studies of melanoma [78], colorectal cancer [79], laryngeal cancer [80], and a variety of thoracic tumors [81] have been reported. These studies showed variable uptake in tumors and low target-to-background for some tumors and locations with high normal tissue uptake, such as the spine or marrow and liver. In all cases, the authors commented that many lesions, especially metastases, were better seen by FDG-PET than by FLT-PET. Dittmann et al [81] noted that spinal metastases from thoracic cancers could be missed because of high background in bone marrow. Francis et al [79] showed that only 34% of colorectal liver metastases were seen by FLT-PET, compared with 97% by FDG-PET. These early results suggest that although FLT-PET may provide specificity for some staging tasks, FLT-PET is unlikely to be of value for cancer staging, especially for tumors with metastases to the marrow and liver, areas of physiologic FLT retention. This echoes results from TdR-PET and is not surprising, because proliferation assays were never intended to stage cancer. The appropriate clinical application of FLT is for characterizing known tumors and assessing their response to treatment through serial imaging studies.

Although preclinical models demonstrate the potential utility of FLT-PET for measuring therapeutic response, limited data are available for this use in humans. Preliminary studies used FLT to monitor neoadjuvant breast cancer treatment [77,82] and showed that FLT could measure changes early in the course of treatment. Studies assessing FLT-PET to measure therapeutic response are underway in many centers and may give rise to multicenter trials in the near future.

Patient imaging with other thymidine analogues

More limited data are available for PET cellular proliferation imaging using thymidine analogues other than FLT. Tjuvajev et al [83] studied brain tumor patients using SPECT and [131I]-IUdR and found that early uptake of IUdR reflected blood–brain barrier breakdown around the brain tumor, but 24-hour uptake reflected IUdR incorporation and tumor clinical and pathologic features. Similar results have been demonstrated for a positron-emitting version of IUdR [84]. These studies support the potential value of longer-lived thymidine analogues for measuring cellular proliferation, but the long half-life of [^{124}I] and its high radiation burden limits its value for serial imaging. Boni et al [85] conducted a pilot study of [^{76}Br]-BrUdR in melanoma patients and found that uptake by PET correlated with in vitro measures of proliferation by BrUdR uptake and Ki-67 immunohistochemistry. The limited clinical use of IUdR and BrUdR as PET imaging agents reflects the limited availability of ^{124}I and ^{76}Br and also the confounding effect of their dehalogenation by in vivo metabolism.

Summary

PET cellular proliferation imaging has its roots in a long history of in vitro cellular proliferation studies to characterize cancer and in the understanding of the biology of thymidine incorporation into DNA gained from these studies. PET imaging represents the logical translation of the in vitro work to measure in vivo tumor proliferation. Preclinical studies of [^{11}C]-thymidine and other PET-labeled thymidine analogues set the stage for early clinical studies that provided very promising results. Recent progress in the application of [^{18}F]-FLT, a clinically practical PET thymidine analogue, to patient studies sets the next stage for clinical PET cellular proliferation imaging. Further mechanistic studies of the imaging agents and well-designed clinical trials will be important in moving PET proliferation imaging into what is likely to be a significant role in the care of cancer patients by providing a quantitative measure of tumor response to cytotoxic or cytostatic therapy.

Acknowledgments

The authors acknowledge John R. Grierson, Janet F. Eary, and Alexander M. Spence for illustrations, patient examples, and helpful discussions; and Mark Muzi and Jeanne M. Link for collaborations and helpful discussions regarding data analysis and metabolite analysis methods.

References

[1] Tannock IF. Cell proliferation. In: Tannock IF, Hill RP, editors. The basic science of oncology. New York: McGraw-Hill; 1992. p. 154–77.

[2] Cleaver JE. Thymidine metabolism and cell kinetics. Front Biol 1967;6:43–100.

[3] Livingston RB, Ambus U, George SL, et al. In vitro determination of thymidine-[H-3] labeling index in human solid tumors. Cancer Res 1974;34:1376–80.

[4] Livingston RB, Hart JS. The clinical applications of cell kinetics in cancer therapy. Ann Rev Toxicol 1977;17:529–43.

[5] Mankoff D, Bellon J. PET imaging of cancer: FDG and beyond. Semin Radiol Oncol 2001;11:16–27.

[6] Christman D, Crawford EJ, Friedkin M, et al. Detection of DNA synthesis in intact organisms with positron-emitting methyl-[C-11]-thymidine. Proc Natl Acad Sci U S A 1972;69:988–92.

[7] Sundoro-Wu BM, Schmall B, Conti PS, et al. Selective alkylation of pyrimidyldianions: synthesis and purification of ^{11}C labeled thymidine for tumor visualization using positron emission tomography. Int J Appl Radiat Isot 1984;35:705–8.

[8] Vander Borght T, Labar D, Pauwels S, et al. Production of [2-^{11}C]thymidine for quantification of cellular proliferation with PET. Int J Rad Appl Instrum [A] 1991;42:103–4.

[9] Link JM, Grierson J, Krohn K. Alternatives in the synthesis of 2-[C-11]-thymidine. J Label Comp Radiopharm 1995;37:610–2.

[10] Poupeye E, Counsell RE, De Leenheer A, et al. Synthesis of ^{11}C-labelled thymidine for tumor visualization using positron emission tomography. Int J Rad Appl Instrum [A] 1989;40:57–61.

[11] Mankoff DA, Shields AF, Graham MM, et al. Kinetic analysis of 2-[carbon-11]thymidine PET imaging studies: compartmental model and mathematical analysis. J Nucl Med 1998;39:1043–55.

[12] Shields AF, Grierson JR, Kozawa SM, et al. Development of labeled thymidine analogs for imaging tumor proliferation. Nucl Med Biol 1996;23:17–22.

[13] Krohn KA, Mankoff DA, Eary JF. Imaging cellular proliferation as a measure of response to therapy. J Clin Pharmacol 2001;41:96S–103S.

[14] Shields AF. PET imaging with ^{18}F-FLT and thymidine analogs: promise and pitfalls. J Nucl Med 2003;44:1432–4.

[15] Shields AF, Larson SM, Grunbaum Z, et al. Short-term thymidine uptake in normal and neoplastic tissues: studies for PET. J Nucl Med 1984;25:759–64.

[16] Belt JA, Marina NM, Phelps DA, et al. Nucleoside transport in normal and neoplastic cells. Adv Enzyme Regul 1993;33:235–52.

[17] Plagemann PGW, Erbe J. Thymidine transport by cultured Novikoff hepatoma cells and uptake by simple diffusion and relationship to incorporation into deoxyribonucleic acid. J Cell Biol 1972;55:161–78.

[18] Wohlhueter RM, Marz R, Plagemann PG. Thymidine

transport in cultured mammalian cells. Kinetic analysis, temperature dependence and specificity of the transport system. Biochim Biophys Acta 1979;553:262–83.

[19] Sherley JL, Kelly TJ. Regulation of human thymidine kinase during the cell cycle. J Biol Chem 1988;263: 8350–8.

[20] Saada A, Ben-Shalom E, Zyslin R, et al. Mitochondrial deoxyribonucleoside triphosphate pools in thymidine kinase 2 deficiency. Biochem Biophys Res Commun 2003;310:963–6.

[21] Kuebbing D, Werner R. A model for compartmentation of de novo and salvage thymidine nucleotide pools in mammalian cells. Proc Natl Acad Sci U S A 1975;72: 3333–6.

[22] Shields AF, Coonrod DV, Quackenbush RC, et al. Cellular sources of thymidine nucleotides: studies for PET. J Nucl Med 1987;28:1435–40.

[23] Miyadera K, Sumizawa T, Haraguchi M, et al. Role of thymidine phosphorylase activity in the angiogenic effect of platelet derived endothelial cell growth factor/thymidine phosphorylase. Cancer Res 1995;55:1687–90.

[24] Goethals P, Lameire N, van Eijkeren M, et al. [Methylcarbon-11] thymidine for in vivo measurement of cell proliferation. J Nucl Med 1996;37:1048–52.

[25] Goethals P, Volders F, Van der Eycken J, et al. Synthesis of 6-methyl[^{11}C]-2′-deoxyuridine and evaluation of its in vivo distribution in Wistar rats. Nucl Med Biol 1997;24:713–8.

[26] Goethals P, van Eijkeren M, Lodewyck W, et al. Measurement of [methyl-carbon-11]thymidine and its metabolites in head and neck tumors. J Nucl Med 1995;36:880–2.

[27] Shields AF, Mankoff D, Graham MM, et al. Analysis of 2-carbon-11-thymidine blood metabolites in PET imaging. J Nucl Med 1996;37:290–6.

[28] Shields AF, Graham MM, Kozawa SM, et al. Contribution of labeled carbon dioxide to PET imaging of carbon-11-labeled compounds. J Nucl Med 1992;33:581–4.

[29] Gunn RN, Yap JT, Wells P, et al. A general method to correct PET data for tissue metabolites using a dual-scan approach. J Nucl Med 2000;41:706–11.

[30] Wells JM, Mankoff DA, Muzi M, et al. Kinetic analysis of 2-[^{11}C]thymidine PET imaging studies of malignant brain tumors: compartmental model investigation and mathematical analysis. Mol Imaging 2002; 1:151–9.

[31] Mankoff DA, Shields AF, Link JM, et al. Kinetic analysis of 2-[^{11}C]thymidine PET imaging studies: validation studies. J Nucl Med 1999;40:614–24.

[32] Shields AF, Mankoff DA, Link JM, et al. Carbon-11-thymidine and FDG to measure therapy response. J Nucl Med 1998;39:1757–62.

[33] Bergstrom M, Lu L, Fasth KJ, et al. In vitro and animal validation of bromine-76-bromodeoxyuridine as a proliferation marker. J Nucl Med 1998;39:1273–9.

[34] Borbath I, Gregoire V, Bergstrom M, et al. Use of 5-[(76)Br]bromo-2′-fluoro-2′-deoxyuridine as a ligand for tumour proliferation: validation in an animal tumour model. Eur J Nucl Med Mol Imaging 2002; 29:19–27.

[35] Guenther I, Wyer L, Knust EJ, et al. Radiosynthesis and quality assurance of 5-[^{124}I]-Iodo-2′-deoxyuridine for functional PET imaging of cell proliferation. Nucl Med Biol 1998;25:359–65.

[36] Ryser JE, Blauenstein P, Remy N, et al. [^{76}Br]Bromo-deoxyuridine, a potential tracer for the measurement of cell proliferation by positron emission tomography, in vitro and in vivo studies in mice. Nucl Med Biol 1999; 26:673–9.

[37] Linden MD, Torres FX, Kubus J, et al. Clinical application of morphologic and immunocytochemical assessments of cell proliferation. Am J Clin Pathol 1992;97:S4–13.

[38] Tjuvajev J, Muraki A, Ginos J, et al. Iododeoxyuridine uptake and retention as a measure of tumor growth. J Nucl Med 1993;34:1152–62.

[39] Flexner C, van der Horst C, Jacobson MA, et al. Relationship between plasma concentrations of 3′-deoxy-3′- fluorothymidine (alovudine) and antiretroviral activity in two concentration-controlled trials. J Infect Dis 1994;170:1394–403.

[40] Grierson JR, Shields AF. Radiosynthesis of 3′-deoxy-3′-[(18)F]fluorothymidine: [(18)F]FLT for imaging of cellular proliferation in vivo. Nucl Med Biol 2000;27: 143–56.

[41] Shields AF, Grierson JR, Dohmen BM, et al. Imaging proliferation in vivo with [F-18]FLT and positron emission tomography. Nat Med 1998;4:1334–6.

[42] Shields AF, Grierson JR, Muzik O, et al. Kinetics of 3′-deoxy-3′-[F-18]fluorothymidine uptake and retention in dogs. Mol Imaging Biol 2002;4:83–9.

[43] Schwartz JL, Tamura Y, Jordan R, et al. Monitoring tumor cell proliferation by targeting DNA synthetic processes with thymidine and thymidine analogs. J Nucl Med 2003;44:2027–32.

[44] Rasey JS, Grierson JR, Wiens LW, et al. Validation of FLT uptake as a measure of thymidine kinase-1 activity in A549 carcinoma cells. J Nucl Med 2002;43:1210–7.

[45] Toyohara J, Waki A, Takamatsu S, et al. Basis of FLT as a cell proliferation marker: comparative uptake studies with [^{3}H]thymidine and [^{3}H]arabinothymidine, and cell-analysis in 22 asynchronously growing tumor cell lines. Nucl Med Biol 2002;29:281–7.

[46] Lu L, Samuelsson L, Bergstrom M, et al. Rat studies comparing ^{11}C-FMAU, ^{18}F-FLT, and ^{76}Br-BFU as proliferation markers. J Nucl Med 2002;43:1688–98.

[47] Sun H, Collins JM, Mangner TJ, et al. Imaging [(18)F]FAU [1-(2′-deoxy-2′-fluoro-beta-D-arabinofuranosyl) uracil] in dogs. Nucl Med Biol 2003;30:25–30.

[48] Conti PS, Alauddin MM, Fissekis JR, et al. Synthesis of 2′-fluoro-5-[^{11}C]-methyl-1-beta-D-arabinofuranosyl-uracil ([^{11}C]-FMAU): a potential nucleoside analog for in vivo study of cellular proliferation with PET. Nucl Med Biol 1995;22:783–9.

[49] Conti P, Alauddin MM, Fissekis JD, et al. Synthesis of [F-18]-2-fluoro-5-methyl-1-β-D-arabinofuranosyluracil ([F-18]FMAU). J Nucl Med 1999;40:83P.

[50] Mangner T, Klecker R, Anderson L, et al. Synthesis of 2′-[18F]fluoro-2′-deoxy-β-D-arabinofuranosyl nucleotides, [18F]FAU, [18F]FMAU, [18F]FBAU and [18F]FIAU, as potential pet agents for imaging cellular proliferation. Nucl Med Biol 2003;30:215–24.

[51] Lu L, Bergstrom M, Fasth KJ, et al. Synthesis of [76Br]bromofluorodeoxyuridine and its validation with regard to uptake, DNA incorporation, and excretion modulation in rats. J Nucl Med 2000;41:1746–52.

[52] Bading JR, Shahinian AH, Bathija P, et al. Pharmacokinetics of the thymidine analog 2′-fluoro-5-[(14)C]-methyl-1- beta-D-arabinofuranosyluracil ([(14)C] FMAU) in rat prostate tumor cells. Nucl Med Biol 2000;27:361–8.

[53] Larson SM, Weiden PL, Grunbaum Z, et al. Positron imaging feasibility studies: I. Characteristics of 3H-thymidine uptake in rodent and canine neoplasms. J Nucl Med 1981;22:869–74.

[54] Sun H, Mangner T, Muzik O, et al. Biodistribution and metabolism of 18F-FMAU: PET studies. J Nucl Med 2001;42:82P–83P.

[55] Shields AF, Mankoff DA, Zheng M, et al. Cardiac retention of labeled thymidine in humans and primates: a new metabolic pathway. J Nucl Med 1995; 36:143P.

[56] Martiat P, Ferrant A, Labar D, et al. In vivo measurement of carbon-11 thymidine uptake in non-Hodgkin's lymphoma using positron emission tomography. J Nucl Med 1988;29:1633–7.

[57] van Eijkeren ME, De Schryver A, Goethals P, et al. Measurement of short-term 11C-thymidine activity in human head and neck tumours using positron emission tomography (PET). Acta Oncol 1992;31:539–43.

[58] van Eijkeren ME, Thierens H, Seuntjens J, et al. Kinetics of [methyl-11C]thymidine in patients with squamous cell carcinoma of the head and neck. Acta Oncol 1996;35:737–41.

[59] O'Sullivan F. Imaging radiotracer model parameters in PET: a mixture analysis approach. IEEE Trans Med Imaging 1993;12:399–412.

[60] Mankoff DA, Shields AF, Graham MM, et al. A graphical analysis method to estimate blood-to-tissue transfer constants for tracers with labeled metabolites. J Nucl Med 1996;37:2049–57.

[61] Wells JM, Mankoff DA, Eary JF, et al. Kinetic analysis of 2-[11C]thymidine PET imaging studies of malignant brain tumors: preliminary patient results. Mol Imaging 2002;1:145–50.

[62] Cornford EM, Oldendorf WH. Independent blood-brain barrier transport systems for nucleic acid precursors. Biochim Biophys Acta 1975;394:211–9.

[63] Wells P, Gunn RN, Alison M, et al. Assessment of proliferation in vivo using 2-[(11)C]thymidine positron emission tomography in advanced intra-abdominal malignancies. Cancer Res 2002;62:5698–702.

[64] De Reuck J, Santens P, Goethals P, et al. [Methyl-11C] thymidine positron emission tomography in tumoral and non-tumoral cerebral lesions. Acta Neurol Belg 1999;99:118–25.

[65] Vander Borght T, Pauwels S, Lambotte L, et al. Brain tumor imaging with PET and 2-[carbon-11]thymidine. J Nucl Med 1994;35:974–82.

[66] Eary JF, Mankoff DA, Spence AM, et al. 2-[C-11] Thymidine imaging of malignant brain tumors. Cancer Res 1999;59:615–21.

[67] Wells P, Aboagye E, Gunn RN, et al. 2-[11C]thymidine positron emission tomography as an indicator of thymidylate synthase inhibition in patients treated with AG337. J Natl Cancer Inst 2003;95:675–82.

[68] Vesselle H, Grierson J, Peterson LM, et al. 18F-Fluorothymidine radiation dosimetry in human PET imaging studies. J Nucl Med 2003;44:1482–8.

[69] Pinder SE, Wencyk P, Sibbering DM, et al. Assessment of the new proliferation marker MIB1 in breast carcinoma using image analysis: associations with other prognostic factors and survival. Br J Cancer 1995;71:146–9.

[70] Vesselle H, Grierson J, Muzi M, et al. In vivo validation of 3′deoxy-3′-[(18)F]fluorothymidine ([(18)F]FLT) as a proliferation imaging tracer in humans: correlation of [(18)F]FLT uptake by positron emission tomography with Ki-67 immunohistochemistry and flow cytometry in human lung tumors. Clin Cancer Res 2002;8:3315–23.

[71] Buck AK, Schirrmeister H, Hetzel M, et al. 3-deoxy-3-[(18)F]fluorothymidine-positron emission tomography for noninvasive assessment of proliferation in pulmonary nodules. Cancer Res 2002;62:3331–4.

[72] Buck AK, Halter G, Schirrmeister H, et al. Imaging proliferation in lung tumors with PET: 18F-FLT versus 18F-FDG. J Nucl Med 2003;44:1426–31.

[73] Wagner M, Seitz U, Buck A, et al. 3′-[18F]fluoro-3′-deoxythymidine ([18F]-FLT) as positron emission tomography tracer for imaging proliferation in a murine B-Cell lymphoma model and in the human disease. Cancer Res 2003;63:2681–7.

[74] Francis DL, Freeman A, Visvikis D, et al. In vivo imaging of cellular proliferation in colorectal cancer using positron emission tomography. Gut 2003;52: 1602–6.

[75] Visvikis D, Francis D, Mulligan R, et al. Comparison of methodologies for the in vivo assessment of (18)FLT utilisation in colorectal cancer. Eur J Nucl Med Mol Imaging 2004;31:169–78.

[76] Muzi MS, Mankoff DA, Grierson JR, et al. The kinetic modeling of FLT (3′-Deoxy-3′-Fluorothymidine) in somatic tumors: mathematical studies. J Nucl Med 2004, in press.

[77] Pio BS, Park CK, Satyamurthy N, et al. PET with fluoro-L-thmyidine allows early prediction of breast cancer response to chemotherapy. J Nucl Med 2003; 44:76P.

[78] Cobben DC, Jager PL, Elsinga PH, et al. 3′-F-fluoro-3′-deoxy-L-thymidine: a new tracer for staging metastatic melanoma? J Nucl Med 2003;44:1927–32.

[79] Francis DL, Visvikis D, Costa DC, et al. Potential impact of [18F]3′-deoxy-3′-fluorothymidine versus [18F]fluoro-2-deoxy-D-glucose in positron emission

tomography for colorectal cancer. Eur J Nucl Med Mol Imaging 2003;30:988–94.

[80] Cobben DC, Van Der Laan BF, Maas B, et al. ^{18}F-FLT PET for visualization of laryngeal cancer: comparison with ^{18}F-FDG PET. J Nucl Med 2004;45:226–31.

[81] Dittmann H, Dohmen BM, Paulsen F, et al. [^{18}F]FLT PET for diagnosis and staging of thoracic tumours. Eur J Nucl Med Mol Imaging 2003;30:1407–12.

[82] Dohmen BM, Shields AF, Dittman H, et al. Use of [^{18}F]FLT for breast cancer imaging. J Nucl Med 2001; 42:29P.

[83] Tjuvajev JG, Macapinlac HA, Daghighian F, et al. Imaging of brain tumor proliferative activity with iodine-131-iododeoxyuridine. J Nucl Med 1994;35: 1407–17.

[84] Blasberg RG, Roelcke U, Weinreich R, et al. Imaging brain tumor proliferative activity with [^{124}I]iododeoxyuridine. Cancer Res 2000;60:624–35.

[85] Boni R, Blauenstein P, Dummer R, et al. Non-invasive assessment of tumour cell proliferation with positron emission tomography and [^{76}Br]bromodeoxyuridine. Melanoma Res 1999;9:569–73.

ELSEVIER
SAUNDERS

Radiol Clin N Am 43 (2005) 169–187

RADIOLOGIC
CLINICS
of North America

Imaging hypoxia and angiogenesis in tumors

Joseph G. Rajendran, MD[a,b,*], Kenneth A. Krohn, PhD[a,b]

[a]*Division of Nuclear Medicine, Department of Radiology, Box 356113, University of Washington, Seattle, WA 98195, USA*
[b]*Department of Radiation Oncology, University of Washington, Seattle, WA, USA*

Advances in molecular imaging are rapidly changing the paradigm for noninvasive diagnostic imaging from largely morphologic methods to ones that include both anatomy and parameters of function, overcoming some of the limitations of previous imaging modalities [1–5]. This paradigm allows clinicians to provide more comprehensive patient evaluation serially and in a noninvasive fashion. Advances in PET imaging instrumentation, coupled with the development of an increasing pharmacopoeia of molecular probes, have been driving forces for the rapid changes that are taking place in molecular medicine [6–9]. These advances are necessary to keep pace with the increasing sophistication of clinical questions asked of imaging specialists.

The physiologic environment for a tumor is different from normal tissue. It exhibits an evolving microenvironment that is largely dictated by abnormal vasculature and metabolism that is disease specific. One of these changes in tissue microenvironment is hypoxia, a state of reduced oxygenation in tissues. Oxygen is an essential metabolic substrate because of its critical role as the terminal electron acceptor in metabolic respiration. Levels of oxygen range through a continuum between normal levels (euoxia or normoxia) and total lack of oxygen (anoxia). The tissue oxygen levels, commonly reported as PO_2 can reach as low as less than 5 mm Hg and cells can still survive and adapt to these circumstances.

Ischemia and hypoxia are not synonymous; the former is a lack of perfusion and can lead to hypoxia, although it may not be evident until the late stages of ischemia. Tissue hypoxia can also be present in the absence of significant ischemia. Many solid tumors develop areas of hypoxia during their evolution. This is primarily caused by unregulated cellular growth, resulting in a greater demand on oxygen for energy metabolism. High interstitial pressure may exacerbate the already inefficient vascularization within the tumor [10]. In addition, other factors, such as low O_2 solubility (anemia), might increase levels of tissue hypoxia. Clinicians owe an understanding of the mechanistic aspects of hypoxia as a variable in response to cancer therapy to Thomlinson and Gray [11], who in the last century showed the impact of a distance greater than 200 μm from a capillary on cell viability and survival (Fig. 1).

Hypoxia-induced changes in tumor biology

Aggressive tumors often have high microvessel density but even higher levels of hypoxia [12]. The attempt by hypoxic cells to use glycolysis to maintain adequate cellular levels of ATP in the absence of oxygen is, however, ineffective compared with oxidative phosphorylation under normoxic conditions. As a consequence of increased glycolysis, cells accumulate lactate, with a consequent change in pH and decreased ATP:ADP ratio. Calcium homeostasis is also impaired. Ca^{++} leaves the mitochondria for the cytosolic space, and ATPase is perturbed with K^+ loss and Na^+ loading. Poor delivery of oxygen to the

This study was supported in part by National Institutes of Health Grant P01 CA42045.

* Corresponding author. Division of Nuclear Medicine, Department of Radiology, Box 356113, University of Washington, Seattle, WA 98195.

E-mail address: rajan@u.washington.edu (J.G. Rajendran).

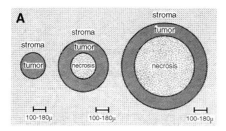

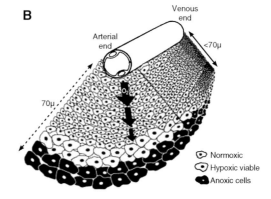

Fig. 1. (*A*) Diagrammatic illustration of the conclusions of Thomlinson and Gray from their study of human bronchogenic carcinoma. The degree of necrosis is a function of the distance from the capillaries. (*B*) Diffusion of oxygen from a capillary through tumor tissue resulting in a gradient of oxygenation and the presence of a sequential range of normoxic to anoxic cells through intermediate hypoxic but viable cells. (*From* Hall EJ. Radiobiology for the radiologist. Philadelphia: Lippincott Williams & Wilkins; 2000. p. 141; with permission.)

tumor eventually leads to a lack of glycolytic activity, even in the presence of hypoxia, a fact that can have profound implications for using fluorodeoxyglucose (FDG) as a surrogate marker for hypoxia (Fig. 2) [13].

Irrespective of the level of perfusion or status of the vasculature in a tumor, hypoxia induces changes that reflect homeostatic attempts to maintain adequate oxygenation by increasing extraction from blood and by inducing cells to adapt by developing more

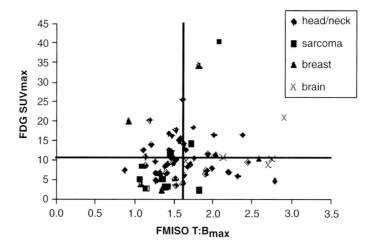

Fig. 2. Graph showing the distribution of FDG and [^{18}F]-fluoromisonidazole (FMISO) uptake (divided into four quadrants based on the median uptake values) in patients with several types of cancer. This shows the heterogeneous correlation between hypoxia and glycolysis.

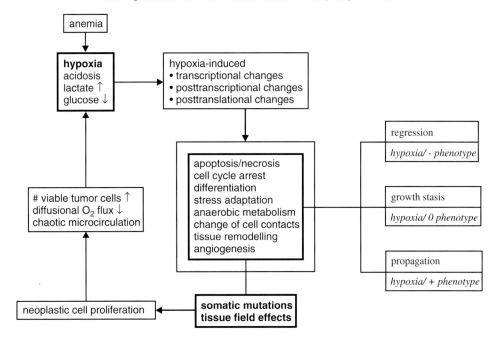

Fig. 3. Hypoxia-induced proteomic changes in cancer cells influencing propagation of cancer. The net result of these effects is manifested by growth, regression, or stable disease. (*From* Hockel M, Vaupel P. Tumor hypoxia: definitions and current clinical, biologic, and molecular aspects. J Natl Cancer Inst 2001;93:266; with permission.)

aggressive survival traits through expression of new proteins. A number of hypoxia-related genes are responsible for these genomic changes and are mediated by downstream transcription factors that have been identified (Figs. 3 and 4) [14–17]. These include expression of endothelial cytokines, such as vascular endothelial growth factor, and signaling molecules, such as interleukin-1, tumor necrosis factor-α, and transforming growth factor-β,and selection of cells with mutant p53 expression [18,19]. Several consequences of this genetic adaptation are relevant to treatment and imaging. For example,

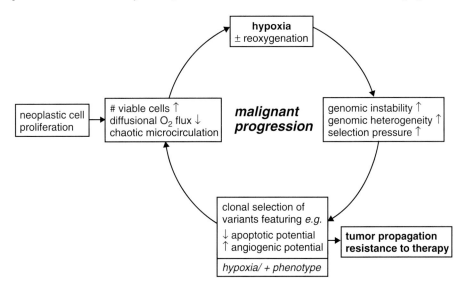

Fig. 4. Progressive genomic changes in a tumor resulting from hypoxia. (*From* Hockel M, Vaupel P. Tumor hypoxia: definitions and current clinical, biologic, and molecular aspects. J Natl Cancer Inst 2001;93:266–76; with permission.)

hypoxic cells do not readily undergo death by apoptosis [20] or arrest in G1 phase of the cell cycle in response to sublethal DNA damage [21,22]. Increased glucose transporter activity is responsible for much of the increased glucose uptake associated with hypoxia, which can be as high as twofold [23,24].

Hypoxia-inducible factor

Mechanistic aspects of tissue oxygen sensing and hypoxia response are areas of active investigation. The primary cellular oxygen-sensing mechanism seems to be mediated by a heme protein that uses O_2 as a substrate to catalyze hydroxylation of proline in a segment of hypoxia-inducible factor (HIF)-1α. This leads to rapid degradation of HIF-1α under normoxic conditions. [25]. In the absence of O_2, HIF-1α accumulates and forms a heterodimer with HIF-1β that is transported to the nucleus and promotes hypoxia-responsive genes, resulting in a cascade of genetic and metabolic events in an effort to mitigate the effects of hypoxia on cellular energetics [21,26]. Stabilization of HIF-1α has been shown to occur early in the process of tumor development [27]. Measurement of overexpressed HIF-1α in tissues by immunocytochemical staining can be used as an indirect measure of hypoxia [28–30] but its heterogeneous expression within a tumor limits the value of immunocytochemical staining.

Angiogenesis

Angiogenesis, the formation of new blood vessels, is an important aspect of the tumor phenotype. It is essential to deliver nutrients for tumor growth, invasion, and metastatic spread. It is an independent prognostic marker and, because vascular endothelial cells are more genetically stable than tumor cells, it is an attractive target for new treatment strategies. In simple terms, angiogenesis is a failure of the balance between proangiogenic and antiangiogenic signals. Angiogenesis that is commonly seen in neoplasia is another consequence of microenvironmental factors. Tumors switch to angiogenesis under a variety of stress signals, which results in tumor growth and metastases. As a general rule, tumors do not grow beyond a size of 1 to 2 mm without producing new blood vessels [31]. The network of blood vessels formed in a tumor can show significant functional deficiencies compared with normal vasculature [10,32] and these distinctions can be exploited for imaging. The angiogenesis trigger in tumor leads to new vessels with capillary endothelial cells with characteristics not found in normal tissues [33].

The emergence of angiogenesis as an important target for cancer therapy has prompted a great deal of new research to understand this molecular process. Gene expression profiling has identified proteins that are selectively expressed by tumor endothelial cells, including a large class of integrins, such as $\alpha_V\beta_3$ and $\alpha_V\beta_5$. These provide the potential for specific targeting of therapeutics [34]. This has coincided with the development of molecular imaging methods that provide the potential to monitor treatment [35,36]. Although angiogenesis is a frequent consequence of hypoxia, some tumors develop extensive angiogenesis without the presence of hypoxia and vice versa. A cause and effect relationship does not always exist. Kourkourakis et al [37] found a U-shaped association between the two phenomena, which was explained mechanistically. Prognosis has been found to be poor when there is poor angiogenesis, perhaps because of the presence of hypoxia or when there is profound angiogenesis, likely because of increased metastatic potential.

One example of de novo angiogenesis is seen in von Hippel-Lindau disease. Spontaneous renal tumors develop with overexpression of HIF-1α, resulting in widespread angiogenesis in the absence of hypoxia. Despite aggressive angiogenesis in many tumors and contrary to expectations, observed blood perfusion rates are lower in the tumor bed than in normal tissue. Moreover, as tumors grow, perfusion is further decreased because of a number of other biophysical parameters [35,38]. Immunocytochemical staining has also been used in evaluating angiogenesis in a tumor that results from some of the previously mentioned molecular changes, specifically the expression of vascular endothelial growth factor [19]. Neither perfusion nor permeability are adequate measure of angiogenesis.

Tumor hypoxia and clinical outcome: what is new?

Radiobiologists have long taught that low levels of intracellular oxygen result in poor response to radiation therapy. Oxygen is important for fixing, in the sense of making permanent, the radiation-induced cytotoxic products in tissues. In its absence, the free radicals formed by ionizing radiation recombine without producing the anticipated cellular damage

[39–41]. As a result, radiation oncologists have been frustrated by the fact that hypoxic tumors are not effectively eradicated with conventional doses of radiation. Clinical and preclinical experience indicates that it can take three times as much photon radiation dose to cause the same cytotoxic effect in hypoxic cells as compared with normoxic cells (Fig. 5) [41–44].

Although all these are established concepts, what is new is that hypoxia results in the development and selection of an aggressive phenotype, resulting in poor response and poor outcome because of increased metastatic potential [20,45–47]. Hypoxia has also been found to promote resistance to a number of chemotherapeutic agents by one or more independent mechanisms: (1) hypoxia can induce slowing of cellular proliferation, (2) changes in perfusion associated with hypoxia may impede delivery of chemotherapy drugs, and (3) gene amplification results in the induction of numerous stress proteins that are factors in limiting response [47,48].

Cancer treatment schemes designed to circumvent the cure-limiting consequences of hypoxia have led, however, to disappointing results [49]. Hyperbaric oxygen, neutron therapy, hyperfractionation, and the use of oxygen-mimetic radiation sensitizers have not had the anticipated clinical benefit. As promising as they may sound, these methods were associated with problems of either lack of widespread availability or serious clinical toxicity or they are simply ineffective in human trials. Authors have suggested several reasons for this lack of benefit. Especially relevant to this article is the probability that an assay is needed to select patients with hypoxia. A benefit in an appropriately selected patient population would be expected and the hypoxia assay could also be used to follow the response to treatment.

Hypoxic cells are attractive targets for hypoxia-activated prodrugs [50,51]. Newer hypoxia-activated prodrugs [52] are less toxic and more effective than their early counterparts, such as mitomycin C [53]. In addition to producing direct cytotoxic effects, these agents exhibit synergistic toxicity when used with radiation and chemotherapy. Although focal hypoxia in a tumor can be treated with boost radiation using intensity-modulated radiotherapy [54,55], more diffuse hypoxia benefits from hypoxic cell toxins and sensitizers. Nuclear imaging with hypoxia-specific tracers should be an important tool for selecting patients who might benefit from this treatment [56].

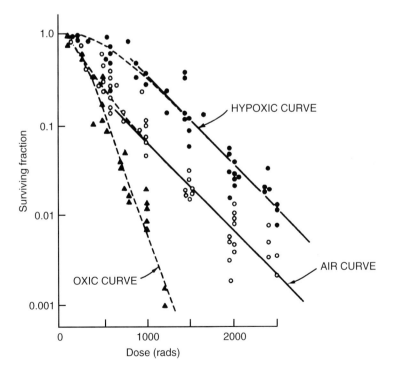

Fig. 5. This illustrates the relative resistance of hypoxic cells to radiation. In comparison with oxygenated cells hypoxic cells require three times more radiation to have the same effect. (*From* Hall EJ. Radiobiology for the radiologist. Philadelphia: Lippincott Williams & Wilkins; 2000. p. 145; with permission.)

The importance of selecting appropriate patients for a hypoxia-directed therapy results in the greatest benefit for the individual patient.

Need to identify hypoxia in tumors

The negative association of hypoxia with response to treatment and clinical outcome strongly implies that evaluating hypoxia helps in identifying tumors with a high hypoxic fraction so that hypoxia-directed treatments can be implemented and treatments that are oxygen dependent can be avoided. Contrary to expectations, there is now abundant evidence that tumor hypoxia does not correlate with tumor size, grade, and extent of necrosis or blood hemoglobin status [57–62]. Moreover, most of the commonly used clinicopathologic parameters for evaluation of tumor hypoxia are not strong indicators of prognosis.

Methods to evaluate tumor hypoxia

Tumor oxygenation has been evaluated by several methods and tumor hypoxia to predicted patient outcome in cancers of the uterine cervix [63], lung [59], head and neck [64–67], and glioma (Fig. 6) [68,69]. Most of these studies, however, have shown widespread heterogeneity in tumor hypoxia within a tumor, between tumors, and between patients with the same tumor type [70]. Although hypoxia generally resolves when a tumor shrinks after treatment with either radiotherapy or chemotherapy, it may show paradoxical results in some tumors, perhaps because of hypoxic cell sparing by the treatment (Fig. 7).

Currently available assays for tumor hypoxia can be categorized as in vivo (invasive and noninvasive) or ex vivo (invasive) biopsy [5,71,72]. A useful assay must distinguish normoxic regions from ones that are hypoxic at a level relevant to cancer, PO_2 in the 5 mm Hg range. Experience has shown that regional levels of hypoxia should be measured for individual patients and tumor sites. To be maximally successful, hypoxia-directed imaging and treatment should target both chronic hypoxia and hypoxia resulting from transient interruption of blood flow (Fig. 8) [73]. The assay should reflect intracellular PO_2 rather than blood flow or some consequence of O_2 on subsequent biochemistry. The observed temporal heterogeneity in tissue PO_2 suggests that a secondary effect, such as intracellular redox status, is not as relevant to cancer

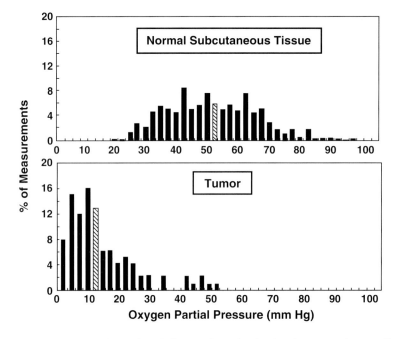

Fig. 6. Oxygen distribution in a metastatic lymph node from a primary head and neck cancer and surrounding normal tissue. These measurements were made with Eppendorf oxygen electrode in a single patient. The median values are represented by hashed bars (*From* Adam M, Gabalski EC, Bloch DA, Ochlert JW, Brown JM, Elsaid AA, et al. Tissue oxygen distribution in head and neck cancer patients. Head Neck 1999;21:146–53; and Brown JM. The hypoxic cell: a target for selective cancer therapy. Eighteenth Bruce F. Cain Memorial Award lecture. Cancer Res 1999;59:5864; with permission.)

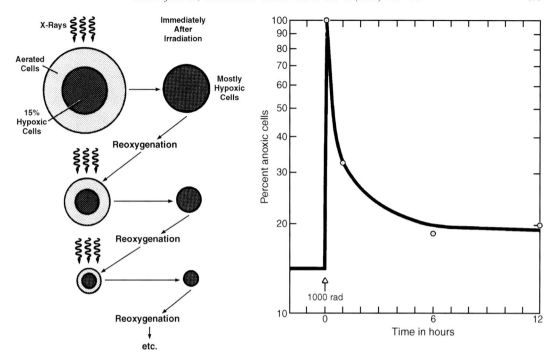

Fig. 7. Reoxygenation in a tumor containing a mixture of aerated and hypoxic cells. This illustrates the changes with each successive fraction of radiation and the sensitivity of oxygenated cells to radiation. (*From* Hall EJ. Radiobiology for the radiologist. Philadelphia: Lippincott Williams & Wilkins; 2000. p. 146–7; with permission.)

treatment outcome as the intracellular partial pressure of O_2. Other desirable characteristics for an ideal clinical hypoxia assay include (1) simple and non-invasive method, (2) nontoxic, (3) rapid and easy to perform with consistency between laboratories, and (4) the ability to quantify without the need for substantial calibration of the detection instrumentation. Location of the tumor in a patient should not be a limiting factor for the assay. Lastly, spatial heterogeneity in the distribution of hypoxia dictates that the ideal assay must provide a complete locoregional evaluation of the tumor. All of these requirements suggest an important role for imaging in evaluating hypoxia.

Polarographic electrode measurements

Early experience evaluating oxygenation of tumors is largely based on direct measurement of O_2 levels using very fine polarographic oxygen electrodes. This assay can be calibrated in units of millimeters of mercury and has been referred to as a gold standard. Heterogeneity of hypoxia within a tumor, which shows a gradient toward the center of the tumor, poses a difficulty for accurately mapping regional PO_2 by this method [58,74]. The electrodes do not provide full maps of a tumor area; they only provide a histogram of the distribution of cell regions as a function of the electrode's reading. There may also be interlaboratory variations in calibration of the electrodes [75]. Polarographic electrodes measure oxygen tension in a group of cells and the readings can be influenced by the presence of blood [76].

Although image-guided sampling can be used to select the path and depth of electrode deployment to avoid blood vessels [77], anatomic imaging methods are notoriously limited in identifying areas of viable tissue within a tumor. Hypodense areas visualized within a tumor on CT (considered necrotic) can indeed have measurable levels of oxygen [76]. Selection of close entry points can reduce sampling error [75], but it also might compromise patient compliance. In addition, electrode measurements are limited by the need for accessible tumor location and difficulties with serial measurements. An accurate value of PO_2 may be less informative than once expected, because cells have different respiratory demand and may not exhibit hypoxic responses at

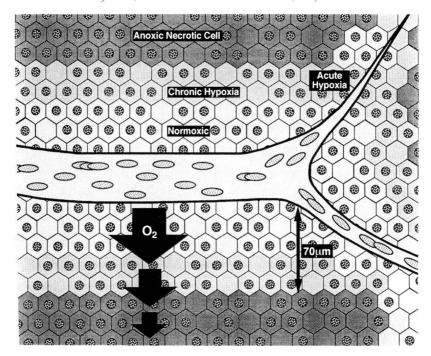

Fig. 8. This diagram illustrates the existence of chronic and acute hypoxia. The former is a result of compromised diffusion of oxygen in actively respiring cells, whereas the latter is a result of acute and temporary blockage of blood vessels in a tumor. (*From* Hall EJ. Radiobiology for the radiologist. Philadelphia: Lippincott Williams & Wilkins; 2000. p. 142; with permission.)

the same levels of tissue oxygenation. Normal cells (eg, cardiomyocytes) experience a level of stress at relatively high PO_2 [78]. Electrode studies commonly report the percentage of readings that fall below some cutoff value that may range from 2.5 to 10 mm Hg, depending on the tumor site. This fractional distribution is a more robust prognostic parameter than absolute PO_2, which is dependent on tissue type and sampling technique, including calibration of the electrode. Also, O_2 is consumed during the electrode assay. The benefit of an absolute value for PO_2 may be less useful and less robust than accurate assessment of the fraction of cells that are hypoxic. For example, it is apparent from Fig. 9 that the distribution of electrode measurements in this tumor is bimodal. The fraction of cells in the hypoxic peak may be much more important than the mean PO_2 or the PO_2 for the nadir separating hypoxia and normoxia. These limitations prompted the search for a noninvasive method that could be done serially to characterize and quantify hypoxia in cancer patients. Imaging methods for hypoxia provide a complete anatomic map of relative oxygenation level in tumor regions with good spatial resolution and in an environment that tends to be highly heterogeneous.

Evaluating angiogenesis

Angiogenesis can be evaluated by either direct or indirect methods. Direct methods were started with largely fluorescent techniques, such as intravital fluorescent video microscopy [79], fluorophore coupling of fibronectin, quenched near-infrared fluorochromes to matrix metalloproteinase-2 substrates, MR imaging [10,80], and color Doppler vascularity index [81–83]. The simplicity of dynamic contrast-enhanced MR imaging has led to fairly widespread use of this technique [84]. It provides a signal that effectively integrates vascular blood flow, blood volume, and vascular permeability.

Noninvasive imaging of the $\alpha_V\beta_3$ integrins that are abundant on vascular endothelium has been attempted by investigators using MR imaging [85], ultrasound [86,87], PET [88–91], and endostatins [92]. The $\alpha_V\beta_3$ integrin is a transmembrane cell adhesion receptor that leads to tumor cells binding of extracellular matrix proteins. The receptor is highly expressed on activated endothelial cells but only weakly expressed in mature endothelium. This has led to $\alpha_V\beta_3$ integrin being evaluated as a target for tumor-specific therapy. The arginine–glycine–

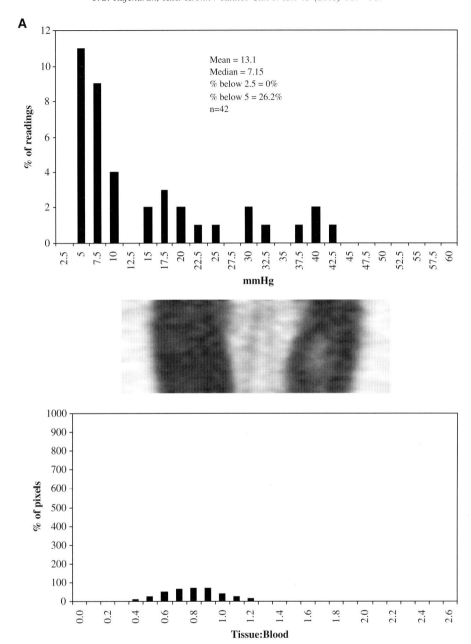

Fig. 9. Comparison of oxygen electrode measurements in a patient with liposarcoma (*A*) and another with osteosarcoma (*B*). Histogram of oxygen electrode PO_2 measurements (*top*), coronal slice of FMISO image (*center*), and tissue:blood histogram of the FMISO uptake into the tumor (*bottom*).

aspartic acid tripeptide recognizes the $\alpha_V\beta_3$ receptor, although it cross-reacts with other integrins. A labeled arginine–glycine–aspartic acid-containing glycopeptide shows great promise as an imaging agent and has also been suggested as a potential therapeutic agent [88–90].

PET and hypoxia imaging

Hypoxia imaging presents the special challenge of making a positive image out of low levels of O_2. Chemists have developed two different imaging agents to address this problem: bioreductive alkyl-

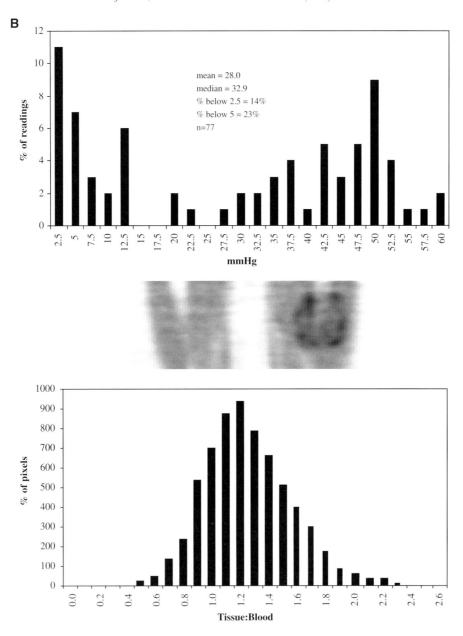

Fig. 9 (*continued*).

ating agents that are O_2-sensitive and metal chelates that are sensitive to the intracellular redox state that develops as a consequence of hypoxia.

Nitroimidazole compounds

Misonidazole, an azomycin-based hypoxic cell sensitizer introduced in clinical radiation oncology nearly three decades ago, binds covalently to intracellular molecules at levels that are inversely proportional to intracellular oxygen concentration below about 10 mm Hg. It is a lipophilic 2-nitroimidazole derivative whose uptake in hypoxic cells is dependent on the sequential reduction of the nitro group on the imidazole ring [93]. This mechanism requires that the cell be alive and undergoing electron transport to provide the electron that initiates the bioreduction step. In the absence of electron transport, the tracer is not reduced and not accumulated. The one-electron reduction product is an unstable radical anion that either gives up its extra electron to O_2 or picks up a second electron. In the presence of O_2, the nitroimidazole simply goes through a futile reduction cycle and is returned to its initial state. In the absence of an alternative electron acceptor, the nitroimidazole continues to accumulate electrons to form the hydroxylamine alkylating agent and become trapped within the alive but O_2-deficient cell (Fig. 10). This unique biochemical mechanism leads to a tracer whose uptake is inversely related to the oxygen tension within the cell. If cells are reoxygenated and then exposed to a new batch of the tracer, it is not accumulated.

[18F]-fluoromisonidazole (FMISO) is an imaging agent derived from misonidazole, one of the earliest radiosensitizers used in clinical radiation therapy. It has a high hypoxia-specific factor, defined as the ratio of uptake in hypoxic cells compared with normoxic cells, which determines the uptake and specificity in vitro. For FMISO the hypoxia-specific factor is between 20 and 50 [94] and is proportional to the magnitude of hypoxic fraction measured by a survival assay. Prodrug imaging agents, such as FMISO, are bioreductively activated in hypoxic tissue but the process is inhibited by the presence of oxygen in tissues. The result is a positive image of the absence of O_2.

FMISO is a highly stable and robust radiopharmaceutical that can be used to quantify tissue hypoxia using PET technology [60,95]. Its easy synthesis and optimal safety profile are responsible for its ready acceptance in the clinic. After extensive clinical validation, FMISO remains the most commonly used agent for hypoxia PET imaging [59,60,96–101]. Its biodistribution and dosimetry

characteristics are ideal for PET imaging [102]. The partition coefficient of FMISO is 0.41 [103], similar to that of the blood flow agent antipyrine, so that initially after injection the tissue distribution reflects blood flow, but after about an hour the distribution reflects its partition coefficient. It is homogeneously distributed with no tissue specificity [78].

The distribution of pixel uptake values after about 90 minutes is narrowly dispersed. This has led to a simple analysis of FMISO PET image by scaling the pixel uptake to plasma concentration. The mean value for this ratio in all tissues is close to unity and almost all normoxic pixels have a value of less than 1.2. The magnitude of the intermediate radical anion product parallels nitroreductase levels, which vary only slightly, so this factor does not affect the imaging analysis of fractional hypoxic volume [96]. The optimum time for imaging seems to be between 90 and 120 minutes and can be adjusted to fit the clinic schedule so that, to the patient or the imaging technologist, the procedure is very similar to a bone scan. Although the tumor:background ratio does not show high contrast, this does not compromise image interpretation. Hypoxia images can be interpreted qualitatively or quantitatively. Qualitative interpretations have been used with a scoring system to grade the uptake in a tumor vis-à-vis normal tissue [56]. After extensive validation studies, the authors prefer a simple but accurate quantitation method using a venous blood sample to calculate a tissue:blood ratio [4,104]. The tumor:plasma ratio has proved useful to estimate the degree of hypoxia in a number of studies, as has the tumor:muscle ratio [101]. The FMISO ratio image provides a reliable and reproducible method that can be introduced readily in the clinic.

Fractional hypoxic volume, defined as the proportion of pixels within the imaged tumor volume having a ratio above some cutoff value, has been used

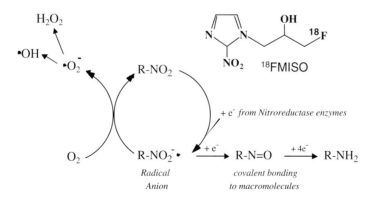

Fig. 10. Structure of misonidazole showing the mechanism of action in the presence and absence of oxygen.

[96] but this requires accurate delineation of tumor margins to define the denominator. The authors prefer the tumor hypoxic volume parameter, which is the total number of pixels with a tissue:blood ratio (T:B) greater than or equal to 1.2. Expressed in milliliters, it is a measure of the extent of tissue hypoxia and obviates the need for stringent demarcation of the tumor boundaries [4]. The advantage of this simple analysis is that it is insensitive to blood flow. It requires only the viability of the hypoxic cell as defined by active electron transport. Mathematic models have been evaluated for more detailed analysis [105], but this level of sophistication is not likely to find a role in routine clinical imaging.

A typical protocol for PET scanning with [^{18}F]-FMISO uses an intravenous administration of a dose of 3.7 mBq (0.1 mCi)/kg, which results in an effective total body dose equivalent of 0.0126 mGy/mBq [102]. Scanning begins after 90 to 120 minutes and lasts for 20 minutes with blood sampling midway during the scan. A transmission scan (20 minutes) is used for attenuation correction of emission data. Typically one axial field of view of 15-cm cranio-caudal dimension is acquired. An FDG scan of the same region is routinely obtained for these patients, with care taken to reposition the patients between images. Addition of FDG imaging data increases the sensitivity of FMISO imaging by indicating the full extent of tumor and helps in correlating metabolic activity and hypoxia in tumor (Figs. 10–15) [13].

Alternative azomycin imaging agents

To improve image contrast, some groups have developed alternative azomycin radiopharmaceuticals for hypoxia imaging by attempting to manipulate the rate of blood clearance [106–108]. Elongation factor-1 was initially developed because of the availability of an antibody stain to verify the distribution in tissue samples [109]. Fluoroerythronitroimidazole was developed as a more hydrophilic derivative of misonidazole that might have more rapid plasma

clearance and this could be an imaging advantage. Fluoroetanidazole has binding characteristics similar to FMISO, but has been reported to have less retention in liver and fewer metabolites in animals [110], but the advantages were not sufficient to carry these derivatives to wide clinical testing. Single-photon emission CT–based hypoxia imaging compounds have been introduced with the hope of taking this technology to gamma camera imaging [111]. The University of Alberta group pioneered the development of iodinated derivatives of nitroimidazoles. Direct halogenation of the imidazole ring does not lead to a stable radiopharmaceutical, so the general approach has been to place sugar residues between the nitroimidazole and the radioiodine to stabilize the molecule. These products exhibit minimal deiodination and two derivatives have been evaluated in patients. Introduction of the sugar results in a more water-soluble molecule than misonidazole. This has two consequences: the hydrophilic product clears more rapidly, but its clearance and its background distribution in normoxic tissues is dependent on blood flow. The resulting images have higher contrast when imaging is typically initiated 110 minutes after injection. A simple ratio analysis to infer hypoxia, however, as used for FMISO images, is not valid.

The success with radioiodinated azomycin arabinosides led to attempts to develop technetium derivatives of 2-nitroimidazole. The practical advantages of a Tc-99m label are well known in the nuclear medicine community and include ready availability at low cost, convenient half-life for hypoxia measurements, and versatile chemistry. Two different approaches have been evaluated: both BMS181321 and HL91 were synthesized and evaluated as hypoxia-based agents. Although both of these molecules involve ligands with potential hypoxia-specific binding characteristics, the reduction chemistry of the metal core is also subject to redox chemistry that can result in separation of the Tc = O core from the ligand [106,112]. The BMS compound was so lipophilic that its background activity was high, especially in the abdomen. A less lipophilic derivative, BMS194796,

FMISO
T:B$_{max}$ = 2.79

FDG
SUV$_{max}$ = 4.5

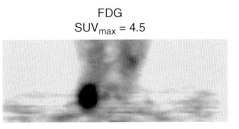

Fig. 11. Corresponding FMISO (*left*) and FDG (*right*) images of a patient with cancer of the larynx with metastatic lymph nodes.

FMISO
T:B$_{max}$ = 2.71

FDG
SUV$_{max}$ = 8.7

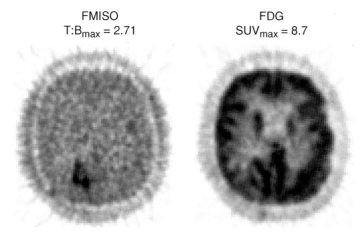

Fig. 12. Corresponding transaxial FMISO (*left*) and FDG (*right*) images of a patient with glioblastoma multiforme in the right occipital region. SUV, standardized uptake value.

has been developed with better clearance properties, especially from the liver [113]. Both of the BMS compounds involve a nitroimidazole group, although it is probably not the dominant influence in determining the biodistribution kinetics of the radiopharmaceutical and its specific localization in hypoxic tissues. The HL91 molecule, TcBnAO, does not include a nitroimidazole; the Tc-ligand coordination chemistry is directly reduced and retained in hypoxic environments [112]. The resulting lack of specificity has led to abandonment of this molecule as a tracer for imaging hypoxia. It also requires a much lower level of O$_2$ for its reduction and uptake, raising concerns for routine clinical applications [114].

Single-photon emission CT radiopharmaceuticals include both the iodinated compounds (eg, [^{123}I] radioiodinated azamycin arabinosides [115]) and technetium-based agents. These radiopharmaceuticals, in contrast to PET agents, suffer from lower image contrast and less potential for quantification [107]. Furthermore, the absence of a gold standard for hypoxia evaluation complicates validation of all

hypoxia markers, including FMISO [94], and treatment outcome studies are urgently needed to provide convincing evidence for the clinical value of hypoxia imaging.

The altered redox environment associated with hypoxia has led to another class of radiopharmaceuticals for imaging hypoxia. Copper bis(thiosemicarbazones) are a class of molecules evaluated as freely diffusible but retained blood flow tracers. The ^{64}Cu-labeled acetyl derivative of pyruvaldehyde bis [N4-methylthiosemicarbazonato] copper (II) complex, Cu-ATSM, has the potential advantage of a longer half-life for practical clinical use [116–118], although the mechanism of retention is less well validated than FMISO. Fujibayashi et al [119] showed that the intracellular retention mechanism was related to the copper-reduction chemistry, Cu^{++} to Cu$^+$, which has a redox potential of −297 mV for Cu-ATSM. Several biologic systems have comparable redox potentials: −315 mV for NADH and −230 mV for glutathione.

Several laboratories showed that Cu-ATSM was retained in hypoxic areas [119]. This radiopharma-

FMISO
T:B$_{max}$ = 2.59

FDG
SUV$_{max}$ = 10.3

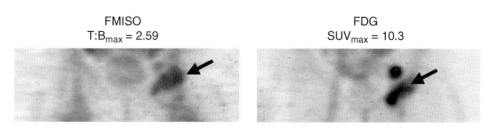

Fig. 13. Corresponding FMISO (*left*) and FDG (*right*) images of a patient with soft tissue sarcoma of the pelvis.

FMISO
T:B$_{max}$ = 2.77

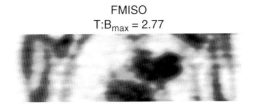

Fig. 14. FMISO image of a patient with a non–small cell lung cancer.

ceutical has rapid washout from normoxic areas. It is a useful imaging agent for identifying regions of tissue that have higher levels of reducing agents, such as NADH, as a consequence of hypoxia. There is ample evidence in the literature that the concentration of NADH is increased under extended hypoxic conditions. This mechanism is distinct from that for the nitroimidazoles, in that the copper agents reflect a consequence of hypoxia rather than the actual PO$_2$. This mechanistic difference might limit the role of Cu-ATSM for measuring a prompt reoxygenation response because the increased levels of NADH persist. Diffusion of NADH-related reducing equivalents might make Cu-ATSM less reflective of the spatial heterogeneity of hypoxia. The same characteristics make the Cu agents preferable for imaging chronic hypoxia, however, where levels of NADH can increase by several fold. There are several useful radionuclides of copper that can be used for imaging [117,120].

PET imaging is likely to become the dominant method for evaluating tumor hypoxia in patients. It simply stands out as the ideal procedure for evaluating tumor hypoxia repeatedly and noninvasively. It has the advantage of evaluating the entire tumor and regional lymph nodes for a patient at the same time in a snapshot fashion. It is less operator-dependent than polarographic oxygen electrodes. Its noninvasiveness and safety profile make it a convenient tool for the follow-up of patients by providing the ability to do repeat imaging [121]. The main advantage of PET is its ability accurately to quantify tissue uptake of the hypoxia tracer, independent of anatomic location of the tumor. Widespread availability of PET scanners (and now PET/CT scanners) and [^{18}F]-labeled hypoxia tracers in the community make this procedure within reach of every community nuclear medicine center. Although the level of pretherapy hypoxia is an important parameter, its change with treatment gives an even better understanding of the effectiveness of treatment.

Hypoxia imaging can be combined with other indicators of tissue hemodynamics and oxygenation, such as perfusion imaging using [^{15}O]water, and tissue markers of proteomic response to hypoxia, such as vascular density and HIF-1α expression using immunocytochemistry, in a complementary fashion. Recently introduced PET/CT scanners provide the opportunity to combine anatomic imaging and functional information. This will not only increase the accuracy of hypoxia imaging but will also allow the images to be incorporated into radiation treatment planning systems to plan and deliver hypoxic subvolume directed radiotherapy boost effectively using intensity-modulated radiotherapy [54,55,122].

Summary

There is a clear need in cancer treatment for a noninvasive imaging assay that evaluates the oxygenation status and heterogeneity of hypoxia and angiogenesis in individual patients. Such an assay could be used to select alternative treatments and to monitor the effects of treatment. Of the several methods available, each imaging procedure has at least one disadvantage. The limited quantitative potential of single-photon emission CT and MR imaging always limits tracer imaging based on these detection systems. PET imaging with FMISO and Cu-ATSM is ready for coordinated multicenter trials,

FMISO
maxT:B 1.53

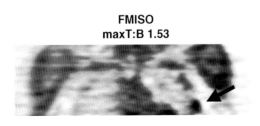

FDG
SUV 5.3

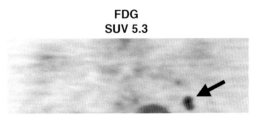

Fig. 15. Corresponding FMISO (*left*) and FDG (*right*) images of a patient with breast cancer.

however, that should move aggressively forward to resolve the debate over the importance of hypoxia in limiting response to cancer therapy. Advances in radiation treatment planning, such as intensity-modulated radiotherapy, provide the ability to customize radiation delivery based on physical conformity [54,55,123,124]. With incorporation of regional biologic information, such as hypoxia and proliferating vascular density in treatment planning, imaging can create a biologic profile of the tumor to direct radiation therapy [124,125]. Presence of widespread hypoxia in the tumor benefits from a systemic hypoxic cell cytotoxin [126]. Angiogenesis is also an important therapeutic target. Imaging hypoxia and angiogenesis complements the efforts in development of antiangiogenesis and hypoxia-targeted drugs. The complementary use of hypoxia and angiogenesis imaging methods should provide the impetus for development and clinical evaluation of novel drugs targeted at angiogenesis and hypoxia [50,127–129]. Hypoxia imaging brings in information different from that of FDG-PET but it will play an important niche role in oncologic imaging in the near future.

FMISO, radioiodinated azamycin arabinosides, and Cu-ATSM are all being evaluated in patients. The Cu-ATSM images show the best contrast early after injection but these images are confounded by blood flow and their mechanism of localization is one step removed from the intracellular O_2 concentration. FMISO has been criticized as inadequate because of its clearance characteristics, but its uptake after 2 hours is probably the most purely reflective of regional PO_2 at the time the radiopharmaceutical is used. The FMISO images show less contrast than those of Cu-ATSM because of the lipophilicity and slower clearance of FMISO but attempts to increase the rate of clearance led to tracers whose distribution is contaminated by blood flow effects. For single-photon emission CT the only option is radioiodinated azamycin arabinosides, because the technetium agents are not yet ready for clinical evaluation. Rather than develop new and improved hypoxia agents, or even quibbling about the pros and cons of alternative agents, the nuclear medicine community needs to convince the oncology community that imaging hypoxia is an important procedure that can lead to improved treatment outcome.

Acknowledgments

The authors appreciate the following individuals for the help they provided. L.M. Peterson, BA, for help with the manuscript, J.F. Eary, MD, for useful critique, and H.S. Vesselle, MD, for help with the oxygen electrode studies.

References

[1] Wahl RL. Anatomolecular imaging with 2-deoxy-2-[18F]fluoro-D-glucose: bench to outpatient center. Mol Imaging Biol 2003;5:49–56.

[2] Herschman HR. Molecular imaging: looking at problems, seeing solutions. Science 2003;302:605–8.

[3] Chapman JD, Bradley JD, Eary JF, Haubner R, Larson SM, Michalski JM, et al. Molecular (functional) imaging for radiotherapy applications: an RTOG symposium. Int J Radiat Oncol Biol Phys 2003;55:294–301.

[4] Rajendran J, Muzi M, Peterson LM, Diaz AZ, Spence AM, Schwartz DS, et al. Analyzing the results of [F-18] FMISO PET hypoxia imaging: what is the best way to quantify hypoxia? J Nucl Med 2002;43:102P.

[5] Peters L, McKay M. Predictive assays: will they ever have a role in the clinic? Int J Radiat Oncol Biol Phys 2001;49:501–4.

[6] Rowland DJ, Lewis JS, Welch MJ. Molecular imaging: the application of small animal positron emission tomography. J Cell Biochem Suppl 2002; 39:110–5.

[7] Maclean D, Northrop JP, Padgett HC, Walsh JC. Drugs and probes: the symbiotic relationship between pharmaceutical discovery and imaging science. Mol Imaging Biol 2003;5:304–11.

[8] Collier TL, Lecomte R, McCarthy TJ, Meikle S, Ruth TJ, Scopinaro F, et al. Assessment of cancer-associated biomarkers by positron emission tomography: advances and challenges. Dis Markers 2002; 18:211–47.

[9] Gambhir SS. Molecular imaging of cancer with positron emission tomography. Nat Rev Cancer 2002;2: 683–93.

[10] Bhujwalla ZM, Artemov D, Aboagye E, Ackerstaff E, Gillies RJ, Natarajan K, et al. The physiological environment in cancer vascularization, invasion and metastasis. Novartis Found Symp 2001;240:23–38 [discussion: 38–45, 152–3].

[11] Thomlinson RH, Gray LH. The histological structure of some human lung cancers and the possible implications for radiotherapy. Br J Cancer 1955;9: 537–49.

[12] Kourkourakis MI, Giotromanolaki A. Cancer vascularization: implications in radiotherapy? Int J Radiat Oncol Biol Phys 2000;48:545–53S.

[13] Rajendran JG, O'Sullivan F, Peterson LM, Schwartz DL, Conrad EU, Spence AM, et al. Hypoxia and glucose metabolism in malignant tumors: evaluation by FMISO and FDG PET imaging. Clin Cancer Res 2004;10:2245–52.

[14] Scandurro AB, Weldon CW, Figueroa YG, Alam J, Beckman BS. Gene microarray analysis reveals a

novel hypoxia signal transduction pathway in human hepatocellular carcinoma cells. Int J Oncol 2001; 19:129–35.

[15] Villaret DB, Wang T, Dillon D, Xu J, Sivam D, Cheever MA, et al. Identification of genes overexpressed in head and neck squamous cell carcinoma using a combination of complementary DNA subtraction and microarray analysis. Laryngoscope 2000; 110:374–81.

[16] Agani F, Semenza GL. Mersalyl is a novel inducer of vascular endothelial growth factor gene expression and hypoxia-inducible factor 1 activity. Mol Pharmacol 1998;54:749–54.

[17] Bae MK, Kwon YW, Kim MS, Bae SK, Bae MH, Lee YM, et al. Identification of genes differentially expressed by hypoxia in hepatocellular carcinoma cells. Biochem Biophys Res Commun 1998;243:158–62.

[18] Dachs GU, Tozer GM. Hypoxia modulated gene expression: angiogenesis, metastasis and therapeutic exploitation. Eur J Cancer 2000;36:1649–60.

[19] Eisma RJ, Spiro JD, Kreutzer DL. Vascular endothelial growth factor expression in head and neck squamous cell carcinoma. Am J Surg 1997;174:513–7.

[20] Hockel M, Schlenger K, Hockel S, Vaupel P. Hypoxic cervical cancers with low apoptotic index are highly aggressive. Cancer Res 1999;59:4525–8.

[21] Guillemin K, Krasnow MA. The hypoxic response: huffing and HIFing. Cell 1997;89:9–12.

[22] Jiang BH, Semenza GL, Bauer C, Marti HH. Hypoxia-inducible factor 1 levels vary exponentially over a physiologically relevant range of O_2 tension. Am J Physiol 1996;271:C1172–80.

[23] Clavo AC, Wahl RL. Effects of hypoxia on the uptake of tritiated thymidine, L-leucine, L-methionine and FDG in cultured cancer cells. J Nucl Med 1996;37: 502–6.

[24] Burgman P, Odonoghue JA, Humm JL, Ling CC. Hypoxia-induced increase in FDG uptake in MCF7 cells. J Nucl Med 2001;42:170–5.

[25] Ivan M, Kondo K, Yang H, Kim W, Valiando J, Ohh M, et al. HIFalpha targeted for VHL-mediated destruction by proline hydroxylation: implications for O_2 sensing. Science 2001;292:464–8.

[26] Huang LE, Arany Z, Livingston DM, Bunn HF. Activation of hypoxia-inducible transcription factor depends primarily upon redox-sensitive stabilization of its alpha subunit. J Biol Chem 1996;271:32253–9.

[27] Bos R, Zhong H, Hanrahan CF, Mommers EC, Semenza GL, Pinedo HM, et al. Levels of hypoxia-inducible factor-1 alpha during breast carcinogenesis. J Natl Cancer Inst 2001;93:309–14.

[28] Zhong H, De Marzo AM, Laughner E, Lim M, Hilton DA, Zagzag D, et al. Overexpression of hypoxia-inducible factor 1alpha in common human cancers and their metastases. Cancer Res 1999;59: 5830–5.

[29] Marxsen JH, Schmitt O, Metzen E, Jelkmann W, Hellwig-Burgel T. Vascular endothelial growth factor gene expression in the human breast cancer cell line MX-1 is controlled by O_2 availability in vitro and in vivo. Ann Anat 2001;183:243–9.

[30] Yaziji H, Gown AM. Immunohistochemical analysis of gynecologic tumors. Int J Gynecol Pathol 2001; 20:64–78.

[31] Folkman J. Tumor angiogenesis: therapeutic implications. N Engl J Med 1971;285:1182–6.

[32] Gullino PM. Angiogenesis and neoplasia. N Engl J Med 1981;305:884–5.

[33] Hood JD, Cheresh DA. Role of integrins in cell invasion and migration. Nat Rev Cancer 2002;2:91–100.

[34] McDonald DM, Teicher BA, Stetler-Stevenson W, Ng SS, Figg WD, Folkman J, et al. Report from the Society for Biological Therapy and Vascular Biology Faculty of the NCI Workshop on Angiogenesis Monitoring. J Immunother 2004;27:161–75.

[35] Costouros NG, Diehn FE, Libutti SK. Molecular imaging of tumor angiogenesis. J Cell Biochem Suppl 2002;39:72–8.

[36] Weber WA, Haubner R, Vabuliene E, Kuhnast B, Wester HJ, Schwaiger M. Tumor angiogenesis targeting using imaging agents. Q J Nucl Med 2001; 45:179–82.

[37] Koukourakis MI, Giatromanolaki A, Sivridis E, Fezoulidis I. Cancer vascularization: implications in radiotherapy? Int J Radiat Oncol Biol Phys 2000; 48:545–53.

[38] Jain RK, Safabakhsh N, Sckell A, Chen Y, Jiang P, Benjamin L, et al. Endothelial cell death, angiogenesis, and microvascular function after castration in an androgen-dependent tumor: role of vascular endothelial growth factor. Proc Natl Acad Sci U S A 1998;95:10820–5.

[39] Hall EJ. Radiobiology for the radiologist. Philadelphia: Lippincott Williams & Wilkins; 2000.

[40] Marples B, Greco O, Joiner MC, Scott SD. Molecular approaches to chemo-radiotherapy. Eur J Cancer 2002;38:231–9.

[41] Overgaard J, Horsman MR. Modification of hypoxia-induced radioresistance in tumors by the use of oxygen and sensitizers. Semin Radiat Oncol 1996;6: 10–21.

[42] Fowler JF. Eighth annual Juan del Regato lecture. Chemical modifiers of radiosensitivity–theory and reality: a review. Int J Radiat Oncol Biol Phys 1985; 11:665–74.

[43] Frommhold H, Guttenberger R, Henke M. The impact of blood hemoglobin content on the outcome of radiotherapy. The Freiburg experience. Strahlenther Onkol 1998;174(Suppl 4):31–4.

[44] Evans SM, Koch CJ. Prognostic significance of tumor oxygenation in humans. Cancer Lett 2003;195:1–16.

[45] Koong AC, Denko NC, Hudson KM, Schindler C, Swiersz L, Koch C, et al. Candidate genes for the hypoxic tumor phenotype. Cancer Res 2000;60: 883–7.

[46] Blancher C, Moore JW, Talks KL, Houlbrook S, Harris AL. Relationship of hypoxia-inducible factor (HIF)-1alpha and HIF-2alpha expression to vascular

endothelial growth factor induction and hypoxia survival in human breast cancer cell lines. Cancer Res 2000;60:7106–13.

[47] Sutherland RM. Tumor hypoxia and gene expression: implications for malignant progression and therapy. Acta Oncol 1998;37:567–74.

[48] Amellem O, Pettersen EO. Cell inactivation and cell cycle inhibition as induced by extreme hypoxia: the possible role of cell cycle arrest as a protection against hypoxia-induced lethal damage. Cell Prolif 1991;24:127–41.

[49] Moulder JE, Rockwell S. Tumor hypoxia: its impact on cancer therapy. Cancer Metastasis Rev 1987;5:313–41.

[50] Blancher C, Harris AL. The molecular basis of the hypoxia response pathway: tumour hypoxia as a therapy target. Cancer Metastasis Rev 1998;17:187–94.

[51] Brown JM. Exploiting the hypoxic cancer cell: mechanisms and therapeutic strategies. Mol Med Today 2000;6:157–62.

[52] Lee DJ, Moini M, Giuliano J, Westra WH. Hypoxic sensitizer and cytotoxin for head and neck cancer. Ann Acad Med Singapore 1996;25:397–404.

[53] Sartorelli AC, Hodnick WF. Mitomycin C: a prototype bioreductive agent. Oncol Res 1994;6:501–8.

[54] Rajendran JG, Schwartz DL, Kinahan PE, Cheng P, Hummel SM, Lewellen B, et al. Imaging with F-18 FMISO-PET permits hypoxia directed radiotherapy dose escalation for head and neck cancer. J Nucl Med 2003;44:415, 127P.

[55] Chao KS, Bosch WR, Mutic S, Lewis JS, Dehdashti F, Mintun MA, et al. A novel approach to overcome hypoxic tumor resistance: Cu-ATSM-guided intensity-modulated radiation therapy. Int J Radiat Oncol Biol Phys 2001;49:1171–82.

[56] Rischin D, Peters L, Hicks R, Hughes P, Fisher R, Hart R, et al. Phase I trial of concurrent tirapazamine, cisplatin, and radiotherapy in patients with advanced head and neck cancer. J Clin Oncol 2001; 19:535–42.

[57] Brown MJ. The hypoxic cell: a target for selective cancer therapy. Eighteenth Bruce F. Cain memorial award lecture. Cancer Res 1999;59:5863–70.

[58] Hockel M, Schlenger K, Knoop C, Vaupel P. Oxygenation of carcinoma of the uterine cervix: evaluation by computerized oxygen tension measurements. Cancer Res 1991;51:6098–102.

[59] Koh WJ, Bergman KS, Rasey JS, Peterson LM, Evans ML, Graham MM, et al. Evaluation of oxygenation status during fractionated radiotherapy in human non small cell lung cancers using [F-18]fluoromisonidazole positron emission tomography. Int J Radiat Oncol Biol Phys 1995;33:391–8.

[60] Rajendran JG, Wilson D, Conrad EU, Peterson LM, Bruckner JD, Rasey JS, et al. F-18 FMISO and F-18 FDG PET imaging in soft tissue sarcomas: correlation of hypoxia, metabolism and VEGF expression. Eur J Nucl Med 2003;30:695–704.

[61] Rajendran JG, Peterson LM, Schwartz DL, Scharnhrost J, Conrad EU, Grierson JR, et al. F-18 FMISO

PET tumor hypoxia imaging: investigating the tumor volume-hypoxia connection. J Nucl Med 2003;44:1340, 1376P.

[62] Adam M, Gabalski EC, Bloch DA, Ochlert JW, Brown JM, Elsaid AA, et al. Tissue oxygen distribution in head and neck cancer patients. Head Neck 1999;21:146–53.

[63] Hockel M, Schlenger K, Knoop C, Vaupel P. Oxygenation of carcinomas of the uterine cervix: evaluation by computerized O_2 tension measurements. Cancer Res 1991;51:6098–102.

[64] Brizel DM, Sibley GS, Prosnitz LR, Scher RL, Dewhirst MW. Tumor hypoxia adversely affects the prognosis of carcinoma of the head and neck. Int J Radiat Oncol Biol Phys 1997;38:285–9.

[65] Lartigau E, Lusinchi A, Weeger P, Wibault P, Luboinski B, Eschwege F, et al. Variations in tumour oxygen tension (PO_2) during accelerated radiotherapy of head and neck carcinoma. Eur J Cancer 1998;34:856–61.

[66] Nordsmark M, Overgaard M, Overgaard J. Pretreatment oxygenation predicts radiation response in advanced squamous cell carcinoma of the head and neck. Radiother Oncol 1996;41:31–9.

[67] Ng P, Peterson LM, Schwartz DL, Scharnhrost J, Krohn KA. Can F-18 fluoromisonidazole PET imaging predict treatment response in head and neck cancer? J Nucl Med 2003;44:416, 128P.

[68] Muzi M, Spence AM, Rajendran JG, Grierson JR, Krohn KA. Glioma patients assessed with FMISO and FDG: two tracers provide different Information. J Nucl Med 2003;44:878, 243P.

[69] Valk P, Mathis C, Prados M, Gilbert J, Budinger T. Hypoxia in human gliomas: demonstration by PET with flouorine-18-fluoromisonidazole. J Nucl Med 1992;33:2133–7.

[70] Rajendran J, Lanell P, Schwartz DS, Muzi M, Scharnhorst JD, Eary JF, et al. [F-18] FMISO PET hypoxia imaging in head and neck cancer: heterogeneity in hypoxia - primary tumor vs lymph nodal metastases. J Nucl Med 2002;43:73P.

[71] Stone HB, Brown JM, Phillips TL, Sutherland RM. Oxygen in human tumors: correlations between methods of measurement and response to therapy. Summary of a workshop held November 19–20, 1992, at the National Cancer Institute, Bethesda, Maryland. Radiat Res 1993;136:422–34.

[72] Hockel M, Vaupel P. Tumor hypoxia: definitions and current clinical, biologic, and molecular aspects. J Natl Cancer Inst 2001;93:266–76.

[73] Rasey JS, Casciari JJ, Hofstrand PD, Muzi M, Graham MM, Chin LK. Determining hypoxic fraction in a rat glioma by uptake of radiolabeled fluoromisonidazole. Radiat Res 2000;153:84–92.

[74] Vaupel P, Kelleher DK, Hockel M. Oxygen status of malignant tumors: pathogenesis of hypoxia and significance for tumor therapy. Semin Oncol 2001;28:29–35.

[75] Nozue M, Lee I, Yuan F, et al. Interlaboratory

variation in oxygen tension measurement by eppendorf "histograph" and comparison with hypoxic marker. J Surg Oncol 1997;66:30–8.

[76] Lartigau E, Le Ridant AM, Lambin P, Weeger P, Martin L, Sigal R, et al. Oxygenation of head and neck tumors. Cancer 1993;71:2319–25.

[77] Brizel DM, Rosner GL, Harrelson J, Prosnitz LR, Dewhirst MW. Pretreatment oxygenation profiles of human soft tissue sarcomas. Int J Radiat Oncol Biol Phys 1994;30:635–42.

[78] Martin GV, Caldwell JH, Graham MM, Grierson JR, Kroll K, Cowan MJ, et al. Noninvasive detection of hypoxic myocardium using fluorine-18-fluoromisonidazole and positron emission tomography. J Nucl Med 1992;33:2202–8.

[79] Jain RK. Angiogenesis and lymphangiogenesis in tumors: insights from intravital microscopy. Cold Spring Harb Symp Quant Biol 2002;67:239–48.

[80] Brasch RC, Li KC, Husband JE, Keogan MT, Neeman M, Padhani AR, et al. In vivo monitoring of tumor angiogenesis with MR imaging. Acad Radiol 2000;7:812–23.

[81] Chen CN, Cheng YM, Lin MT, Hsieh FJ, Lee PH, Chang KJ. Association of color Doppler vascularity index and microvessel density with survival in patients with gastric cancer. Ann Surg 2002;235:512–8.

[82] Cheng WF, Lee CN, Chu JS, Chen CA, Chen TM, Shau WY, et al. Vascularity index as a novel parameter for the in vivo assessment of angiogenesis in patients with cervical carcinoma. Cancer 1999;85:651–7.

[83] Cheng WF, Chen TM, Chen CA, Wu CC, Huang KT, Hsieh CY, et al. Clinical application of intratumoral blood flow study in patients with endometrial carcinoma. Cancer 1998;82:1881–6.

[84] Stevenson JP, Rosen M, Sun W, Gallagher M, Haller DG, Vaughn D, et al. Phase I trial of the antivascular agent combretastatin A4 phosphate on a 5-day schedule to patients with cancer: magnetic resonance imaging evidence for altered tumor blood flow. J Clin Oncol 2003;21:4428–38.

[85] Sipkins DA, Cheresh DA, Kazemi MR, Nevin LM, Bednarski MD, Li KC. Detection of tumor angiogenesis in vivo by alphaVbeta3-targeted magnetic resonance imaging. Nat Med 1998;4:623–6.

[86] Leong-Poi H, Christiansen JP, Klibanov AL, Kaul S, Lindner JR. Noninvasive assessment of angiogenesis by contrast ultrasound imaging with microbubbles targeted to alpha-V integrins. J Am Coll Cardiol 2003;41:430–1.

[87] Leong-Poi H, Christiansen J, Klibanov AL, Kaul S, Lindner JR. Noninvasive assessment of angiogenesis by ultrasound and microbubbles targeted to alpha(v)-integrins. Circulation 2003;107:455–60.

[88] Haubner R, Wester HJ, Weber WA, Mang C, Ziegler SI, Goodman SL, et al. Noninvasive imaging of alpha(v)beta3 integrin expression using 18F-labeled RGD-containing glycopeptide and positron emission tomography. Cancer Res 2001;61:1781–5.

[89] Haubner R, Wester HJ, Burkhart F, Senekowitsch-Schmidtke R, Weber W, Goodman SL, et al. Glycosylated RGD-containing peptides: tracer for tumor targeting and angiogenesis imaging with improved biokinetics. J Nucl Med 2001;42:326–36.

[90] Ogawa M, Hatano K, Oishi S, Kawasumi Y, Fujii N, Kawaguchi M, et al. Direct electrophilic radiofluorination of a cyclic RGD peptide for in vivo alpha(v)-beta3 integrin related tumor imaging. Nucl Med Biol 2003;30:1–9.

[91] Blankenberg FG, Eckelman WC, Strauss HW, Welch MJ, Alavi A, Anderson C, et al. Role of radionuclide imaging in trials of antiangiogenic therapy. Acad Radiol 2000;7:851–67.

[92] Barthel H. Endostatin imaging to help understanding of antiangiogenic drugs. Lancet Oncol 2002;3:520.

[93] Prekeges JL, Rasey JS, Grunbaum Z, Krohn KH. Reduction of fluoromisonidazole, a new imaging agent for hypoxia. Biochem Pharmacol 1991;42:2387–95.

[94] Chapman JD, Engelhardt EL, Stobbe CC, Schneider RF, Hanks GE. Measuring hypoxia and predicting tumor radioresistance with nuclear medicine assays. Radiother Oncol 1998;46:229–37.

[95] Grierson JR, Link JM, Mathis CA, Rasey JS, Krohn KA. Radiosynthesis of fluorine-18 fluoromisonidazole. J Nucl Med 1989;30:343–50.

[96] Rasey JS, Wui-Jin K, Evans ML, Peterson LM, Lewellen TK, Graham MM, et al. Quantifying regional hypoxia in human tumors with positron emission tomography of [18F]fluoromisonidazole: a pretherapy study of 37 patients. Int J Radiat Oncol Biol Phys 1996;36:417–28.

[97] Rajendran J, Lanell P, Schwartz DS, Scharnhorst JD, Koh WJ, Eary JF, et al. PET imaging in head and neck cancer with [F-18]FMISO and [F-18] FDG: evaluating different aspects of tumor biology - hypoxia and metabolism. Proc Am Assoc Cancer Res 2002;43:758P.

[98] Liu RS, Chu LS, Yen SH, Chang CP, Chou KL, Wu LC, et al. Detection of anaerobic odontogenic infections by fluorine-18 fluoromisonidazole. Eur J Nucl Med 1996;23:1384–7.

[99] Bentzen L, Keiding S, Horsman MR, Falborg L, Hansen SB, Overgaard J. Feasibility of detecting hypoxia in experimental mouse tumours with 18F-fluorinated tracers and positron emission tomography: a study evaluating [18F]Fluoro-2-deoxy-D-glucose. Acta Oncol 2000;39:629–37.

[100] Read SJ, Hirano T, Abbott DF, Sachinidis JI, Tochon-Danguy HJ, Chan JG, et al. Identifying hypoxic tissue after acute ischemic stroke using PET and 18F-fluoromisonidazole. Neurology 1998;51:1617–21.

[101] Yeh SH, Liu RS, Wu LC, Yang DJ, Yen SH, Chang CW, et al. Fluorine-18 fluoromisonidazole tumour to muscle retention ratio for the detection of hypoxia in nasopharyngeal carcinoma. Eur J Nucl Med 1996;23:1378–83.

[102] Graham MM, Peterson LM, Link JM, Evans ML, Rasey JS, Koh WJ, et al. Fluorine-18-fluoromisoni-

dazole radiation dosimetry in imaging studies. J Nucl Med 1997;38:1631–6.

[103] Rasey JS, Koh WJ, Grierson JR, Grunbaum Z, Krohn KA. Radiolabelled fluoromisonidazole as an imaging agent for tumor hypoxia. Int J Radiat Oncol Biol Phys 1989;17:985–91.

[104] Koh WJ, Rasey JS, Evans ML, Grierson JR, Lewellen TK, Graham MM, et al. Imaging of hypoxia in human tumors with [F-18]fluoromisonidazole. Int J Radiat Oncol Biol Phys 1992;22:199–212.

[105] Casciari JJ, Graham MM, Rasey JS. A modeling approach for quantifying tumor hypoxia with [F-18]fluoromisonidazole PET time-activity data. Med Phys 1995;22:1127–39.

[106] Chapman JD, Schneider RF, Urbain JL, Hanks GE. Single-photon emission computed tomography and positron-emission tomography assays for tissue oxygenation. Semin Radiat Oncol 2001;11:47–57.

[107] Nunn A, Linder K, Strauss HW. Nitroimidazoles and imaging hypoxia. Eur J Nucl Med 1995;22:265–80.

[108] Biskupiak JE, Krohn KA. Second generation hypoxia imaging agents [editorial; comment]. J Nucl Med 1993;34:411–3.

[109] Kachur AV, Dolbier Jr WR, Evans SM, Shiue CY, Shiue GG, Skov KA, et al. Synthesis of new hypoxia markers EF1 and [18F]-EF1. Appl Radiat Isot 1999;51:643–50.

[110] Tewson TJ. Synthesis of [18F]fluoroetanidazole: a potential new tracer for imaging hypoxia. Nucl Med Biol 1997;24:755–60.

[111] Wiebe LI, Stypinski D. Pharmacokinetics of SPECT radiopharmaceuticals for imaging hypoxic tissues. Q J Nucl Med 1996;40:270–84.

[112] Siim BG, Laux WT, Rutland MD, Palmer BN, Wilson WR. Scintigraphic imaging of the hypoxia marker (99m)technetium-labeled 2,2′-(1,4-diaminobutane)-bis(2-methyl-3-butanone) dioxime (99mTc-labeled HL-91; prognox): noninvasive detection of tumor response to the antivascular agent 5,6-dimethylxanthenone-4-acetic acid. Cancer Res 2000;60:4582–8.

[113] Rumsey WL, Kuczynski B, Patel B, Bauer A, Narra RK, Eaton SM, et al. SPECT imaging of ischemic myocardium using a technetium-99m-nitroimidazole ligand. J Nucl Med 1995;36:1445–50.

[114] Zhang X, Melo T, Ballinger JR, Rauth AM. Studies of 99mTc-BnAO (HL-91): a non-nitroaromatic compound for hypoxic cell detection. Int J Radiat Oncol Biol Phys 1998;42:737–40.

[115] Stypinski D, Wiebe LI, McEwan AJ, Schmidt RP, Tam YK, Mercer JR. Clinical pharmacokinetics of 123I-IAZA in healthy volunteers. Nucl Med Commun 1999;20:559–67.

[116] Shelton ME, Green MA, Mathias CJ, Welch MJ,

Bergmann SR. Assessment of regional myocardial and renal blood flow with copper-PTSM and positron emission tomography. Circulation 1990;82:990–7.

[117] Lewis JS, McCarthy DW, McCarthy TJ, Fujibayashi Y, Welch MJ. Evaluation of Cu-64-ATSM in vitro and in vivo in a hypoxic model. J Nucl Med 1999;40:177–83.

[118] Dehdashti F, Mintun MA, Lewis JS, Bradley J, Govindan R, Laforest R, et al. In vivo assessment of tumor hypoxia in lung cancer with 60Cu-ATSM. Eur J Nucl Med Mol Imaging 2003;30:844–50.

[119] Fujibayashi Y, Taniuchi H, Yonekura Y, Ohtani H, Konishi J, Yokoyama A. Copper-62-ATSM: a new hypoxia imaging agent with high membrane permeability and low redox potential. J Nucl Med 1997;38:1155–60.

[120] Ballinger JR. Imaging hypoxia in tumors. Semin Nucl Med 2001;31:321–9.

[121] Gabalski EC, Adam M, Pinto H, Brown JM, Bloch DA, Terris DJ. Pretreatment and midtreatment measurement of oxygen tension levels in head and neck cancers. Laryngoscope 1998;108:1856–60.

[122] Klabbers BM, Lammertsma AA, Slotman BJ. The value of positron emission tomography for monitoring response to radiotherapy in head and neck cancer. Mol Imaging Biol 2003;5:257–70.

[123] Alber M, Paulsen F, Eschmann SM, Machulla HJ. On biologically conformal boost dose optimization. Phys Med Biol 2003;48:N31–5.

[124] Ling CC, Humm J, Larson S, Amols H, Fuks Z, Leibel S, et al. Towards multidimensional radiotherapy (MD-CRT): biological imaging and biological conformality. Int J Radiat Oncol Biol Phys 2000;47:551–60.

[125] Tome WA, Fowler JF. Selective boosting of tumor subvolumes. Int J Radiat Oncol Biol Phys 2000;48:593–9.

[126] Peters LJ. Targeting hypoxia in head and neck cancer. Acta Oncol 2001;40:937–40.

[127] Solomon B, McArthur G, Cullinane C, Zalcberg J, Hicks R. Applications of positron emission tomography in the development of molecular targeted cancer therapeutics. BioDrugs 2003;17:339–54.

[128] Klimas MT. Positron emission tomography and drug discovery: contributions to the understanding of pharmacokinetics, mechanism of action and disease state characterization. Mol Imaging Biol 2002;4:311–37.

[129] Hammond LA, Denis L, Salman U, Jerabek P, Thomas Jr CR, Kuhn JG. Positron emission tomography (PET): expanding the horizons of oncology drug development. Invest New Drugs 2003;21:309–40.

ELSEVIER
SAUNDERS

Radiol Clin N Am 43 (2005) 189–204

RADIOLOGIC
CLINICS
of North America

Monitoring response to treatment in patients utilizing PET

Norbert E. Avril, MD[a],*, Wolfgang A. Weber, MD[b]

[a]Division of Nuclear Medicine, Department of Radiology, University of Pittsburgh Medical Center, 200 Lothrop Street,
Pittsburgh, PA 15213, USA
[b]Department of Medical and Molecular Pharmacology, University of California at Los Angeles, 10833 Le Conte Avenue,
AR 193 CHS, Los Angeles, CA 90095, USA

The treatment of cancer patients is constantly evolving, striving for more efficient therapies with fewer side effects. Chemotherapy and radiation therapy are still the major therapeutic modalities besides surgery. Because a single treatment modality alone frequently does not provide a cure, multimodality treatment regimens are often being applied. In addition, new chemotherapeutic agents are continuously being developed and evaluated in clinical trials. The technology of radiation therapy has advanced with optimization of dose levels and fractionation schedules. In addition, the delivery of more targeted radiation is now possible by using inverse dose planning and intensity modulation radiation therapy techniques. New therapeutic strategies are on the horizon, such as biologic therapies, therapies based on gene transfer and the modulation of gene expression, and therapies targeting tumor angiogenesis. Biologic therapies or immunotherapies are already considered a fourth modality of cancer treatment (eg, interferon and monoclonal antibodies for the treatment of non-Hodgkin's lymphoma and breast cancer have become part of standard cancer treatment). Many types of immunotherapy, however, such as cancer vaccines, remain experimental. The use of antiangiogenic drugs is a typical example of a new therapeutic approach that does not result in immediate cell death and dissolution of tumor masses. Although inhibiting the growth of new blood vessels in cancer tissue, the actual tumor mass often

remains stable, requiring new surrogate end points for monitoring therapeutic effects.

The ultimate goal of cancer treatment is to achieve a complete remission. The current end point for assessing response to therapy in solid tumors is by measuring the change in tumor size [1]. Anatomic imaging modalities, predominantly CT, MR imaging, and ultrasound, are used to obtain unidimensional or bidimensional measurements of reference tumor lesions from pretreatment scans relative to follow-up. Important limitations of anatomic imaging-based assessment of treatment response, however, have to be taken into consideration. Several criteria to define tumor response have been developed; of these the World Health Organization criteria are most frequently used. Generally, a tumor is classified as responding when the product of two perpendicular diameters of a mass has decreased by at least 50%. In cases with multiple lesions, the summation of the products should decrease by more than 50% [2]. More recently the World Health Organization criteria have been changed to unidimensional tumor diameter measurements. The new RECIST (response evaluation criteria in solid tumors) criteria define tumor response as a decrease of the maximum tumor diameter by at least 30% [1]. For a spherical tumor, a decrease of its diameter by 30% corresponds to a decrease of the product of two perpendicular diameters by 50%. The RECIST criteria have been primarily designed to simplify and standardize the tumor size measurement and have not changed the threshold values for definition of a tumor response. Despite the widely accepted practice of using these criteria, it is important to note that a 50% or 30%

* Corresponding author.
E-mail address: AvrilNE@upmc.edu (N.E. Avril).

decrease of tumor size is a more or less arbitrary convention, which is not based on outcome studies. In fact, the correlation between radiologic tumor response and patient outcome is frequently weak. Tumor response as defined by morphologic imaging techniques is frequently not accepted as a surrogate end point for the evaluation of new anticancer drugs [3]. Furthermore, dissolving and shrinkage of a tumor mass is the final step in a complex cascade of cellular and subcellular changes after initiation of treatment. Frequently, several cycles of chemotherapy or other treatments need to be applied before treatment response can be assessed by current anatomic imaging modalities. Even the evaluation of response after completion of treatment can pose a challenge. If a residual mass is present, it is difficult to differentiate viable tumor tissue from posttreatment changes, such as scarring and fibrosis.

It is becoming increasingly important in the current clinical setting to identify response to therapy as early as possible so that ineffective therapies can be discontinued. In particular, early identification of nonresponse is crucial to avoid ineffective treatment, unnecessary side effects, and costs. This goal becomes particularly important in solid tumor treatment, because most conventional chemotherapies in these tumors do not result in a complete anatomic response. Therapeutic approaches can be modified on an individual basis, however, and there is clearly a need for modalities that allow assessment and prediction of treatment response early in the course of therapy. Ideally, this modality should be noninvasive and provide accurate information about treatment response of different tumor sites for individual patients.

PET imaging and image analysis

PET is a noninvasive imaging technique that measures the concentration of positron-emitting radiopharmaceuticals in the body. Depending on the radiolabeled tracer used, PET can be used to determine various physiologic and biochemical processes in vivo. PET is highly sensitive, with the capacity to detect subnanomolar concentrations of radiotracer, and provides superior image resolution to conventional nuclear medicine imaging with gamma cameras. Currently, PET imaging can target several biologic features of tumors including glucose metabolism, cell proliferation, perfusion, and hypoxia. Following malignant transformation, various tumors are characterized by elevated glucose consumption

and subsequent increased uptake of the glucose analogue fluorine-18 fluorodeoxyglucose ([^{18}F-FDG). PET imaging using FDG has been applied for staging of cancer patients for about a decade now. It is generally accepted that imaging the metabolic activity of tumor tissue provides more sensitive and more specific information about the extent of disease than morphologic-anatomic imaging alone. FDG-PET has become a standard imaging procedure for staging and restaging of many types of cancer and in the United States; insurance coverage currently includes head and neck cancer, thyroid cancer, solitary pulmonary nodules, lung cancer, breast cancer, esophageal cancer, colorectal cancer, lymphoma, and melanoma. The metabolic activity of cancer tissue measured by PET offers additional information about cancer biology and can be used to determine tumor aggressiveness and also help to assess response to treatment. PET imaging in cancer patients is frequently performed as a "torso scan" covering an area from the base of the skull to the groin by acquiring emission data from multiple bed positions over a period of 20 to 40 minutes. The area covered by one bed-position is determined by the field of view of the PET scanner and is in the range of 15 cm for most devices; the time to acquire emission data for one bed-position is typically between 3 and 5 minutes. In addition, a transmission scan with radioactive sources that are integrated into the scanner is required for correction of photon attenuation and is also essential for subsequent quantification of tracer uptake in tissue.

The uptake mechanism and biochemical pathway of FDG has been extensively studied in vitro and in vivo. The transport of the radiotracer through the cell membrane by glucose transport proteins and subsequent intracellular phosphorylation by hexokinase have been identified as key steps for subsequent tissue accumulation [4]. Because FDG-6-phosphate is not a suitable substrate for glucose-6-phosphate isomerase, and the enzyme level of glucose-6-phosphatase is generally low in tumors, FDG-6-phosphate accumulates in cells and is visualized by PET.

Attenuation-corrected PET images provide quantitative information about the tracer concentration in tissue, which is particularly important for monitoring therapeutic response. Various approaches of different complexity can be applied for quantitative PET analysis. Standardized uptake values (SUVs) are frequently being calculated providing a semiquantitative measure of FDG accumulation in tissue by normalizing the tissue radioactivity concentration measured with PET to injected dose and patient's body weight [5]. The radioactivity concentration in the body also depends on the time interval between FDG injection and imaging. Because FDG uptake in fat is lower than in muscle, the lean body weight or the body surface area have been proposed as alternatives [5]. Following intravenous administration of the radiotracer there is an increase in FDG uptake in tissue over time; PET imaging for follow-up comparison must be acquired at the same time interval after tracer injection as the baseline scan. Many institutions use a 60-minute uptake period where the patient is resting in a quiet room before acquiring the PET scan. There is an inverse relationship between FDG uptake (SUV) and blood glucose level that has to taken into account for the interpretation of follow-up PET scans. The SUV measurements are also affected by the size of a lesion. Partial volume effects cause significant underestimation of isotope concentration in structures smaller than two times the scanner resolution at full width half maximum. Appropriate recovery coefficients, which represent the ratio of apparent to true isotope concentration in the structure of interest, can be used to correct for partial volume effects. SUVs are obtained by placing a region of interest on the PET images. The size of the region of interest affects the radioactivity measurements: the larger the region of interest, the lower the mean SUV. In the clinical setting, the maximum SUV within the region of interest, which represents the highest radioactivity concentration in one voxel within the tumor, is frequently being used for comparison between PET studies.

Previous studies have demonstrated that SUV and simplified tracer kinetic modeling, using the Patlak-Gjedde analysis, provide highly reproducible parameters of tumor glucose use [6,7]. Weber et al [7] studied 16 patients twice within 10 days with FDG-PET while they were receiving no therapy. FDG net influx constants (Ki), SUVs, normalized to blood glucose (SUV-gluc and Ki-gluc) were determined for 50 separate lesions. The precision of repeated measurements was determined on a lesion-by-lesion and a patient-by-patient basis. None of the parameters showed a significant increase or decrease between the two PET scans. The differences of repeated measurements were approximately normally distributed for all parameters with a standard deviation of the mean percentage difference of about 10%. Changes of a parameter of more than 20% are outside the 95% range for spontaneous fluctuations and can be considered to reflect true changes in glucose metabolism of a tumor mass. The absolute value of the change must also be considered. According to the

findings in this study, SUV changes of ± 0.9 or changes in Ki of ± 0.7 mL/100 g/min are outside the 95% range for spontaneous fluctuations of the respective parameter. Analysis on a patient-by-patient basis yielded almost identical results indicating that the main source of variability was the measurement of individual lesions. There was no clear advantage in using tracer kinetic approaches compared with SUV measurements. It seems feasible to use SUV measurements for the evaluation of therapy response. The patients were imaged under stable clinical conditions, however, with no signs of tumor progression, infection, or changes in laboratory abnormalities. Furthermore, no patients with overt diabetes mellitus were included. Because diabetes mellitus may affect the blood clearance and whole-body distribution of FDG by multiple mechanisms, tracer kinetic approaches may be preferable to SUV measurements in this group of patients [8]. The use of SUVs for serial measurements of short-term changes in tumor glucose use during therapy is also supported by a recent study in patients with advanced non–small cell lung cancer [9]. In this study 57 patients were studied by FDG-PET before platinum-based chemotherapy and 3 weeks after initiation of therapy. Changes in the SUV of the primary tumor were closely correlated with changes of the FDG-net influx as determined by Patlak analysis. In addition, changes of both parameters 3 weeks after initiation of chemotherapy were significantly correlated with subsequent reduction of tumor size and patient survival. Failure to achieve a measurable reduction in tumor FDG-uptake after 3 weeks of therapy was associated with 96% risk of not achieving an objective response with the first-line chemotherapy regimen. Nonresponders in FDG-PET were characterized by a three times shorter time to tumor progression and a 1.7 times shorter overall survival.

Although these and other studies indicate that SUVs may be used to determine quantitatively changes in tumor glucose use over time, it is important to note that a strict PET protocol is required to minimize the variation between FDG-PET studies. The time between FDG injection and imaging needs to be standardized and should vary less than 5 minutes between baseline and follow-up. The radioactivity in the syringe should be measured before and after injection and appropriately corrected for radioactive decay to determine accurately the dose of FDG injected. Extravasation of the radiotracer during injection also influences quantification. Finally, the patient's blood glucose levels should be comparable between the scans and ideally less than 150 mg/dL at the time of tracer injection. The specific method for calculation of SUVs (eg, normalization to body weight or the lean body mass) is less important for the purpose of therapy monitoring because intra-individual comparisons of SUVs are being made. When FDG-PET is used for early assessment of therapy response, significant changes in body weight influencing the results of the SUV calculation are unlikely. In contrast, normalization to body surface area or lean body mass is preferable for interindividual comparison of SUVs, especially if the study population includes obese patients.

Prediction of treatment response after initiation of therapy

Ten years ago, little was known about changes in tumor glucose metabolism in the course of chemotherapy or radiation therapy. Most in vitro and in vivo studies in tumor-bearing animals suggested a good correlation between tumor viability and FDG uptake. Other nonhuman studies, however, found an increase in FDG uptake of tumor cells after initiation of therapy. The concept of using FDG-PET for monitoring therapeutic response is based on the decrease of tumor glucose use and its correlation with the effectiveness of treatment and ultimately with the reduction of viable tumor cells. In tumors responding to treatment a reduction of glucose use occurs early in the course of therapy. Serial PET scans during treatment should allow prediction of response.

In 1993, Wahl et al [10] studied 11 women with newly diagnosed locally advanced primary breast cancers undergoing chemohormotherapy with sequential FDG-PET imaging. Patients underwent a baseline and four follow-up PET scans during the first three cycles of treatment. Tumor response was determined histopathologically after nine cycles of treatment. The FDG uptake in eight patients with partial or complete pathologic responses decreased

promptly with treatment, whereas the tumor diameter did not significantly decrease. On day 8 of therapy, tumor FDG uptake was 78% of baseline and decreased further to 68% at day 21, 60% at day 42, and 52% at day 63. In contrast, three patients with nonresponding tumors did not show a significant decrease in FDG uptake. The authors concluded that FDG-PET has substantial promise as an early non-invasive metabolic marker of the efficacy of cancer treatment. Similar findings were also observed by Jansson et al [11] in 12 patients with locally advanced or metastatic breast cancer treated with chemotherapy. Romer et al [12] studied the changes in metabolic activity over time in non-Hodgkin's lymphoma and compared pretreatment FDG-PET with day 7 and day 42 after initiation of therapy. In successfully treated patients, FDG uptake decreased by 60% to 67% from baseline to day 7. This study showed that in responding non-Hodgkin's lymphoma, two thirds of the metabolic effect of chemotherapy occurred within the first 7 days of treatment. In addition, the long-term prognosis could be predicted early after initiation of chemotherapy by the change in glucose metabolism. These studies suggest that serial FDG-PET imaging can be a valuable tool for monitoring response to therapy early in the course of treatment and numerous studies have proved the hypothesis that changes in tumor glucose metabolism predict the outcome of therapy. The results of these studies are summarized in Table 1.

Lymphoma

Lymphomas are a heterogeneous group of malignancies of the lymphoid system and include Hodgkin's lymphoma and non-Hodgkin's lymphoma. Lymphomas are usually highly sensitive to chemotherapy and radiation therapy and patients who do not achieve a complete remission after initial treatment clearly benefit from a more aggressive therapeutic approach (eg, high-dose chemotherapy with stem cell

Table 1
Early prediction of treatment response by fluorodeoxyglucose-PET

| | | | | | Median survival | | |
Study	Tumor type	Year	N	Criterion	Responder	Nonresponder	P value
Kostakoglu et al, 2002 [32]	Lymphoma	2002	30	Visual	>24	5	<0.001
Weber et al, 2001 [20]	Esophagus	2001	37	−35% SUV	>48	20	0.04
Wieder et al, 2004 [53]	Esophagus	2004	22	−30% SUV	>38	18	0.011
Ott et al, 2003 [21]	Gastric	2002	35	−35% SUV	>48	17	0.001
Brun et al, 2002 [74]	Head/neck	2002	47	Median	>120	40	0.004
Weber et al, 2003 [9]	Lung	2003	57	−20% SUV	9	5	0.005

transplantation). Generally, CT provides a poor characterization of early treatment response because several cycles of chemotherapy are required before masses involved with lymphoma decrease substantially in size.

One of the first reports on therapy-induced changes in glucose metabolism of lymphoma includes two patients with non-Hodgkin's lymphoma [13]. Persisting FDG uptake during the first two cycles of chemotherapy in one patient predicted treatment failure, whereas a substantial reduction of FDG uptake was found in the other patient responding to treatment. Jerusalem et al [14] studied 28 patients with FDG-PET after a median of three cycles of chemotherapy and correlated the presence of abnormal FDG uptake with the clinical outcome. Five of the 28 patients still had increased FDG uptake in one or more sites and only one patient remained in complete remission. In contrast, among the 23 patients with a negative FDG-PET scan, all but two who died from toxicity of chemotherapy achieved clinical complete remission. Although promising, a weakness of this study is the heterogeneous patient population including primary and relapsed lymphoma patients. In another study, including 30 patients imaged with a dual-head coincidence gamma camera at baseline and after one cycle of chemotherapy, the FDG uptake obtained after the first cycle of chemotherapy correlated better with the progression-free survival than those after completion of chemotherapy [15]. This study, although limited by using coincidence gamma camera imaging specifically for restaging after completion of chemotherapy, clearly shows the prognostic information based on changes of tumor glucose metabolism between baseline and the first cycle of chemotherapy. In a series of 70 patients with newly diagnosed aggressive non-Hodgkin's lymphoma, Spaepen et al [16] studied the diagnostic information of FDG-PET for midtreatment evaluation. Presence or absence of abnormal FDG uptake was related to progression-free survival and overall survival. Thirty-three patients showed persistent abnormal FDG uptake at midtreatment and none of these patients achieved a complete remission. Thirty-one out of 37 patients with a negative PET scan, however, remained in complete remission. Recently, Torizuka et al [17] reported on 20 lymphoma patients who underwent FDG-PET imaging at baseline and after one to two cycles of chemotherapy. Ten patients achieved complete remission after completion of chemotherapy, whereas the other 10 patients did not respond to chemotherapy. The FDG uptake between baseline and follow-up decreased by 81% in responders compared with 35% in nonresponders. By

using a 60% reduction of SUVs as a cutoff value, the responders were clearly separated from all but one of the nonresponders.

Gastric and esophageal carcinoma

Most patients with gastric or esophageal cancer present with locally advanced disease. To improve the rate of curative surgical resections, preoperative (neoadjuvant) chemotherapy or chemoradiotherapy has been evaluated over several years. There is still no consensus, however, as to whether neoadjuvant therapy improves patient survival [18,19]. Nevertheless, data suggest that in patients responding to preoperative chemotherapy or chemoradiotherapy survival was significantly improved compared with surgical treatment alone. This beneficial effect seems to be outweighed by the poor prognosis of nonresponding patients. Early prediction of tumor response is of particular importance in patients with esophageal and gastric cancer. Weber et al [20] studied 40 patients with locally advanced adenocarcinomas of the esophagogastric junction who underwent preoperative (neoadjuvant) chemotherapy. FDG-PET imaging was performed at baseline and on day 14 of the first cycle of chemotherapy. Changes in tumor FDG uptake were correlated with clinical and histopathologic response after 3 months of chemotherapy. In clinical responders, defined by a decrease of tumor length and wall-thickness by more than 50%, FDG uptake measured at day 14 had decreased by 54% compared with baseline. In contrast, in nonresponding tumors FDG uptake decreased by only 15%. Using a threshold of 35% decrease of baseline metabolic activity allowed predicting subsequent clinical response with a sensitivity and specificity of 93% and 95%, respectively [20]. For prediction of histopathologic response sensitivity and specificity were 89% and 75%, respectively. The 2-year survival of patients responding on FDG-PET imaging was 49%, compared with only 9% for patients who did not respond. In a more recent study the same group has prospectively applied a threshold of 35% SUV decrease from baseline in patients with gastric cancer [21]. Forty-four patients with locally advanced gastric cancer underwent serial FDG-PET imaging; nine patients were excluded from further analysis because of low tumoral FDG-uptake in the baseline scan. In the remaining 35 patients the sensitivity and specificity of FDG-PET for prediction of histopathologic response were 77% and 86%, respectively. The 2-year survival was 90% for patients responding according the PET criterion of a SUV decrease of more than 35% compared with 25% for PET nonresponders.

These data suggest that changes in tumor metabolic activity may be used to individualize the use of chemotherapy in patients with esophageal and gastric cancer. PET nonresponders identified after initiation of chemotherapy may undergo salvage therapy; alternative therapeutic options include the use of different chemotherapy regimens, chemoradiotherapy, or immediate surgical resection. Such an approach could significantly reduce the side effects and costs of ineffective therapies in nonresponding patients. Furthermore, disease progression during chemotherapy with an ineffective drug regimen has been discussed as one reason for the poor survival of patients with histopathologically nonresponding tumors. Individualized chemotherapy monitored by PET may improve overall survival by reducing the time period of ineffective therapy. This hypothesis can only be evaluated in randomized trials because failure to respond to chemotherapy may also be a marker for a biologically more aggressive tumor, which is associated with a poor prognosis irrespective of the applied therapy.

Breast cancer

Primary (neoadjuvant) chemotherapy is increasingly used to treat patients with locally advanced breast cancer. Because of the preoperative reduction of tumor volume, the rate of breast-preserving surgery has increased. Additionally, patients with complete pathologic response have significantly higher disease-free and overall survival rates than nonresponders [22,23]. Approximately 70% of the patients undergoing primary chemotherapy show clinical response, but only 20% to 30% have partial or complete regression in histopathologic tissue analysis. The therapeutic effectiveness of neoadjuvant chemotherapy cannot be determined accurately until definitive breast surgery is performed. Considering the side effects of chemotherapy, there is a need for early identification of nonresponding patients. There are several studies available addressing the role of FDG-PET in predicting response early in the course of therapy.

Following the encouraging results from Wahl et al [10], other groups have had similar results. In 30 patients with noninflammatory, large (>3 cm), or locally advanced breast cancers who received eight doses of primary chemotherapy the mean reduction in FDG uptake after the first cycle of chemotherapy was significantly higher in lesions with partial, complete macroscopic, or complete microscopic response

assessed by histopathologic examination [24]. After a single cycle of chemotherapy, PET predicted complete pathologic response with a sensitivity of 90% and specificity of 74%. In other study, Schelling et al [25] compared results from PET imaging with pathologic response using distinct histopathologic criteria, namely minimal residual disease and gross residual disease, previously identified to provide prognostic information [22,23]. FDG uptake in breast cancer after the first and second cycle of chemotherapy was compared with baseline PET. Patients classified as a responder by histopathology had a significantly more pronounced decrease of FDG uptake than nonresponding patients. As early as after the first course of therapy, responding and nonresponding tumors could be differentiated by PET. By a threshold defined as a SUV decrease below 55% compared with the baseline, all responders were correctly identified after the first course (sensitivity 100%, specificity 85%). Accuracy to predict histopathologic response was 88% and 91% after the first and second course of therapy. In the clinical setting FDG-PET may be helpful in improving patient management by avoiding ineffective chemotherapy and unnecessary side effects, and supporting the decision to continue dose-intensive preoperative chemotherapy in responding patients. In contrast, in 35 patients with breast cancer Mankoff et al [26] found a large overlap between changes in metabolic activity in histopathologic responders and nonresponders. This discrepant finding may be explained by the different timing of the PET scans comparing baseline with PET 2 months after completion of chemotherapy. After that period of time histopathologic nonresponding tumors may demonstrate a relatively large decrease in tumor size and FDG-PET may be unable to differentiate between small absolute differences in the amount of viable tumor cells. Consistent with this explanation, Smith et al [24] also observed a higher accuracy of FDG-PET for prediction of tumor response after the first cycle of chemotherapy than at later points in time.

It is important to note that a transient increase in glucose use has been found in responding tumors treated with hormonotherapy. In a first series, Dehdashti et al [27] performed FDG-PET in 11 women before and 7 to 10 days after initiation of therapy with tamoxifen. In all patients, clinical and radiologic follow-up was performed with a median interval of 12 months. Seven patients responded and all showed an increase of FDG uptake 1 week after therapy. This metabolic flare effect is a recognized side effect of antiestrogen therapy, which is clinically characterized by pain and erythema in soft tissue lesions and increased pain in osseous metastases. An explanation for this metabolic flare effect is that antiestrogen therapy first has an agonist effect before the antagonist effect overrules. This agonist effect occurs within 7 to 10 days after the beginning of a treatment and is usually followed by disease re-mission. Recently, the same group confirmed their findings in a larger series including 40 patients [28]. In the responders, the tumor FDG uptake increased after tamoxifen by 28.4% with only five of these patients having evidence of a clinical flare reaction. In nonresponders, there was no significant change in tumor FDG uptake from baseline. There are no reports so far about metabolic flare in more aggres-sive chemotherapeutic regimes.

Gastrointestinal stromal tumors

Gastrointestinal stromal tumors are mesenchymal spindle cell (70%–80%) or epithelioid (20%–30%) neoplasms. "Gastrointestinal stromal tumor" is a relatively new terminology and includes such tumors as leiomyomas, leiomyoblastomas, or leiomyosarco-mas characterized by a positive immunohistochemis-try staining for C-kit (CD117), which is a tyrosine kinase growth factor receptor. Constitutive activation of kit receptor tyrosine kinase is critical in the pathogenesis of these tumors. Imatinib mesylate is a selective tyrosine kinase inhibitor, which has been shown to be effective in these tumors in preclinical models and in clinical studies. In a randomized multicenter trial, 79 patients (53.7%) had a partial response, 41 patients (27.9%) had stable disease, and in 7 patients (4.8%) response could not be evaluated [29]. Inhibition of the kit signal-transduction pathway has evolved as a new form of treatment for gastro-intestinal stromal tumors, which resist conventional chemotherapy [29]. FDG-PET imaging has been shown to be highly effective to evaluate treatment response in these patients. Imatinib caused a rapid decrease in FDG uptake in responding tumors, whereas major changes in tumor volume tend to occur later after the start of treatment. Stroobants et al [30] studied 21 patients with gastrointestinal stromal tumors and related tumors with FDG-PET before and 8 days after the start of treatment. Response by FDG-PET was observed in 13 patients of whom 11 had a complete response and 2 had a partial response in follow-up. PET response was associated with a longer progression-free survival, 92% versus 12% after 1 year. FDG-PET seems to be an early and sensitive method to evaluate response of gastrointestinal stromal tumor to imatinib treatment.

Fluorine-18-fluorodeoxyglucose-PET for assessment of treatment response

Restaging after completion of treatment is essen-tial to verify response and to determine the need for subsequent additional therapy. Conventional ana-tomic imaging modalities often reveal residual masses where cancer was present. It is very difficult to assess if this represents viable tumor or fibrotic scar tissue. This is of particular importance in patients with Hodgkin's or high-grade non-Hodgkin's lym-phoma after completion of chemotherapy. The ability accurately to monitor response to treatment is crucial to select patients who need more intensive or salvage treatment. Even biopsy may be inaccurate because residual masses frequently contain a mixture of viable tumor cells and scar tissue, which can lead to false-negative results. In the past, gallium-67 (^{67}Ga) single-photon emission computed tomography (SPECT) has been used for the evaluation of residual masses following chemotherapy in lymphoma patients [31]. Few studies exist that directly compare [^{67}Ga]-SPECT with FDG-PET [32,33]. The inherent superior resolution of PET and the higher tumor-to-back-ground ratio provided by FDG uptake results in a clear superior sensitivity of FDG-PET compared with [^{67}Ga]-SPECT. In addition, the relatively high radi-ation exposure from ^{67}Ga, the hepatobiliary excretion, and the need to obtain multiple images 2 to 5 days after administration of the radiopharmaceutical has made [^{67}Ga]-SPECT almost obsolete when PET is available. The largest experience for assessment of tumor response by FDG-PET has been obtained in patients with lymphoma. The prognostic relevance of FDG-PET after completion of chemotherapy or chemoradiotherapy is summarized in Table 2.

Lymphoma

A group from Bologna, Italy, studied 44 patients with Hodgkin's disease or aggressive non-Hodgkin's lymphoma presenting with abdominal involvement and compared the results of CT and PET at the end of chemotherapy or radiation therapy [34]. After treat-ment seven patients were PET- and CT-negative; none of them relapsed. The remaining 37 patients had residual masses on CT but only 13 patients of these also had increased FDG uptake. All 13 patients with positive FDG-PET relapsed; however, there was only one relapse among the 24 patients who were positive on CT but PET-negative. The 2-year relapse-free survival rate was 95% for those with negative FDG-PET. A positive FDG-PET scan was highly predictive of residual disease. Jerusalem et al [35] found similar

Table 2
Prognostic relevance of fluorodeoxyglucose-PET after completion of chemotherapy or chemoradiotherapy

Authors	Tumor type	Year	N	Criterion	Responder	Nonresponder	P value
Jerusalem et al, 1999 [35]	Lymphoma	1999	54	Visual	>40	3	<0.001
Spaepen et al, 2001 [39]	Lymphoma	2001	93	Visual	>46	7	<0.001
Cremerius et al, 2001 [78]	Lymphoma	2001	15	Visual	>40	3	0.003
Weihrauch et al, 2001 [37]	Lymphoma	2001	28	Visual	>50	3	0.004
Naumann et al, 2001 [76]	Lymphoma	2001	15	SUV	>48	10	0.002
Bruecher et al, 2001 [40]	Esophagus	2001	24	SUV	>22	7	<0.001
Flamen et al, 2002 [41]	Esophagus	2002	36	Visual	>34	7	0.005
Downey et al, 2003 [42]	Esophagus	2003	17	SUV	>50	30	0.08
Brun et al, 2002 [74]	Head/neck	2002	47	SUV	>72	42	0.004
Kunkel et al, 2003 [79]	Head/neck	2003	35	SUV	>60	18	0.02

results in 54 patients with Hodgkin's disease or intermediate-grade to high-grade non-Hodgkin's lymphoma. Residual masses on CT were present in 24 patients, with 5 patients out of this group also having positive FDG uptake. One patient was PET-positive with no mass seen on CT. All six patients with a positive FDG-PET scan relapsed, as did 5 of 19 patients with residual masses on CT but negative on FDG-PET, and 3 of 29 patients with a negative CT and a negative PET scan. The authors pointed out that a positive FDG-PET scan predicts early progression but a negative PET scan cannot exclude the presence of minimal residual disease, possibly leading to a later relapse.

The treatment and prognosis of Hodgkin's disease and non-Hodgkin's lymphoma are clearly different, and recently PET studies have been published taking these differences into account. De Wit et al [36] compared PET with CT in 37 patients after treatment for Hodgkin's lymphoma. A total of 50 PET and CT scans were performed; CT showed 39 residual masses from which 8 relapsed during follow-up. In addition, 3 out of 11 patients who had a negative CT relapsed. The sensitivity to predict disease-free survival with CT was 72%, the specificity 21%. Twenty-two PET scans were positive with 10 subsequent recurrences, compared with only 1 relapse out of 28 negative PET scans. The sensitivity of FDG-PET to predict disease-free survival was 91%, and the specificity 69%. The number of false-positive PET results is surprisingly high in this study; however, six patients underwent additional radiotherapy after the PET scan who might have had residual disease but were negative in follow-up. Another study included 28 patients with a residual mediastinal mass of at least 2 cm after initial therapy or after salvage chemotherapy of Hodgkin's lymphoma [37]. A PET-negative mediastinal tumor was observed in 19 patients, of whom

16 remained in remission and 3 patients relapsed. In 6 out of 10 patients with a positive PET, progression of disease or relapse occurred, whereas 4 patients remained in remission. The negative predictive value of FDG-PET at 1 year was 95%, and the positive predictive value was 60%. The disease-free survival for PET-negative and PET-positive patients at 1 year was 95% and 40%, respectively. This study clearly indicates that in Hodgkin's patients with a residual mediastinal mass, which is negative on FDG-PET, patients unlikely relapse within the first year. A positive PET result, however, indicates a high risk of relapse and requires further diagnostic procedures and a close follow-up.

Several studies also addressed the role of FDG-PET for treatment evaluation in non-Hodgkin's lymphoma. Mikhaeel et al [38] reported on 49 patients with aggressive non-Hodgkin's lymphoma with all patients being positive on pretreatment FDG-PET. The result of posttreatment PET scans seemed to predict disease outcome, with relapse rates of 100% (9 of 9) for positive PET scans and only 17% (6 of 36) when the PET was negative. In a subgroup of 33 patients the direct comparison of posttreatment PET with CT showed that PET was more accurate than CT in assessing remission status following treatment. Relapse rate was 100% for positive PET and only 18% for negative PET, compared with 41% and 25% for patients with positive and negative CT, respectively. PET was particularly useful in the assessment of residual masses seen on CT. In a larger series, including 93 patients with non-Hodgkin's lymphoma, Spaepen et al [39] evaluated PET in detecting residual disease and, consequently, predicting relapse after first-line treatment. A normal FDG-PET scan was found in 67 patients and within a median follow-up of 653 days, 56 out of 67 remained in complete remission; 11 of 67 patients relapsed with a median progression-free survival of 404 days. Persistent abnormal FDG uptake was seen in 26 patients, and all of them relapsed with a median progression-free survival of only 73 days.

Persistent increased FDG uptake in initially involved tumor sites in patients with Hodgkin's disease or non-Hodgkin's lymphoma is highly predictive for residual or recurrent disease. If PET shows areas of increased FDG outside the initially involved sites the differential diagnosis includes inflammation, bone marrow stimulation, or thymic hyperplasia. Minimal residual disease can still be present in patients with a negative PET scan and result in subsequent late relapses. It is important to note that the previously discussed studies included patients with aggressive disease and the FDG uptake in low-grade lymphomas is generally lower and FDG-PET might be of less value in these patients.

Esophageal cancer

Initial studies evaluating tumor response by FDG-PET in patients with esophageal and gastric cancer have also yielded encouraging results. Residual FDG-uptake after completion of chemoradiotherapy seems to be a specific marker for viable residual tumor tissue and is associated with a poor prognosis. Brucher et al [40] studied 27 patients with locally advanced squamous cell carcinomas of the esophagus before neoadjuvant chemoradiotherapy and 3 to 4 weeks after completion of therapy. Therapy-induced reduction of tumor FDG uptake was 72% for histopathologic responders compared with 42% for nonresponders. Using a threshold of 51% SUV decrease of baseline resulted in a sensitivity of 100% and a specificity of 52% for PET assessment of tumor response. Tumor response assessed by PET was also a strong prognostic factor. Median survival of PET-responders was 23 months compared with just 9 months in PET nonresponders. Similar results were found by Flamen et al [41] who studied 36 patients with esophageal cancer before and 3 to 4 weeks after preoperative chemoradiotherapy. Using a visual analysis of FDG-PET scans this group obtained a sensitivity of 71% and specificity of 81% for PET assessment of histopathologic response. Patients classified as nonresponders in FDG-PET had a median survival of only 8 months compared with more than 24 months for PET responders. In a relatively small group of 17 patients studied before and after neoadjuvant chemoradiotherapy the 2-year survival rate of PET responders, defined as greater than 60% decrease in FDG uptake, was 63% compared with 38% in PET nonresponders [42].

Other tumors

FDG-PET has also been evaluated for monitoring treatment effects in patients with sarcomas. Histopathologic tumor regression, defined by less than 10% viable tumor tissue, is one of the most important prognostic factors in patients with osteosarcoma and Ewing's sarcoma [43]. Conventional radiographic imaging does not reliably discriminate between responding and nonresponding osseous tumors. Hawkins et al [44] studied 33 pediatric patients with osteosarcoma or Ewing's sarcoma with FDG-PET before preoperative chemotherapy and before surgery. SUVs before (SUV1) and after (SUV2) chemotherapy were correlated with response assessed by histopathology in surgically excised tumors. The ratio of SUV2 to SUV1 significantly correlated with the percentage of tumor necrosis. The authors concluded that changes in tumor FDG uptake could potentially be used as a noninvasive surrogate to predict response in these patients. In 27 patients with osteosarcoma, Schulte et al [45] also observed a significant correlation between histopathologic tumor regression and changes in FDG uptake. The tumor-to-background ratios for FDG uptake were determined before and after neoadjuvant chemotherapy. Changes in FDG uptake were compared with the histologic grade of tumor regression in the resected specimen revealing 17 responders and 10 nonresponders. The therapy-related decrease of FDG uptake in osteosarcomas was closely correlated with the percentage of tumor necrosis induced by chemotherapy. By using a cutoff level of 0.6, expressed as a quotient of post-therapeutic and pretherapeutic tumor-to-background ratios, all responders and 8 of 10 nonresponders were identified by PET.

In rectal cancer, preoperative chemoradiotherapy is increasingly used to allow sphincter-preserving tumor resection. Amthauer et al [46] studied 22 patients with locally advanced rectal cancer before and after preoperative chemoradiotherapy. The reduction in tumor FDG uptake was compared with histopathologic tumor response. Using a posttherapeutic reduction in SUV of greater than 36% to define response, FDG-PET revealed a sensitivity of 100% compared with 33% for endorectal ultrasound and a specificity of 86% versus 80% in response prediction. In a similar study design Calvo et al [47] also observed a significant correlation between changes in tumor FDG uptake and tumor response.

In lung cancer, 73 patients were prospectively evaluated for tumor response to chemoradiotherapy by CT and FDG-PET [48]. Complete response in FDG-PET was defined as normalization of all sites

Table 3
Assessment of response to chemotherapy in patients with lymphoma by PET and CT

Study	Year	N	PET (%)		CT (%)	
			Sensitivity	Specificity	Sensitivity	Specificity
Jerusalem et al, 1999 [35]	1999	54	57	100	71	65
de Wit et al, 2001 [36]	2001	37	91	69	72	21
Spaepen et al, 2001 [39]	2000	93	84	100	35	83
Hueltenschmidt et al, 2001 [75]	2001	63	95	89	95	39
Naumann et al, 2001 [76]	2001	58	88	68	NA	NA

Abbreviation: NA, not applicable.

with abnormal FDG uptake and partial response as a significant reduction in FDG uptake of all known lesions without the appearance of new lesions. Tumor response assessed by FDG-PET predicted better patient survival than response by CT criteria, the pretreatment tumor stage, or patient performance status.

In patients with relapsed metastatic germ cell tumors, Bokemeyer et al [49] evaluated FDG-PET for assessment of response to salvage high-dose chemotherapy. Findings in FDG-PET were compared with established means of tumor response assessment including CT, MR imaging, and changes in serum tumor markers. FDG-PET, CT, and tumor markers were obtained after two to three cycles of induction chemotherapy, before the start of high-dose chemotherapy. The outcome of high-dose chemotherapy was correctly predicted by FDG-PET in 91% of the cases, by CT in 59%, and serum tumor markers in 48%. Eight patients with a favorably predicted outcome by CT and serum tumor marker but a positive FDG-PET scan before high-dose chemotherapy failed treatment. FDG-PET had a higher sensitivity and specificity (100% and 78%) compared with CT and MR imaging (43% and 78%) and tumor markers (15% and 100%).

In seminoma, De Santis et al [50] studied FDG-PET as a predictor for viable residual tumor after chemotherapy. Fifty-six FDG-PET scans of 51 patients were assessable and correlated with either the histology of the resected mass or the clinical outcome. FDG-PET correctly predicted all 19 cases with

residual lesions larger than 3 cm and 35 (95%) of 37 with residual lesions less than 3 cm in size. Table 3 summarizes the accuracy of FDG-PET for assessment of histopathologic response after completion of therapy. The prognostic relevance of residual FDG-uptake after completion of therapy is shown in Table 4.

Timing of serial PET imaging

The timing between the last treatment and FDG-PET imaging for assessment of tumor response is of crucial importance. There are no clinical data indicating that chemotherapy causes a metabolic flare phenomenon of tumor tissue, which would lead to an initial increase in FDG uptake after initiation of therapy as it was indicated by in vitro results [51,52]. In these in vitro studies, the FDG uptake was assayed in surviving cells after chemotherapy or radiation therapy. This differs from the clinical situation, where the PET signal in a mass is determined by a combination of decreased FDG uptake because of tumor necrosis and cancer cell death plus potentially increased FDG uptake by surviving tumor cells. In most of the clinical studies published so far, the specificity of FDG-PET for detection of viable residual tumor tissue after completion of chemotherapy has been found to be higher than the sensitivity. Of note, as described previously a metabolic flare phenomenon has been observed in

Table 4
Assessment of response to chemotherapy in patients with solid tumors

Study	Tumor type	Year	N	PET (%)	
				Sensitivity	Specificity
Lowe et al, 1997 [77]	Head/neck	1997	28	90	83
Schulte et al, 1999 [45]	Osterosarcoma	1999	27	80	100
Bruecher et al, 2001 [40]	Esophagus	2001	27	55	100
Flamen et al, 2002 [41]	Esophagus	2002	36	71	82
Kollmansberger et al, 2002 [49]	Germ cell	2002	45	59	92
De Santis et al, 2004 [50]	Seminoma	2004	51	80	100

metastatic breast cancer as an indicator of good response to antiestrogen therapy [27,28].

Radiotherapy often causes a severe inflammatory reaction, which has raised concerns about using FDG-PET for assessment of tumor response to radiotherapy or chemoradiotherapy. It has frequently been recommended that FDG-PET should only be performed several months after completion of radiotherapy. There is a surprising lack of data, however, to support this recommendation. Although there is no doubt that radiation-induced inflammation accumulates FDG, the intensity of FDG uptake is often considerably lower than of the untreated primary tumors. Furthermore, the configuration of increased FDG uptake in radiation-induced inflammation is frequently markedly different from the configuration seen in a malignant tumor. In the clinical setting it is often possible to differentiate between radiation-induced inflammation and residual tumor tissue, especially when comparing a pretreatment with a posttreatment PET scan. Wieder et al [53] systematically studied the time course of changes in tumor FDG uptake in 38 patients with locally advanced squamous cell carcinomas of the esophagus treated by preoperative chemoradiotherapy. Patients were imaged before chemoradiotherapy, 2 weeks after initiation of therapy, at completion of therapy, and another 4 weeks later before surgery. None of the serial PET scans demonstrated an increase in tumor FDG uptake indicating that radiation-induced inflammatory reactions are quantitatively less relevant than the decrease of FDG uptake in viable tumor cells. Of note, the decrease in FDG uptake after 2 weeks of therapy was significantly correlated with subsequent histopathologic tumor regression and patient survival [53]. In addition, there are now several studies in head and neck cancer [54], lung cancer [48], and in esophageal cancer [40–42] showing a high specificity of FDG-PET for detection of viable tumor tissue following chemoradiotherapy. In contrast, Arslan et al [55] found that in patients with esophageal cancer radiation-induced inflammation could not be differentiated from viable tumor tissue. It is important to note, however, that this study included less advanced tumors, which accordingly demonstrated relatively low FDG uptake in the baseline scan. Even in responding tumors relative changes in tumor FDG uptake are necessarily smaller than in tumors with higher FDG uptake in the baseline scan.

Using FDG-PET for restaging after completion of treatment relies on the metabolic activity of tumor tissue. As a result of treatment, only small amounts of residual viable tumor may be present and lead to disease recurrence. Metabolic stunning of tumor cells by chemotherapy or radiotherapy has to be taken into account in which tumor cells are still viable, but exhibit a low metabolic activity because of the recent treatment. To achieve the highest sensitivity for detection of residual tumor tissue FDG-PET should be performed as late as possible after completion of therapy to enhance the detection of residual tumor tissue. In the authors' experience, a waiting period of 4 to 6 weeks after completion of therapy is a reasonable compromise. Imaging at later time points probably improves the accuracy of FDG-PET for detection of residual tumor tissue and short-term follow-up is recommended in equivocal cases.

Recent advances in PET imaging

PET and CT

There are exiting new developments in the field of PET instrumentation and PET tracers. PET-CT is a new imaging modality that allows the acquisition of spatially registered PET and CT data in one imaging procedure [56]. This hardware solution overcomes limitations of software fusion methods, such as alignment problems caused by internal organ movement, variations in scanner bed profile, and positioning of the patient for the scan, improving sensitivity and specificity of PET imaging. PET-CT is unique because it provides combined anatomic and functional imaging information, which allows tissue characterization and assessment of the exact localization and the extent of tumor tissue. Using a combined PET-CT scanner for monitoring therapeutic effects rather than separate conventional PET and CT scanners could have several advantages. It allows the assessment of tumor size (volume) and metabolic activity at the same time in one co-registered imaging procedure. Because partial volume effects play an important role in limiting the measurement of the true tracer concentration in small tumor masses, the use of PET-CT allows more accurate quantification of FDG uptake in the course of therapy. To date, there have been no studies evaluating the role of FDG-PET–CT to predict response early during the course of therapy but with the increasing availability of PET-CT combined PET and CT criteria should be established for prediction and assessment of therapy response.

Imaging cell proliferation

Increased cell proliferation is an essential characteristic of malignant tumors. The number of clonogenic cells in the S-phase represents the growth fraction of a tumor, which constitutes approximately 3% to 15% of the total cell mass for most tumors. The higher the tumor growth fraction, the more rapidly the effects of therapy is manifest at the tumor volumetric level. Alternatively, a quantitative estimate of tumor proliferation activity obtained through noninvasive imaging could predict or allow for rapid monitoring of response to therapy. DNA synthesis is tightly regulated through the cell cycle and the use of radiolabeled precursors of DNA synthesis has been shown to allow for noninvasive imaging and measurement of cell proliferation. Several PET tracers have been developed to image cell proliferation. The major limitation of C-11 labeled thymidine is its rapid degradation in blood and the number of radioactive metabolites confound the interpretation of the PET images [57]. Several ^{18}F-labeled thymidine analogues resistant to degradation in vivo have been developed. Fluorothymidine (3′-deoxy-3′-fluorothymidine) was initially developed for the treatment of HIV infections. The radiolabeled derivative, 3-deoxy-3-[^{18}F]–fluorothymidine (FLT), can be labeled at high specific activity and is resistant to degradation in blood. Following transmembrane transport of FLT into the cell, the intracellular accumulation of FLT is dependent on cellular thymidine kinase-1 activity. FLT is phosphorylated at approximately 30% of the rate of thymidine and FLT-monophosphate accumulates as a membrane-impermeable metabolite in the cell [58]. Because FLT is a chain terminator in DNA synthesis, very little is integrated into DNA. Thymidine kinase-1 is expressed only in cells undergoing DNA replication during the S phase of the cell cycle; the intracellular accumulation of FLT is hypothesized to reflect cell replication. Increased [^{18}F]-FLT uptake has been observed in tumor tissue but also in other rapidly proliferating normal cells, such as bone marrow. Initial studies in untreated patients demonstrated increased FLT uptake in different types of malignant thoracic tumors and colorectal carcinoma [59–62].

Radiolabeled amino acids

Cellular amino acid uptake is mediated by a complex system of sodium-dependent and sodium-independent carrier proteins. The increased pooling of amino acids observed in malignant tumors seems to be caused mainly by increased expression and activity of the L-type sodium-independent transporter system. The fraction of radiolabeled amino acids that is incorporated into proteins is small compared with

the total amount that is taken up by cells. PET imaging using radiolabeled amino acids reflects the sum of both fractions, and generally tracer uptake is related to tumor cell proliferation. To date, several amino acids have been radiolabeled for PET imaging; however, given their ease of synthesis and limited formation of metabolites in vivo, carbon-11 ([^{11}C])-methyl-methionine (MET) and [^{11}C]-tyrosine have been most extensively studied [63].

In a series of 21 lung cancer patients, Kubota et al [64] compared MET uptake with CT tumor volume before and within 2 weeks after radiotherapy or chemoradiotherapy. Patients with early recurrence had a significant lower decrease in MET uptake compared with baseline than patients with no or late recurrence in follow-up. Although MET-PET clearly distinguished the early recurrence group from the late-recurrence group, the late-recurrence group was indistinguishable from patients who had no recurrence. MET-PET seemed to be helpful in this study, however, for evaluating tumor viability when a residual mass was present on CT. Wieder et al [65] studied the use of MET-PET for therapy monitoring in 15 patients with rectal cancer undergoing preoperative chemoradiotherapy. All tumors were visualized on the baseline PET scan and had a significantly higher MET uptake than normal rectum. MET uptake decreased during therapy in all tumors; however, changes in MET uptake did not correlate with histopathologic tumor response. The authors concluded that MET-PET might not be suitable for assessment of the response to therapy in patients with rectal cancer. Similar results were found in previously untreated head and neck cancer [66]. Fifteen patients underwent MET-PET before external-beam radiotherapy and after a median dose of 24 Gy. A total of 13 primary tumors and 12 metastatic lymph nodes were identified on MET-PET. MET uptake in head and neck cancer showed a significant decrease during the first 2 to 3 weeks of radiotherapy. The decrease in MET uptake was comparable in relapsing patients and those who remain locally controlled, however, and the use of MET-PET for prediction of response to radiotherapy was limited. Using a 3.1 SUV cutoff value, MET-PET allowed one to distinguish between complete responders (<3.1) and nonresponders. After completion of radiotherapy, Lindholm et al [67] found significantly lower MET uptake in tumors showing a histopathologic response than in those that did not respond. Although changes in MET uptake were shown to reflect response to radiotherapy treatment in patients suffering from various tumors, the clinical relevance of these findings currently still seems controversial.

Imaging hypoxia

Several studies have indicated that tumor hypoxia may be a limiting factor for treatment success, specifically in radiotherapy. Reduced hemoglobin levels and low tumor-oxygen tension are associated with higher treatment failure rates. Improvements in local tumor control could be achieved by the use of hypoxic cell radiosensitizer or hyperbaric oxygen. Identification and quantification of tumor hypoxia may predict outcome and may identify patients who might benefit from concomitant radiosensitizing therapy to overcome the hypoxia effect.

For the purpose of hypoxia imaging, PET and SPECT tracers have been developed. The 2-nitro-imidazole moiety present in radiopharmaceuticals, such as [18F]-misonidazole (MISO), acts as a bio-reductive molecule, accepting a single electron and producing a free radical anion that, after further reduction, is incorporated into cells under hypoxic conditions. More recently copper-64 ([64Cu]–labeled bis(thiosemicarbazone) complexes ([64Cu]-ATSM) have also been introduced for imaging of hypoxia [68].

Koh et al [69] reported the first experience with 18F–labeled MISO for therapy monitoring in eight patients with different cancers, mainly of the head and neck. All patients underwent PET imaging before primary radiotherapy and six of eight studies revealed significant MISO accumulation in tumor tissue at 2 hours after injection. Toward the end of fractionated radiotherapy, MISO-PET was repeated in three patients with head-and-neck carcinoma who had initially positive scans. MISO uptake decreased below the threshold previously identified suggesting reoxygenation of tumor tissue. The same group also reported on seven patients with locally advanced non–small cell lung cancer [70]. Patients underwent sequential MISO-PET while receiving primary radiotherapy. The authors concluded that, although there was a general tendency toward improved oxygenation in human tumors during fractionated radiotherapy, these changes were unpredictable and may be insufficient in extent and timing to overcome the negative effects of existing pretreatment hypoxia. MISO-PET might appropriately allow for the selection of patients with radioresistant hypoxic cancers through single pretreatment evaluation of tumor hypoxia. Rasey et al [71] studied 37 patients with different tumors, 36 of which showed increased MISO uptake. The tumor fractional hypoxic volume ranged from 0% to 94.7% and no correlation to tumor size was observed. The extent of hypoxia varied markedly between tumors in the same site or of the same histology. Hypoxia, identified by MISO-PET, was distributed heterogeneously between regions within a single tumor and the results from MISO-PET imaging were consistent with O_2 electrode measures with other types of human tumors. ^{64}Cu-ATSM has shown encouraging results for defining the hypoxic tumor volume for radiotherapy planning [72] and the uptake of ^{64}Cu-ATSM was inversely related to progression-free survival and overall survival in patients with cervical cancer [73].

Summary

Establishing new surrogate end points for monitoring response to treatment is needed for current therapy modalities and for new therapeutic strategies including molecular targeted cancer therapies. PET as a functional imaging technology provides rapid, reproducible, noninvasive in vivo assessment and quantification of several biologic processes targeted by these therapies. PET is useful in a variety of clinical relevant applications, including distinguishing between radiation necrosis and tumor recurrence, determining the resectability of recurrent tumor, and evaluating response to therapy. FDG-PET has demonstrated efficacy for monitoring therapeutic response in a wide range of cancers, including breast, esophageal, lung, head and neck, and lymphoma. FDG-PET can assess tumor glucose use with high reproducibility. Following therapy, the decrease of glucose use correlates with the reduction of viable tumor cells. FDG-PET allows the prediction of therapy response early in the course of therapy and determining the viability of residual masses after completion of treatment. The molecular basis for the success of FDG-PET is the rapid reduction of tumor glucose metabolism in effective therapies. Of even higher clinical relevance is the accurate identification of nonresponders in patients without a significant change in tumor glucose metabolism after initiation of therapy. PET imaging can easily visualize these changes in metabolic activity and indicate, sometimes within hours of the first treatment, whether or not a patient will respond to a particular therapy. In contrast to CT, MR imaging, or ultrasound, PET imaging allows identification of responding and nonresponding tumors early in the course of therapy. With this information, physicians can rapidly modify ineffective therapies for individual patients and thereby potentially improve patient outcomes and reduce cost.

One of the major limitations for the routine application of FDG-PET imaging for therapy monitoring is that no generally accepted cutoff values

have been established to differentiate optimally between responders and nonresponders. The patient series are still relatively small and frequently consist of
different tumor types and different therapy regimens.

Prospective studies including a sufficient number
of patients are needed to define cutoff values to
differentiate between responder and nonresponder for
different tumors and different treatment regimes. In
the future, PET imaging can also serve in the evaluation of new therapeutic agents, new experimental
treatments, and specifically in monitoring clinical
phase II studies.

References

[1] Therasse P, Arbuck SG, Eisenhauer EA, et al. New
    guidelines to evaluate the response to treatment in solid
    tumors. European Organization for Research and
    Treatment of Cancer, National Cancer Institute of the
    United States, National Cancer Institute of Canada. J
    Natl Cancer Inst 2000;92:205–16.

[2] Miller AB, Hoogstraten B, Staquet M, et al. Reporting
    results of cancer treatment. Cancer 1981;47:207–14.

[3] Buyse M, Thirion P, Carlson RW, et al. Relation
    between tumour response to first-line chemotherapy
    and survival in advanced colorectal cancer: a meta-
    analysis. Meta-Analysis Group in Cancer. Lancet
    2000;356:373–8.

[4] Avril N. GLUT1 expression in tissue and [F-18]FDG
    uptake. J Nucl Med 2004;45:930–2.

[5] Zasadny KR, Wahl RL. Standardized uptake values of
    normal tissues at PET with 2-[fluorine- 18]-fluoro-2-
    deoxy-D-glucose: variations with body weight and a
    method for correction. Radiology 1993;189:847–50.

[6] Minn H, Zasadny KR, Quint LE, et al. Lung cancer:
    reproducibility of quantitative measurements for eval-
    uating 2-[F-18]-fluoro-2-deoxy-D-glucose uptake at
    PET. Radiology 1995;196:167–73.

[7] Weber WA, Ziegler SI, Thodtmann R, et al. Reprodu-
    cibility of metabolic measurements in malignant
    tumors using FDG PET. J Nucl Med 1999;40:1771–7.

[8] Torizuka T, Clavo AC, Wahl RL. Effect of hyper-
    glycemia on in vitro tumor uptake of tritiated FDG,
    thymidine, L-methionine and L-leucine. J Nucl Med
    1997;38:382–6.

[9] Weber WA, Petersen V, Schmidt B, et al. Positron
    emission tomography in non-small-cell lung cancer:
    prediction of response to chemotherapy by quantitative
    assessment of glucose use. J Clin Oncol 2003;21:
    2651–7.

[10] Wahl RL, Zasadny K, Helvie M, et al. Metabolic
    monitoring of breast cancer chemohormonotherapy
    using positron emission tomography: initial evaluation.
    J Clin Oncol 1993;11:2101–11.

[11] Jansson T, Westlin JE, Ahlstrom H, et al. Positron
    emission tomography studies in patients with locally

advanced and/or metastatic breast cancer: a method
    for early therapy evaluation? J Clin Oncol 1995;13:
    1470–7.

[12] Romer W, Hanauske AR, Ziegler S, et al. Positron
    emission tomography in non-Hodgkin's lymphoma:
    assessment of chemotherapy with fluorodeoxyglucose.
    Blood 1998;91:4464–71.

[13] Hoekstra OS, van Lingen A, Ossenkoppele GJ, et al.
    Early response monitoring in malignant lymphoma
    using fluorine-18 fluorodeoxyglucose single-photon
    emission tomography. Eur J Nucl Med 1993;20:
    1214–7.

[14] Jerusalem G, Beguin Y, Fassotte MF, et al. Persistent
    tumor 18F-FDG uptake after a few cycles of poly-
    chemotherapy is predictive of treatment failure in non-
    Hodgkin's lymphoma. Haematologica 2000;85:613–8.

[15] Kostakoglu L, Coleman M, Leonard JP, et al. PET
    predicts prognosis after 1 cycle of chemotherapy in
    aggressive lymphoma and Hodgkin's disease. J Nucl
    Med 2002;43:1018–27.

[16] Spaepen K, Stroobants S, Dupont P, et al. Early
    restaging positron emission tomography with (18)F-
    fluorodeoxyglucose predicts outcome in patients with
    aggressive non-Hodgkin's lymphoma. Ann Oncol
    2002;13:1356–63.

[17] Torizuka T, Nakamura F, Kanno T, et al. Early therapy
    monitoring with FDG-PET in aggressive non-Hodg-
    kin's lymphoma and Hodgkin's lymphoma. Eur J Nucl
    Med Mol Imaging 2004;31:22–8.

[18] Medical Research Council Oesophageal Cancer Work-
    ing Group. Surgical resection with or without preopera-
    tive chemotherapy in oesophageal cancer: a randomised
    controlled trial. Lancet 2002;359:1727–33.

[19] Kelsen DP, Ginsberg R, Pajak TF, et al. Chemotherapy
    followed by surgery compared with surgery alone for
    localized esophageal cancer. N Engl J Med 1998;339:
    1979–84.

[20] Weber WA, Ott K, Becker K, et al. Prediction of
    response to preoperative chemotherapy in adenocarci-
    nomas of the esophagogastric junction by metabolic
    imaging. J Clin Oncol 2001;19:3058–65.

[21] Ott K, Fink U, Becker K, et al. Prediction of response
    to preoperative chemotherapy in gastric carcinoma by
    metabolic imaging: results of a prospective trial. J Clin
    Oncol 2003;21:4604–10.

[22] Machiavelli MR, Romero AO, Perez JE, et al.
    Prognostic significance of pathological response of
    primary tumor and metastatic axillary lymph nodes
    after neoadjuvant chemotherapy for locally advanced
    breast carcinoma. Cancer J Sci Am 1998;4:125–31.

[23] Honkoop AH, van Diest PJ, de Jong JS, et al.
    Prognostic role of clinical, pathological and biological
    characteristics in patients with locally advanced breast
    cancer. Br J Cancer 1998;77:621–6.

[24] Smith IC, Welch AE, Hutcheon AW, et al. Positron
    emission tomography using [(18)F]-fluorodeoxy-D-
    glucose to predict the pathologic response of breast
    cancer to primary chemotherapy. J Clin Oncol 2000;
    18:1676–88.

[25] Schelling M, Avril N, Nährig J, et al. Positron emission tomography using [F-18] fluorodeoxyglucose for monitoring primary chemotherapy in breast cancer. J Clin Oncol 2000;18:1689–95.

[26] Mankoff DA, Dunnwald LK, Gralow JR, et al. Changes in blood flow and metabolism in locally advanced breast cancer treated with neoadjuvant chemotherapy. J Nucl Med 2003;44:1806–14.

[27] Dehdashti F, Flanagan FL, Mortimer JE, et al. Positron emission tomographic assessment of "metabolic flare" to predict response of metastatic breast cancer to antiestrogen therapy. Eur J Nucl Med 1999;26:51–6.

[28] Mortimer JE, Dehdashti F, Siegel BA, et al. Metabolic flare: indicator of hormone responsiveness in advanced breast cancer. J Clin Oncol 2001;19:2797–803.

[29] Demetri GD, von Mehren M, Blanke CD, et al. Efficacy and safety of imatinib mesylate in advanced gastrointestinal stromal tumors. N Engl J Med 2002; 347:472–80.

[30] Stroobants S, Goeminne J, Seegers M, et al. 18FDG-positron emission tomography for the early prediction of response in advanced soft tissue sarcoma treated with imatinib mesylate (Glivec). Eur J Cancer 2003; 39:2012–20.

[31] Kaplan WD, Jochelson MS, Herman TS, et al. Gallium-67 imaging: a predictor of residual tumor viability and clinical outcome in patients with diffuse large-cell lymphoma. J Clin Oncol 1990;8:1966–70.

[32] Kostakoglu L, Leonard JP, Kuji I, et al. Comparison of fluorine-18 fluorodeoxyglucose positron emission tomography and Ga-67 scintigraphy in evaluation of lymphoma. Cancer 2002;94:879–88.

[33] Shen YY, Kao A, Yen RF. Comparison of 18F-fluoro-2-deoxyglucose positron emission tomography and gallium-67 citrate scintigraphy for detecting malignant lymphoma. Oncol Rep 2002;9:321–5.

[34] Zinzani PL, Magagnoli M, Chierichetti F, et al. The role of positron emission tomography (PET) in the management of lymphoma patients. Ann Oncol 1999; 10:1181–4.

[35] Jerusalem G, Beguin Y, Fassotte MF, et al. Whole-body positron emission tomography using 18F-fluorodeoxyglucose for posttreatment evaluation in Hodgkin's disease and non-Hodgkin's lymphoma has higher diagnostic and prognostic value than classical computed tomography scan imaging. Blood 1999;94: 429–33.

[36] de Wit M, Bohuslavizki KH, Buchert R, et al. 18FDG-PET following treatment as valid predictor for disease-free survival in Hodgkin's lymphoma. Ann Oncol 2001;12:29–37.

[37] Weihrauch MR, Re D, Scheidhauer K, et al. Thoracic positron emission tomography using 18F-fluorodeoxyglucose for the evaluation of residual mediastinal Hodgkin disease. Blood 2001;98:2930–4.

[38] Mikhaeel NG, Timothy AR, O'Doherty MJ, et al. 18-FDG-PET as a prognostic indicator in the treatment of aggressive non-Hodgkin's lymphoma-comparison with CT. Leuk Lymphoma 2000;39:543–53.

[39] Spaepen K, Stroobants S, Dupont P, et al. Prognostic value of positron emission tomography (PET) with fluorine-18 fluorodeoxyglucose ([18F]FDG) after first-line chemotherapy in non-Hodgkin's lymphoma: is [18F]FDG-PET a valid alternative to conventional diagnostic methods? J Clin Oncol 2001;19:414–9.

[40] Brucher B, Weber W, Bauer M, et al. Neoadjuvant therapy of esophageal squamous cell carcinoma: response evaluation by positron emission tomography. Ann Surg 2001;233:300–9.

[41] Flamen P, Van Cutsem E, Lerut A, et al. Positron emission tomography for assessment of the response to induction chemotherapy in locally advanced esophageal cancer. Ann Oncol 2002;13:361–8.

[42] Downey RJ, Akhurst T, Ilson D, et al. Whole body 18FDG-PET and the response of esophageal cancer to induction therapy: results of a prospective trial. J Clin Oncol 2003;21:428–32.

[43] Salzer-Kuntschik M, Delling G, Beron G, et al. Morphological grades of regression in osteosarcoma after polychemotherapy: study COSS 80. J Cancer Res Clin Oncol 1983;106:21–4.

[44] Hawkins DS, Rajendran JG, Conrad III EU, et al. Evaluation of chemotherapy response in pediatric bone sarcomas by [F-18]-fluorodeoxy-D-glucose positron emission tomography. Cancer 2002;94:3277–84.

[45] Schulte M, Brecht-Krauss D, Werner M, et al. Evaluation of neoadjuvant therapy response of osteogenic sarcoma using FDG PET. J Nucl Med 1999; 40:1637–43.

[46] Amthauer H, Denecke T, Rau B, et al. Response prediction by FDG-PET after neoadjuvant radiochemotherapy and combined regional hyperthermia of rectal cancer: correlation with endorectal ultrasound and histopathology. Eur J Nucl Med Mol Imaging 2004;31(6):811–9.

[47] Calvo FA, Domper M, Matute R, et al. 18F-FDG positron emission tomography staging and restaging in rectal cancer treated with preoperative chemoradiation. Int J Radiat Oncol Biol Phys 2004;58:528–35.

[48] Mac Manus MP, Hicks RJ, Matthews JP, et al. Positron emission tomography is superior to computed tomography scanning for response-assessment after radical radiotherapy or chemoradiotherapy in patients with non-small-cell lung cancer. J Clin Oncol 2003;21:1285–92.

[49] Bokemeyer C, Kollmannsberger C, Oechsle K, et al. Early prediction of treatment response to high-dose salvage chemotherapy in patients with relapsed germ cell cancer using [(18)F]FDG PET. Br J Cancer 2002;86:506–11.

[50] De Santis M, Becherer A, Bokemeyer C, et al. 2–18fluoro-deoxy-D-glucose positron emission tomography is a reliable predictor for viable tumor in postchemotherapy seminoma: an update of the prospective multicentric SEMPET trial. J Clin Oncol 2004;22:1034–9.

[51] Higashi K, Clavo AC, Wahl RL. In vitro assessment of 2-fluoro-2-deoxy-D-glucose, L-methionine and thymidine as agents to monitor the early response of a

human adenocarcinoma cell line to radiotherapy. J Nucl Med 1993;34:773–9.

[52] Haberkorn U, Morr I, Oberdorfer F, et al. Fluorodeoxy-glucose uptake in vitro: aspects of method and effects of treatment with gemcitabine. J Nucl Med 1994; 35:1842–50

[53] Wieder H, Brucher BL, Zimmerman F, et al. Time course of tumor metabolic activity during chemoradio-therapy of esophageal squamous cell carcinoma and response to treatment. J Clin Oncol 2004;22:900–9.

[54] Greven KM, Williams III DW, McGuirt Sr WF, et al. Serial positron emission tomography scans following radiation therapy of patients with head and neck cancer. Head Neck 2001;23:942–6.

[55] Arslan N, Miller TR, Dehdashti F, et al. Evaluation of response to neoadjuvant therapy by quantitative 2-deoxy-2-[18F]fluoro-D-glucose with positron emission tomography in patients with esophageal cancer. Mol Imaging Biol 2002;4:301–10.

[56] Townsend DW, Carney JP, Yap JT, et al. PET/CT today and tomorrow. J Nucl Med 2004;45:4S–14S.

[57] Shields AF, Mankoff D, Graham MM, et al. Analysis of 2-carbon-11-thymidine blood metabolites in PET imaging. J Nucl Med 1996;37:290–6.

[58] Mier W, Haberkorn U, Eisenhut M. [18F]FLT: portrait of a proliferation marker. Eur J Nucl Med Mol Imaging 2002;29:165–9.

[59] Shields AF, Grierson JR, Kozawa SM, et al. Development of labeled thymidine analogs for imaging tumor proliferation. Nucl Med Biol 1996;23:17–22.

[60] Vesselle H, Grierson J, Muzi M, et al. In vivo validation of 3′deoxy-3′-[(18)F]fluorothymidine ([(18)F]FLT) as a proliferation imaging tracer in humans: correlation of [(18)F]FLT uptake by positron emission tomography with Ki-67 immunohistochem-istry and flow cytometry in human lung tumors. Clin Cancer Res 2002;8:3315–23.

[61] Francis DL, Visvikis D, Costa DC, et al. Potential impact of [(18)F]3′-deoxy-3′-fluorothymidine versus [(18)F]fluoro-2-deoxy- D-glucose in positron emission tomography for colorectal cancer. Eur J Nucl Med Mol Imaging 2003;30(7):988–94.

[62] Buck AK, Schirrmeister H, Hetzel M, et al. 3-deoxy-3-[(18)F]fluorothymidine-positron emission tomography for noninvasive assessment of proliferation in pulmo-nary nodules. Cancer Res 2002;62:3331–4.

[63] Jager PL, Vaalburg W, Pruim J, et al. Radiolabeled amino acids: basic aspects and clinical applications in oncology. J Nucl Med 2001;42:432–45.

[64] Kubota K, Yamada S, Ishiwata K, et al. Evaluation of the treatment response of lung cancer with positron emission tomography and L-[methyl-11C]methionine: a preliminary study. Eur J Nucl Med 1993;20:495–501.

[65] Wieder H, Ott K, Zimmermann F, et al. PET imaging with [11C]methyl-L-methionine for therapy monitoring in patients with rectal cancer. Eur J Nucl Med Mol Imaging 2002;29:789–96.

[66] Nuutinen J, Jyrkkio S, Lehikoinen P, et al. Evaluation of early response to radiotherapy in head and neck cancer measured with [11C]methionine-positron emis-sion tomography. Radiother Oncol 1999;52:225–32.

[67] Lindholm P, Leskinen-Kallio S, Grenman R, et al. Evaluation of response to radiotherapy in head and neck cancer by positron emission tomography and [11C]methionine. Int J Radiat Oncol Biol Phys 1995; 32:787–94.

[68] Lewis JS, McCarthy DW, McCarthy TJ, et al. Evaluation of 64Cu-ATSM in vitro and in vivo in a hypoxic tumor model. J Nucl Med 1999;40:177–83.

[69] Koh WJ, Rasey JS, Evans ML, et al. Imaging of hypoxia in human tumors with [F-18]fluoromisonida-zole. Int J Radiat Oncol Biol Phys 1992;22:199–212.

[70] Koh WJ, Bergman KS, Rasey JS, et al. Evaluation of oxygenation status during fractionated radiotherapy in human non small cell lung cancers using [F-18]fluo-romisonidazole positron emission tomography. Int J Radiat Oncol Biol Phys 1995;33:391–8.

[71] Rasey JS, Koh WJ, Evans ML, et al. Quantifying regional hypoxia in human tumors with positron emission tomography of [18F]fluoromisonidazole: a pretherapy study of 37 patients. Int J Radiat Oncol Biol Phys 1996;36:417–28.

[72] Chao KS, Bosch WR, Mutic S, et al. A novel approach to overcome hypoxic tumor resistance: Cu-ATSM-guided intensity-modulated radiation therapy. Int J Radiat Oncol Biol Phys 2001;49:1171–82.

[73] Dehdashti F, Grigsby PW, Mintun MA, et al. Assessing tumor hypoxia in cervical cancer by positron emission tomography with 60Cu-ATSM: relationship to thera-peutic response-a preliminary report. Int J Radiat Oncol Biol Phys 2003;55:1233–8.

[74] Brun E, Kjellen E, Tennvall J, et al. FDG PET studies during treatment: prediction of therapy outcome in head and neck squamous cell carcinoma. Head Neck 2002;24(2):127–35.

[75] Hueltenschmidt B, Sautter-Bihl ML, Lang O, et al. Whole body positron emission tomography in the treatment of Hodgkin disease. Cancer 2001;91(2): 302–10.

[76] Naumann R, Vaic A, Beuthien-Baumann B, et al. Prognostic value of positron emission tomography in the evaluation of post-treatment residual mass in patients with Hodgkin's disease and non-Hodgkin's lymphoma. Br J Haematol 2001;115:793–800.

[77] Lowe VJ, Dunphy FR, Varvares M, et al. Evaluation of chemotherapy response in patients with advanced head and neck cancer using [F-18]fluorodeoxyglucose positron emission tomography. Head Neck 1997;19: 666–74.

[78] Cremerius U, Fabry U, Neuerburg J, et al. Prognostic significance of positron emission tomography using fluorine-18-fluorodeoxyglucose in patients treated for malignant lymphoma. Nuklearmedizin 2001;40:23–30.

[79] Kunkel M, Forster GJ, Reichert TE, et al. Radiation response non-invasively imaged by [18F]FDG-PET predicts local tumor control and survival in advanced oral squamous cell carcinoma. Oral Oncol 2003;39: 170–7.

ELSEVIER
SAUNDERS

Radiol Clin N Am 43 (2005) 205 – 220

RADIOLOGIC
CLINICS
of North America

MR techniques for in vivo molecular and cellular imaging

Edward J. Delikatny, PhD*, Harish Poptani, PhD

*Molecular Imaging Laboratory, Department of Radiology, University of Pennsylvania School of Medicine,
B6 Blockley Hall, 423 Guardian Drive, Philadelphia, PA 19104, USA*

MR imaging is routinely used in the clinic for diagnostic imaging and is often the technique of choice for anatomic imaging of the brain and other soft tissues. It has the advantage of providing exquisite anatomic resolution, routinely down to 1 to 2 mm in plane at clinical field strengths of 1.5 T, and is the only imaging modality that can provide an assessment of function or molecular expression in tandem with anatomic detail. For these reasons, MR imaging is becoming a powerful modality in experimental molecular imaging. The design and implementation of specific molecular contrast agents targeting cell-surface receptors, enzyme activity, or measuring gene expression is beginning to allow the distinction of a range of biologic and physiologic processes related to cancer and other pathologies. Because of the high resolution attainable, MR imaging is also used increasingly to provide adjunct locator images for other imaging modalities with poorer intrinsic resolution, such as positron emission tomography and optical imaging [1].

The signal to noise in an MR image depends on the density of protons present in the region of interest and the degree of polarization of the nuclear spin states. In the case of soft tissues with high water content, sufficient spin density is present to obtain high-quality images in short time periods, even though the induced spin polarization for protons is only on the order of five excess spins in the ground state per 10^6 spins at magnetic field strengths of 1.5 T. The practical outcome is that the temporal resolution of MR imaging can be limited compared with other imaging modes, and a full MR imaging examination can sometimes be a lengthy procedure, exceeding 1 hour. Another factor to consider is that the minimum detectable concentration of molecular probes or contrast agents can be orders of magnitude greater than those required by other imaging modalities. Changes induced by exogenous paramagnetic contrast agents or xenobiotics detectable by MR imaging or spectroscopic methods rely on the delivery of micromolar concentrations to the tissues of interest to be observed. This means that the use of MR imaging for detection of gene expression or cell surface receptors presents a challenge because these molecules are usually present in low concentrations: 10^{-9}-10^{-12} mol/g tissue [2]. Strategies to overcome these limitations are discussed later in this article.

Basis of MR imaging contrast

The normal contrast in MR images depends on proton spin density and on the T1 and T2 (T2*) relaxation times of the tissue. T1 is called the spin-lattice or longitudinal relaxation time and is the characteristic time for magnetization to return to the main magnetic field (z) axis after the application of radiofrequency pulses. T2 is defined as the spin-spin or transverse relaxation time and is the time for spin magnetization to dephase in the transverse (xy) plane. T2* is the transverse relaxation time measured in the presence of magnetic field inhomogeneities. In

The authors acknowledge the support of the University of Pennsylvania Research Foundation, the National Institutes of Health (NIH Grants R21-CA-79718 and R21-EB-002537), and the Small Animal Imaging Resource Program at the University of Pennsylvania (R24-CA83105).

* Corresponding author.
E-mail address: delikatn@mail.med.upenn.edu
(E.J. Delikatny).

general, T1s are longer than T2s, and this difference is greater in solids and in tissues with low water content. By systematically varying acquisition parameters, such as the repetition time (TR) or the echo time (TE) in an MR spin-echo or gradient-echo imaging experiment, one can generate contrast that is weighted either toward T1 or T2. Short TR and short TE experiments lead to images with T1-weighted contrast, whereas T2-weighted images result from sequences using longer TR and TE. The result of this is that tissues with higher water content (eg, synovial fluid, cerebrospinal fluid, and regions of edema) appear hypointense (dark) on T1-weighted images and hyperintense (bright) on T2-weighted images relative to surrounding tissues. The opposite is true in tissues with low water content (muscle, brain, liver), which appear hyperintense when a T1-weighted sequence is used and hypointense on T2-weighted images [3].

In soft tissues, where the spin density of water protons is relatively high, differences in local relaxation times are usually sufficient to provide interorgan contrast [2]. However, the determination of differences between normal and pathologic tissues, where relaxation times are often similar, is more difficult and is enhanced by the administration of a paramagnetic or superparamagnetic contrast agent. Interaction of the contrast agents with adjacent water molecules leads to a local reduction in T1 or T2 relaxation times of water. Two general types of contrast agents exist: those that primarily decrease water T1, leading to increased signal on T1-weighted images, and those that predominantly decrease T2, leading to a reduction of signal on T2-weighted images [3]. One major class of contrast agents affecting T1 is the gadolinium-based paramagnetic chelates, whereas T2 agents consist of superparamagnetic complexes, such as the iron oxide nanoparticles.

In molecular imaging, additional signal contrast is provided through these contrast agents targeted to a biochemical or physiologic property of interest. The design of specific targeted contrast agents is often based on chemical modification of existing contrast agents to include receptor or organelle targeting moieties, or regions that act as specific enzyme substrates, or respond to changes in gene expression.

Basis of MR imaging contrast agents

The level of induced contrast by a paramagnetic contrast agent depends on its relaxivity, which is defined by the expression $1/T_{1,2obs} = 1/T_{1,2d} + r_1$ [CA], where $1/T_{1,2\ obs}$ is the observed T1 or T2 in an MR imaging experiment; $1/T_{1,2d}$ is the diamagnetic contribution to the T1 or T2; [CA] is the concentration of the contrast agent; and r_1 is the relaxivity and is equal to $1/T_{1,2p}$, the paramagnetic contribution to the relaxation rate [4]. Relaxivity is defined as the relaxation rate of water protons in a 1-mmol/L solution of contrast agent and is expressed in mmol/$L^{-1}sec^{-1}$. The increase in relaxation rate induced by any given contrast agent is linearly dependent on the local concentration of the paramagnetic compound. It is also a function of the effective correlation time, τ_c, of the complex, which in turn depends on the correlation time of the unpaired electron spins in the metal (τ_S); on the residence time of the water molecule in the hydration spheres (τ_M); and on the reorientational correlation time of the molecule or complex (τ_R) [2,4]: $1/\tau_c = 1/\tau_S + 1/\tau_R + 1/\tau_M$.

In the case of soluble paramagnetic chelates or complexes, the hydration sphere component is often further separated into a dominant inner sphere and secondary outer sphere contribution. The particular relevance of the second equation lies in the fact that the relaxivity of paramagnetic compounds can be increased either by restricting the rotational molecular motion of the complex, or by allowing increased access of water molecules to the paramagnetic core. As is seen later, the increase in relaxivity induced by polymerization or coagulation, or by increasing the molecular weight of the complex, is an important consideration used in the development of smart contrast agents. Moreover, the design of capped gadolinium complexes that permit increased water access as a result of enzymatic activity or in the presence of specific ions has greatly increased the scope for the design of targeted functional contrast agents.

In the case of superparamagnetic iron-oxide (SPIO) particles, the increased relaxivity leading to hypointense changes observed in T2- and T2*-weighted images is induced primarily by local magnetic susceptibility effects that lead to dephasing of nearby protons [5,6]. These susceptibility changes result from the large microscopic field gradients, created by the aligned magnetic moments of the superparamagnetic particles. Because the relative changes in T2 relaxivity induced by iron oxide nanoparticles depend on the size of the particles and the effective iron concentration, the modulation of these parameters can be exploited in the design of functional contrast agents.

One important consideration in the development and application of MR imaging contrast agents is the limits of sensitivity of contrast agents introduced into cells or tissues. Aime et al [7] have reviewed the sensitivity limits for paramagnetic contrast agents and calculated that a minimum of 2×10^9 gadolinium chelates with relaxivities on the order of 5 to 7 mmol/ L^{-1} sec^{-1} must be present per cell for significant changes in MR imaging contrast to be observed, consistent with an internal concentration of 10 to 100 µmol/L. Because the theoretical limit of gadolinium relaxivity is around 100 mmol/L^{-1} sec^{-1} [4], this highlights the need for the development of contrast agents with higher native or inducible relaxivity to increase the limits of detection. Moreover, the formulation of contrast agents in the form of multisite ligands or by encapsulation to deliver high local concentration provides an additional method for increasing sensitivity.

Superparamagnetic agents generally induce larger changes in T2 relaxivities than paramagnetic compounds do, leading to increased contrast-to-noise changes. The size and effective concentration of iron oxide particle per cell determines the T2* relaxivities of these compounds. SPIO particles (7–30 nm) exhibit a relaxivity of about 250 mmol/L^{-1} sec^{-1} at 4.7 T, whereas micron-sized nanoparticles may

exhibit relaxivities as high as 360 mmol/L^{-1} sec^{-1} at these magnetic fields [8]. At clinical field strengths of 1.5 T, it has been reported that about 0.9×10^6 SPIO-labeled cells can be detected by MR imaging [9], whereas single cells can be detected at 11.7 T [8].

Gadolinium chelates

Gadolinium is the most commonly used paramagnetic atom for MR imaging contrast and a series of clinically approved chelates of gadolinium exist (Fig. 1). Gadolinium complexes have a number of favorable properties for use as MR imaging relaxation contrast agents. These complexes tend to be highly soluble, and have a high and relatively uniform relaxivity, on the order of 3.5 to 4 mmol/ L^{-1} sec^{-1} [10]. The induced changes in relaxivity appear as an increase in signal intensity on T1-weighted images. Although gadolinium ions are toxic, a number of chelates have been synthesized

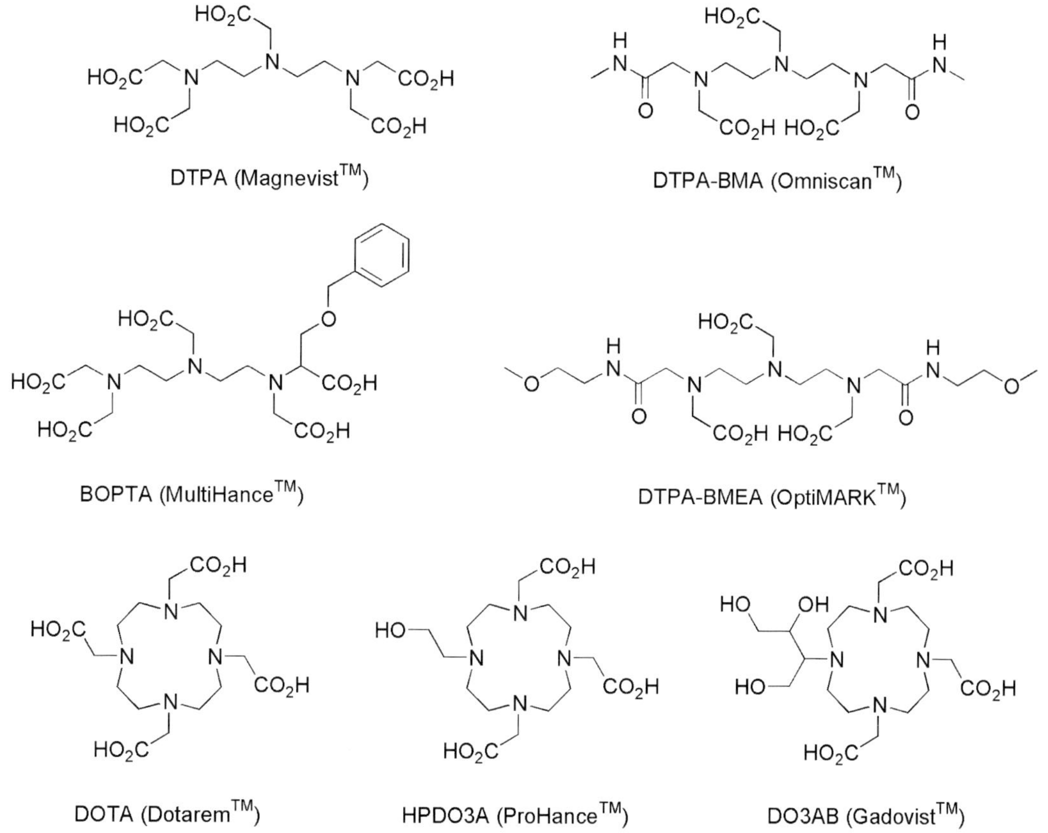

Fig. 1. Ligands of clinically approved gadolinium-based MR imaging contrast agents. (*From* Jacques V, Desreux J-F. New classes of MRI contrast agents. In: Krause W, editor. Contrast agents I: magnetic resonance imaging. Topics in current chemistry, vol. 221. Heidelberg: Springer-Verlag; 2002. p. 126; with permission.)

that are chemically inert and thermodynamically stable. Many currently used gadolinium complexes are octadentate ligand chelates. These are generally small hydrophilic molecules that can pass freely from the vasculature into the interstitial space, but are impermeable to the plasma membrane and are excluded from cells and remain extracellular. These compounds tend to have pharmacokinetic half-lives on the order of 1 to 2 hours, and because of their chemical stability are excreted unchanged, predominantly through the kidneys [10]. These agents are widely used as intravenous contrast agents to provide contrast in neoplastic and inflammatory lesions in brain and soft tissues, but also to assess damage after myocardial ischemia and as a probe into renal function [10]. The most commonly used gadolinium chelate is gadolinium–diethylenetriamine pentaacetic acid (Gd-DTPA). This molecule is an octadentate chelate, coordinating gadolinium to three tertiary amide groups and to five terminal carboxyls. One coordination site remains open to interact with adjacent water molecules, leading to enhanced relaxation of the proton water spins. The chemical structures of this and other clinically approved octadentate gadolinium chelates are given in Fig. 1.

Methods of increasing gadolinium-induced contrast

Because signal to noise is a crucial limitation for MR in molecular imaging, a number of elegant experimental protocols have been devised to enhance and amplify the contrast available from contrast agents. These schemes generally fall into one of three categories: (1) the synthesis or trapping of multiple paramagnetic centers as a single contrast agent that can be delivered as a bolus; (2) the oligomerization, self-assembly, or binding of a number of paramagnetic centers in response to a particular stimulus, such as the presence of a specific protein or nucleic acid sequence; or (3) the activation of a pro-contrast agent by a conformational change or the enzymatic removal of a side chain, with subsequent increase in relaxivity arising because of the restriction of molecular motion, or from the exposure of the paramagnetic center to water.

An increase in gadolinium concentration in a single contrast agent has been accomplished by linking multiple gadolinium chelates to polylysine or polyornithine [11] or to polysaccharides [12]. Such strategies using polylysine-linked Gd-DTPA have also been used as blood pool contrast agents. An alternate approach is to encapsulate multiple soluble gadolinium chelates in liposomes, protein aggregates, or nanoparticles. In one example of this approach, up to 10 molecules of GdHPDO3A were trapped in the central cavity of apoferritin (Fig. 2) using a low pH dissociation and a neutral pH reassembly protocol [7] leading to a 20-fold increase in relaxivity [13]. Sipkins et al [14] used antibody-conjugated paramagnetic polymerized liposomes targeted to intercellular adhesion molecule-1 to show a significant increase in T1-weighted images in a mouse model of autoimmune encephalitis. Paramagnetic polymerized liposomes containing gadolinium chelate and coated with antibodies to the endothelial integrin $\alpha_v\beta_3$ have also been used to measure angiogenesis in a rabbit tumor model [15]. An alternate approach is to use perfluorocarbon nanoparticles containing 50 to 90,000 gadolinium chelates and encapsulated by lipid-surfactant monolayers to target $\alpha_v\beta_3$ in tumors [16], atherosclerosis [17], or plaque formation [18].

A concerted effort has gone into the development of gadolinium complexes bound to larger proteins or polymers that can be used as blood pool agents. The large size of these compounds prevents their crossing from the vasculature into the interstitial space, such that these agents are suitable for MR angiography including assessment of regional blood flow in areas of ischemia and microvascular perfusion [19]. This increased size, however, also leads to reduced molecular motion resulting in an increase in relaxivity by an order of magnitude or greater relative to Gd-DTPA [20,21]. Because many of the blood pool agents also include multiple paramagnetic centers, these contrast agents exhibit a high sensitivity suitable for dynamic contrast angiography. Examples of blood pool agents include those with paramagnetic centers bound to proteins or polypeptides, such as Gd-DTPA–albumin and Gd-DTPA–polylysine, those attached to dendrimers, or those incorporated into micelles or liposomes. A similar approach with gadolinium dendrimers has also been used to image the lymphatic system in mice [22,23]. The interested reader is referred to a number of excellent review articles on the subject [19,21,24].

The second approach for improving contrast involves polymerization of paramagnetic centers into oligomers or binding of contrast agents to substrates or target sites, such that the resulting restriction of motion leads to a higher relaxivity and greater MR imaging contrast. In one example of this, Bogdanov et al [25] demonstrated polymerization of gadolinium bound to phenols during peroxidase-induced reduction of hydrogen peroxide. This approach was used successfully to image endothelial cell surface E-selectin probed with an antiselectin-peroxidase com-

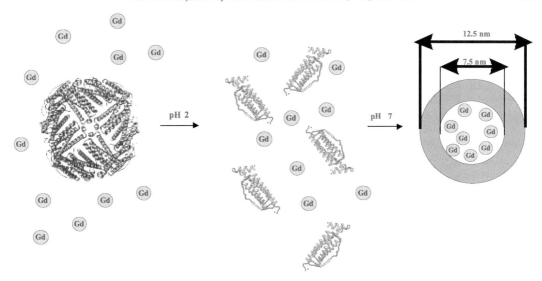

Fig. 2. Schematic representation of the trapping of gadolinium complexes in the center of apoferritin. The scheme relies on the dissociation of apoferritin into subunits at pH 2 and reformation at pH 7. (*From* Aime S, Frullano L, Geninatti Crich S. Compartmentalization of a gadolinium complex in the apoferritin cavity: a route to obtain high relaxivity contrast agents for magnetic resonance imaging. Angew Chem Int Ed Engl 2002;41:1018; with permission.)

plex. Aime et al [7,26] have reported a similar enzyme-catalyzed approach whereby the actions of peroxidase on the side groups of a gadolinium chelate cause a condensation into oligomers. Increased relaxivity through binding of gadolinium compounds to proteins has been accomplished using gadolinium-labeled substrate analogues targeting the active site of galactose regulatory protein [27]. An alternate approach relies on enzymatic transformation of a gadolinium-containing complex to a form that has a high affinity to serum albumin, and subsequent binding leads to increased relaxivity [28].

Activation of pro-contrast agents has been shown in a seminal study in which the ninth coordination site of a gadolinium chelate is exposed as a result of enzymatic removal of a galactose cap by the commonly used marker enzyme, β-galactosidase, leading to an irreversible increase in relaxivity (Fig. 3) [29,30]. This system was used to follow the expression of β-galactosidase after microinjection of β-gal mRNA or a *LacZ* construct into *Xenopus* embryos [30]. A similar approach was used to design an MR imaging contrast agent sensitive to calcium. The calcium chelator BAPTA (1,2-bis[*o*-aminophenoxy]ethane-N,N,N',N'-tetraacetic acid) was linked to gadolinium to produce an indicator in which the terminal carboxyl residues of BAPTA were coordinated to the ninth gadolinium site through weak electrostatic interactions. The presence of calcium induced a conformational change exposing the

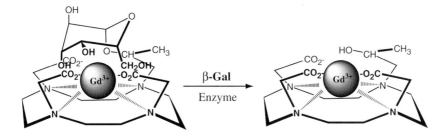

Fig. 3. Structure of the Egad-Gd complex, a derivative of Gd-HPDO3A. The complex contains a β-galactose moiety that prevents the access of water to the paramagnetic center. The diagram shows the transition from a weak to a strong relaxivity state. Cleavage of the sugar residue by β-galactosidase allows the inner sphere coordination site of the Gd(III) ion to become accessible to water, increasing the relaxivity. (*From* Louie AY, Huber MM, Ahrens ET, Rothbacher U, Moats R, Jacobs RE, et al. In vivo visualization of gene expression using magnetic resonance imaging. Nat Biotechnol 2000;18:322; with permission.)

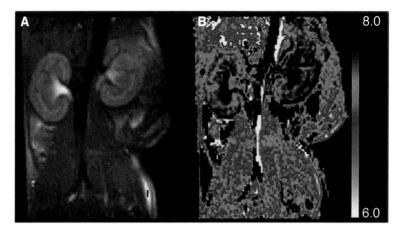

Fig. 4. The pH image of an acetazolamide-treated mouse. (*A*) T1-weighted postcontrast reference anatomic image showing the kidneys and nearby tissues. The cortex, medulla, calyx, and proximal segments of both ureters are visible. (*B*) Corresponding calculated pH image. A pH of 8.2 was measured in a urine sample collected immediately following the imaging experiment. (*From* Raghunand N, Howison C, Sherry AD, Zhang S, Gillies RJ. Renal and systemic pH imaging by contrast-enhanced MRI. Magn Res Med 2003;49:256; with permission.)

gadolinium to water molecules leading to a twofold increase in relaxivity [31].

Recently, gadolinium-containing contrast agents have also been synthesized to measure pH. Various approaches have been used including direct detection of changes in T1-relaxation rate resulting from protonation of chelator side arms [32]. This method has been used to detect increased pH in rat kidneys after administration of carbonic anhydrase inhibitors (Fig. 4) [33]. An alternate strategy uses compounds in which the protonation of a sulfonamide ion at low pH prevents the chelation of an adjacent amide ligand to the gadolinium center in a DO3A derivative, increasing relaxivity through increased water access [34]. Another approach relies on changes in the saturation transfer rate of the slow chemically exchanging protons on amine groups in the ligands of paramagnetic chelates. Irradiation of the mobile water protons leads to a direct pH-dependent decrease in the intensity of the water signal that is not dependent on the concentration of the contrast agent [7,13,35].

In summary, a number of ingenious strategies have been created for the development of gadolinium-based contrast agents and modulation of their relaxivities in response to specific molecular stimuli leading to increased sensitivity for detection. One great advantage to the paramagnetic agents is that increases in T1 contrast lead to a positive hyper-intensity on MR images resulting in a high contrast-to-noise ratio compared with surrounding host tissue or organ system. Overall, paramagnetic contrast agents hold great promise for future applications in MR imaging–based molecular imaging.

Iron oxide nanoparticles

An alternate method of generating sensitivity-enhanced MR imaging contrast has been developed using SPIO nanoparticles or monocrystalline iron oxide nanoparticles (MIONs) [5]. Because of their small crystal size (4–6 nm), these particles exhibit magnetic moments that are unaffected by the lattice orientation. When placed in a magnetic field, these particles align in a way so as to create extremely large

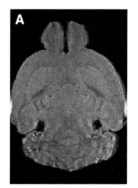
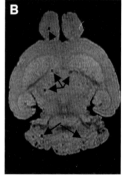

Fig. 5. Representative high-resolution gradient echo images of mouse brain: control animal (*A*) shows the normal anatomic details of the brain. The animal injected neonatally with superparamagnetic iron oxide–labeled C17.2 neural stem cells and imaged 7 weeks later (*B*) shows extensive regions of hypointensity (*arrows*) depicting the presence of SPIO-labeled stem cells (S. Magnitsky, D.J. Watson, R.M. Walton, J.W.M. Bulte, J.H. Wolfe, H. Poptani, unpublished data, 2004.)

microscopic field gradients that dephase the neighboring water protons, reducing the T2 (T2*) relaxation time [6]. This leads to a substantial reduction in signal on T2*-weighted gradient echo images. The degree of signal decrease caused by SPIO or monocrystalline iron oxide nanoparticles can be used as a semiquantitative measure of particle accumulation or

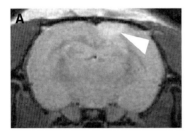
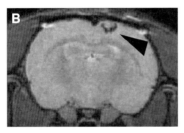
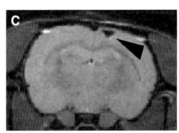
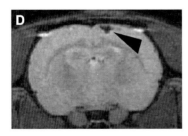
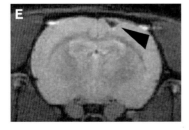

concentration within a specified region of interest [5,6]. To avoid uncontrolled aggregation of magnetic crystals in the tissue, these particles are generally coated with low-molecular-weight polymers leading to clusters of electron-dense crystal cores covered with the polymer. The effective particle size depends on the choice of size of iron particle and the attached surface coating. In general, the mean diameter of these particles is in the order of 10 to 20 nm. Hinds et al [8], however, have recently reported the use of micron-sized iron oxide particles for detection of single cells. These agents have been primarily used as blood pool agents [21], for detection of lymph nodes [36] and lymph node metastases [37], for the detection of liver metastases [38], and for brain tumor delineation [39]. The sensitivity of detection of these contrast agents depends on the size of the nanoparticle used and the effective iron concentration per cell.

Magnetic susceptibility contrast induced by iron oxide particles has successfully been used for high-resolution single-cell imaging [8,40], T lymphocyte [41], and stem cell tracking [6]. The applicability of iron oxide particles as MR imaging contrast agents has been demonstrated in phantom studies [9,42], cells [8,40,41,43,44], and in ex vivo tissue samples (Fig. 5) [42,45]. In vivo the potentially most important application of iron oxide–based nanoparticles has been their use in cell tracking of implanted hemapoietic, neuroprogenitor stem cells or monocytes [6,40,42–44,46–51]. Because stem cells migrate and differentiate into cells similar to the host cells, it is necessary to label the donor stem cells with a contrast agent that distinguishes them from host cells. The contrast produced by the label must be sufficient to detect small clusters of cells by high-resolution MR imaging [45]. In these applications, iron oxide particles linked to targeting moieties are introduced to cells ex vivo. Labeled cells are then

Fig. 6. T2-weighted images of a rat brain with a cortical photochemical lesion and mesenchymal stem cells injected into the femoral vein. The upper images (lesion) show photochemical lesions (*arrowhead*) 12 hours after thrombosis evoked by dye-light interaction, before any cell implantation (*A*). A hypointense signal (*arrowhead*) was observed 6 days after intravenous injection (*B*), which was further enhanced 13 (*C*) and 29 (*D*) days postinjection, and this hypointensity persisted for 47 days (*E*). (*From* Jendelova P, Herynek V, DeCroos J, Glogarova K, Andersson B, Hajek M, et al. Imaging the fate of implanted bone marrow stromal cells labeled with superparamagnetic nanoparticles. Magn Reson Med 2003;50:773; with permission.)

injected to animals and their bio-distribution is tracked with T2-weighted imaging (Fig. 6).

Various techniques of labeling iron oxide nanoparticles have been reported including dextran coating to facilitate chemical attachment of proteins for surface targeting and cytoplasmic internalization [46]. Cell surface labeling can present challenges for long-term in vivo experiments, because of the rapid reticuloendothelial recognition and clearance of labeled cells from the bloodstream. A number of elegant labeling strategies have been used for intracellular delivery of iron-oxide particles including linking to dendrimers for nonspecific phagocytic internalization [6], receptor-mediated endocytosis of nanoparticles through an engineered transferrin receptor [52,53], or synthesis of monocrystalline iron oxide nanoparticles coupled to the HIV-tat nuclear

targeting domain peptide [46] for nuclear delivery (Fig. 7). Tat peptide targeting has also been used successfully in the delivery of paramagnetic contrast agents [54]. One potential limitation of nuclear targeting is the possibility of particle degradation and subsequent toxic effects of free iron-oxide particles. For cytoplasmic or lysosomal localization, the internalization of these particles is often mediated by fluid-phase or receptor-mediated endocytosis [6,8,9,40,42–45,50] or by lipofection [44,49,51]. The iron-oxide particles clustered within the endosomal compartments can later be released and reused in normal iron metabolism pathways reducing the potential for any deleterious toxic effects on the cell. Although most of these agents are not commercially available [6,8,9,40,41,45,48,55–58], clinically approved iron oxide particles bound to commercially

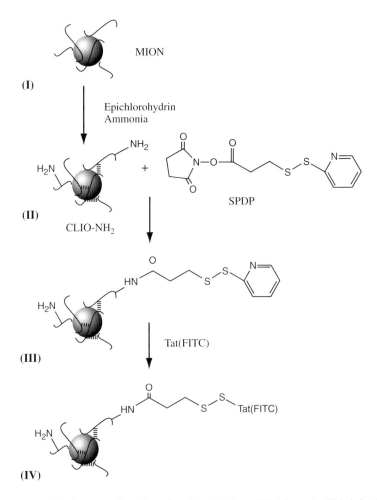

Fig. 7. Synthetic scheme of SPIO-Tat peptide. (*From* Josephson L, Tung CH, Moore A, Weissleder R. High-efficiency intracellular magnetic labeling with novel superparamagnetic-Tat peptide conjugates. Bioconjug Chem 1999;10:188; with permission.)

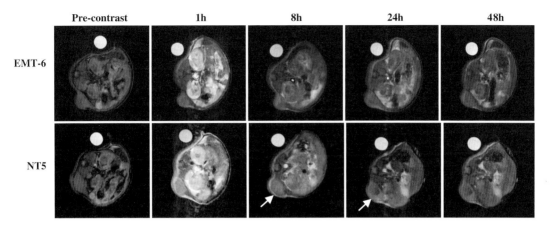

Fig. 8. T1-weighted MR images of EMT-6 and NT-5 tumors obtained before administration of the avidin-GdDTPA conjugate and at 1, 8, 24, and 48 hours after contrast injection. The arrows show enhanced signal from the tumor at the 8- and 24-hour time points for the HER-2/*neu* expressing NT-5 tumor. (*From* Artemov D, Mori N, Ravi R, Bhujwalla ZM. Magnetic resonance molecular imaging of the Her-2/neu receptor. Cancer Res 2003;63:2725; with permission.)

available transfection agents, such as Superfect, lipofectamine, or poly-L-lysine, have recently been introduced for endocytotic labeling of stem cells [44,50,51]. The advantage of using these agents is their simplicity in synthesis and their availability [44,49–51].

Recent publications have shown advancement in targeting of MR imaging contrast agents to cell-surface receptors, gene expression, or enzymatic activity. Tumors expressing an engineered transferrin receptor have been imaged by MR imaging using an SPIO-labeled transferrin receptor ligand [48,53,59]. A potential drawback may be the ectopic over-expression of the transferrin receptor and accumulation of SPIO particles, which may alter the target cell physiology [47,48]. An alternative method of imaging gene expression uses tyrosinase activity of melanoma cells. This results in the production of

melanin, which binds to iron, producing a bright signal on T1-weighted images [60,61]. The Her-2/*neu* receptor, a tyrosine kinase from the *EGFR* family that is amplified in many cancers, was targeted in vitro using streptavidin-conjugated SPIO nanoparticles [62,63] in breast cancer cells and in vivo using an avidin gadolinium complex in NT-5 cells over-expressing Her-2/*neu*. These experiments require pretreatment of the cells with a biotinylated antibody to facilitate binding to the avidin-conjugated contrast agent (Fig. 8). Another example of targeting contrast agents is for the detection the alterations in cellular architecture specific to programmed cell death. Apoptosis has been detected in drug-treated EL-4 tumors in vivo after an intravenous administration of a SPIO bound to synaptotagmin I, a protein that binds to the phosphatidylserine exposed on the cell surface during the early stages of apoptosis (Fig. 9) [64]. Similar

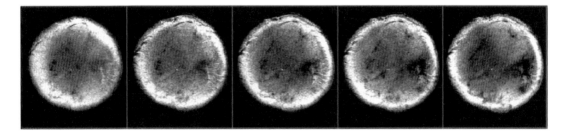

Fig. 9. T2-weighted MR images (TE = 30 ms) of a tumor in a mouse treated with cyclophosphamide and etoposide before and after injection of C2–superparamagnetic iron oxide (20 mg Fe/kg tissue). The first image was acquired before injection of the contrast agent and the following images were acquired at 11 min, 47 min, 77 min, and 107 min after injection. The hypointense regions within the images appear as the degree of apoptosis increases. (*From* Zhao M, Beauregard DA, Loizou L, Davletov B, Brindle KM. Non-invasive detection of apoptosis using magnetic resonance imaging and a targeted contrast agent. Nat Med 2001;7:1243; with permission.)

results have been reported using annexin V–labeled iron oxide nanoparticles [65].

A recent report demonstrates that the actions of proteases on biotinylated target recognition sequences in vitro can decrease the clustering of avidin-labeled iron oxide nanoparticles resulting in changes in T2* proportional to the degree of protease activity present (Fig. 10) [66]. Similarly, Perez et al [67] have reported enzyme-sensitive nanoassemblies of iron oxide nanoparticles that undergo cleavage in the presence of the proapoptotic protease caspase-3, causing an increase in T2. In the same study, dextran-coated SPIO linked to oligonucleotides were shown to self-polymerize into particles of four to five subunits in the presence of specific DNA sequences, resulting in a substantial decrease in T2 [67]. A similar approach has been used to detect the presence of virus particles in serum through T2 changes

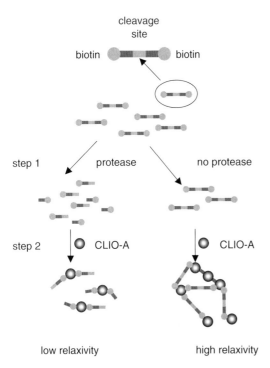

Fig. 10. Schematic view of the MR spectroscopy assay using bi-biotinylated peptides. The bi-biotinylated peptide substrates contain a central sequence with a cleavage site and flanking terminal biotins. The presence of avidin-labeled cross-linked iron oxide nanoparticles induces formation of a cluster resulting in increased T2 relaxivity. The actions of a protease converts the bi-biotinylated peptides into mono-biotinylated fragments, with accompanying low T2 relaxivity. (*From* Zhao M, Josephson L, Tang L, Weissleder R. Magnetic sensors for protease arrays. Angew Chem Int Ed Engl 2003;42:1376; with permission.)

resulting from the polymerization of viral antibodies attached to dextran-coated SPIO [68].

These reports suggest that there is a substantial interest in the development of specifically targeted contrast agents for MR imaging. A number of strategies are emerging for the introduction and implementation of these techniques in cell and animal model systems, with the long-term goal of specific noninvasive disease reporters for clinical applications. Improving the sensitivity and specificity of contrast agents is an important consideration for future progress, as is the discovery of more sophisticated targeting mechanisms leading to specific intracellular accumulation. One potential method of improving specificity is to take advantage of the inherent ability of MR imaging to discriminate between chemical moieties through alterations in the chemical shift of these moieties in the contrast agents. The implementation of chemical shift–sensitive targeted contrast agents will facilitate the use of MR spectroscopic techniques in molecular imaging studies.

MR spectroscopy

In vivo MR spectroscopy is a well-developed technique that has been used extensively in the detection and staging of tumors and in monitoring response to therapy. MR spectroscopy detects changes in the local distribution of MR visible metabolites other than water. Many potentially relevant nuclei can be used in the study of biologic systems, notably hydrogen (^{1}H), carbon-13 (^{13}C), fluorine-19 (^{19}F), and phosphorous-31 (^{31}P). Proton is the most widely used nucleus because it has 100% natural abundance and a large magnetic moment leading to high intrinsic sensitivity. This high sensitivity translates into greater spatial resolution and reduced scan time for in vivo MR experiments. The proton also has a magnetic spin quantum number of one half, which results in simpler spectra because of the absence of any quadripolar interactions inherent to nuclei with higher spin. A number of naturally occurring metabolites are routinely observed using proton MR spectroscopy including resonances arising from the methyl groups of amino acids, lactate, *N*-acetylaspartate (in brain), creatine, and choline, and the methyl and methylene groups of fatty acyl chains in mobile neutral lipids. Although proton is generally the nucleus of choice for MR imaging, proton MR spectroscopy has yet to play a strong role in molecular imaging, because of the lack of spectroscopically detectable contrast agents. The future development of proton-based probes will provide spectroscopic imaging at higher spatial and temporal resolution.

[19]F is also a spin one-half nucleus with 100% natural abundance and a relatively high sensitivity of 0.83 compared with the proton. Because there are no naturally occurring fluorine-containing metabolites, background ^{19}F signals in cells and tissues are low, making this nucleus a potential candidate for the development of contrast agents for molecular imaging studies. In one example of the use of ^{19}F MR to monitor enzyme activity associated with gene therapy, murine tumors expressing L6 antigens were treated with L6 monoclonal antibodies conjugated to the microbial enzyme cytosine deaminase. The subsequent conversion of the prodrug 5-fluorocytosine to the cytotoxic agent 5-fluorouracil could then be followed with in vivo ^{19}F spectroscopy [69]. This approach has been subsequently verified using colon cells stably transfected with yeast cytosine deaminase [70], and in colon tumor xenografts directly injected with attenuated *Salmonella* bacteria overexpressing cytosine deaminase (Fig. 11) [71].

[31]P is also spin one-half and 100% naturally abundant but is markedly less sensitive than the proton, because of its smaller magnetic moment. This nucleus has been used extensively, for studies of energy and phospholipid metabolism and intracellular pH because of the visibility in cells and tissues of resonances arising from NTP, NDP, phospholipid metabolites, and intracellular phosphate [72,73]. Some elegant approaches using ^{31}P spectroscopy have been applied to visualize enzyme activity or gene expression. For example, the expression of creatine kinase in mouse liver leads to the appearance of ^{31}P MR resonances arising from phosphocreatine in mice fed with creatine, which can be used as a measure of transgenic gene expression or of the success of gene therapy (Fig. 12) [74–76]. A similar approach has been used to observe phosphoarginine in the skeletal muscle of mice in which the invertebrate enzyme arginine kinase has been expressed [77].

Finally, ^{13}C, which is spin one-half but combines a smaller magnetic moment with 1.08% natural abundance, has relatively poor sensitivity but is practical for enrichment studies. Carbon-13 has found great use in tracer studies for delineation of metabolic pathways [78–80], but has also been used to detect labeled drug uptake and distribution [81] and changes in energy metabolism in tumors [82]. Recent developments have shown that it is possible to prepare highly spin polarized molecules chemically through partial reduction of ^{13}C-labeled alkynes with para-hydrogen [83], or through dynamic nuclear polarization in the solid state in the presence of an organic free radical [84,85]. The demonstration that these compounds can be used to substantially improve signal to noise in MR angiography studies in vivo [83,85] indicates a possible future role for ^{13}C MR in molecular imaging.

MR spectroscopy is generally less sensitive than MR imaging, because spectroscopy assesses intracellular metabolites in the millimolar concentration range, as opposed to imaging, which relies on the detection of tissue water at much higher concentrations. As such the spatial resolution obtained in

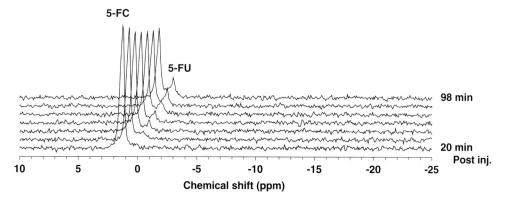

Fig. 11. Serial ^{19}F MR spectroscopy spectra (13-minute time resolution) showing the conversion of 5-fluorocytosine to 5-fluorouracil in the presence of cytosine deaminase in a murine tumor. The tumor was treated with an attenuated *Salmonella typhimurium* strain recombinant to provide cytosine deaminase, followed 1 day later by intratumoral injection with 5-fluorocytosine. (*From* Dresselaers T, Theys J, Nuyts S, Wouters B, de Bruijn E, Anne J, et al. Non-invasive 19F MR spectroscopy of 5-fluorocytosine to 5-fluorouracil conversion by recombinant Salmonella in tumours. Br J Cancer 2003;89: 1798; with permission.)

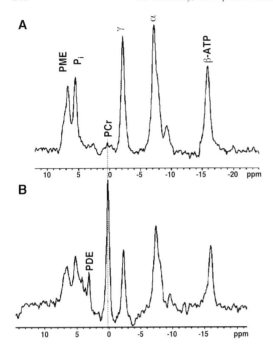

Fig. 12. In vivo ^{31}P MR spectra of murine livers transduced with the creatine kinase-B gene. (*A*) Spectrum from the liver of control mice. (*B*) Spectrum from the liver of creatine kinase transduced animals showing a strong phosphocreatine resonance. NTP, resonances of nucleoside triphosphate (γ, α, and β); P_i, inorganic phosphate; PDE, phosphodiesters, PME, phosphomonoesters. (*From* Auricchio A, Zhou R, Wilson JM, Glickson JD. In vivo detection of gene expression in liver by 31P nuclear magnetic resonance spectroscopy employing creatine kinase as a marker gene. Proc Natl Acad Sci U S A 2001;98:5206; with permission.)

single or multivoxel spectroscopic measurements is much less, with voxel sizes ranging from 8 to 64 mm^3 in small animal studies and on the order of 1 cm^3 in humans for protons. For less sensitive nuclei like ^{31}P, voxels on the order of 27 cm^3 are normally achievable in humans. In mice, the size of the animal and sensitivity limitations may preclude the use of localized pulse sequences and as a result unlocalized ^{31}P spectra are often acquired.

Despite these limitations, spectroscopy offers a greater potential for delineation of multiple molecular pathways, relying on discrimination provided by resonances from different chemical compounds at different chemical shifts. The challenge lies in designing smart contrast agents with unique chemical shift signatures that can be delivered at sufficient concentrations to be observed using in vivo spectroscopy.

Summary

MR-based molecular imaging is a science in infancy. Current clinical contrast agents are often geared toward the assessment of gross physiologic function, rather than targeting specific biochemical pathways. The development of specific targeted smart contrast agents for Food and Drug Administration approval or clinical trials has only begun. The fact that MR imaging can obtain images of extremely high resolution, coupled with its ability to simultaneously assess structure and function through the use of targeted contrast agents indicates that MR will play a pivotal role in clinical molecular imaging of the future. Many of the challenges that face MR imaging and spectroscopy are inherent to all modalities in the rapidly growing field of molecular imaging. The development of smart contrast agents to report on receptor function, and to monitor gene expression or the results of gene therapy in humans is paramount. These compounds need to undergo rigorous testing to be approved for clinical use: the assessment of acute toxicity, pharmacokinetics, long-term accumulation, and subsequent chronic effects. For receptor-targeted contrast agents, the degree of receptor occupancy and the intrinsic agonist or antagonist properties of the probe that may affect normal cellular function need to be determined to avoid undesired side effects.

The particular problems that face MR imaging, those of sensitivity and target specificity, need to be overcome. Signal amplification achieved through high relaxivity contrast agents containing multiple paramagnetic centers, or of larger superparamagnetic particles, is the first step in this direction. The modulation of relaxivity through oligomerization, or other modifications that cause restriction of rotational motions, shows great promise for improving the discriminative powers of MR imaging, and may permit multiple targets to be assessed simultaneously. Moreover, the introduction of smart indicators that lead to changes in spectroscopic properties will allow further discrimination to be achieved through the implementation of chemical shift or spectroscopic imaging. The growing number of MR imaging applications in this rapidly expanding field point to a bright future for MR imaging in molecular imaging.

References

[1] Jacobs RE, Cherry SR. Complementary emerging techniques: high-resolution PET and MRI. Curr Opin Neurobiol 2001;11:621–9.

[2] Jacques V, Desreux J-F. New classes of MRI contrast agents. In: Krause W, editor. Contrast agents I: magnetic resonance imaging. Topics in current chemistry, vol. 221. Heidelberg: Springer-Verlag; 2002. p. 123–64.

[3] Wehrli FW, McGowan JC. The basis of MR contrast. In: Atlas SW, editor. Magnetic resonance imaging of the brain and spine. Philadelphia: Lippincott-Raven; 1996. p. 29–47.

[4] Tóth E, Helm L, Merbach AE. Relaxivity of MRI contrast agents. In: Krause W, editor. Contrast agents I: magnetic resonance imaging. Topics in current chemistry, vol. 221. Heidelberg: Springer-Verlag; 2002. p. 61–101.

[5] Bulte JW, Duncan ID, Frank JA. In vivo magnetic resonance tracking of magnetically labeled cells after transplantation. J Cereb Blood Flow Metab 2002; 22:899–907.

[6] Bulte JW, Douglas T, Witwer B, Zhang SC, Strable E, Lewis BK, et al. Magnetodendrimers allow endosomal magnetic labeling and in vivo tracking of stem cells. Nat Biotechnol 2001;19:1141–7.

[7] Aime S, Cabella C, Colombatto S, Geninatti Crich S, Gianolio E, Maggioni F. Insights into the use of paramagnetic Gd(III) complexes in MR-molecular imaging investigations. J Magn Reson Imaging 2002;16: 394–406.

[8] Hinds KA, Hill JM, Shapiro EM, Laukkanen MO, Silva AC, Combs CA, et al. Highly efficient endosomal labeling of progenitor and stem cells with large magnetic particles allows magnetic resonance imaging of single cells. Blood 2003;102:867–72.

[9] Fleige G, Seeberger F, Laux D, Kresse M, Taupitz M, Pilgrimm H, et al. In vitro characterization of two different ultrasmall iron oxide particles for magnetic resonance cell tracking. Invest Radiol 2002;37: 482–8.

[10] Gries H. Extracellular MRI contrast agents based on gadolinium. In: Krause W, editor. Contrast agents I: magnetic resonance imaging, vol. 221. Heidelberg: Springer-Verlag; 2002. p. 1–24.

[11] Aime S, Botta M, Geninatti Crich S, Giovenzana G, Palmisano G, Sisti M. Novel paramagnetic macromolecular complexes derived from the linkage of a macrocyclic Gd(III) complex to polyamino acids through a squaric acid moiety. Bioconjug Chem 1999;10:192–9.

[12] Armitage FE, Richardson DE, Li KC. Polymeric contrast agents for magnetic resonance imaging: synthesis and characterization of gadolinium diethylenetriamine pentaacetic acid conjugated to polysaccharides. Bioconjug Chem 1990;1:365–74.

[13] Aime S, Frullano L, Geninatti Crich S. Compartmentalization of a gadolinium complex in the apoferritin cavity: a route to obtain high relaxivity contrast agents for magnetic resonance imaging. Angew Chem Int Ed Engl 2002;41:1017–9.

[14] Sipkins DA, Gijbels K, Tropper FD, Bednarski M, Li KC, Steinman L. ICAM-1 expression in autoimmune encephalitis visualized using magnetic resonance imaging. J Neuroimmunol 2000;104:1–9.

[15] Sipkins DA, Cheresh DA, Kazemi MR, Nevin LM, Bednarski MD, Li KC. Detection of tumor angiogenesis in vivo by alphaVbeta3-targeted magnetic resonance imaging. Nat Med 1998;4:623–6.

[16] Winter PM, Caruthers SD, Kassner A, Harris TD, Chinen LK, Allen JS, et al. Molecular imaging of angiogenesis in nascent Vx-2 rabbit tumors using a novel alpha(v)beta3-targeted nanoparticle and 1.5 tesla magnetic resonance imaging. Cancer Res 2003;63: 5838–43.

[17] Winter PM, Morawski AM, Caruthers SD, Fuhrhop RW, Zhang H, Williams TA, et al. Molecular imaging of angiogenesis in early-stage atherosclerosis with alpha(v)beta3-integrin-targeted nanoparticles. Circulation 2003;108:2270–4.

[18] Flacke S, Fischer S, Scott MJ, Fuhrhop RJ, Allen JS, McLean M, et al. Novel MRI contrast agent for molecular imaging of fibrin: implications for detecting vulnerable plaques. Circulation 2001;104:1280–5.

[19] Clarkson RB. Blood-pool MRI contrast agents: properties and characterization. In: Krause W, editor. Contrast agents I: magnetic resonance imaging. Topics in current chemistry, vol. 221. Heidelberg: Springer-Verlag; 2002. p. 201–35.

[20] Saeed M, Wendland MF, Engelbrecht M, Sakuma H, Higgins CB. Value of blood pool contrast agents in magnetic resonance angiography of the pelvis and lower extremities. Eur Radiol 1998;8:1047–53.

[21] Saeed M, Wendland MF, Higgins CB. Blood pool MR contrast agents for cardiovascular imaging. J Magn Reson Imaging 2000;12:890–8.

[22] Kobayashi H, Kawamoto S, Star RA, Waldmann TA, Tagaya Y, Brechbiel MW. Micro-magnetic resonance lymphangiography in mice using a novel dendrimer-based magnetic resonance imaging contrast agent. Cancer Res 2003;63:271–6.

[23] Kobayashi H, Kawamoto S, Choyke PL, Sato N, Knopp MV, Star RA, et al. Comparison of dendrimer-based macromolecular contrast agents for dynamic micro-magnetic resonance lymphangiography. Magn Reson Med 2003;50:758–66.

[24] Kroft LJ, de Roos A. Blood pool contrast agents for cardiovascular MR imaging. J Magn Reson Imaging 1999;10:395–403.

[25] Bogdanov Jr A, Matuszewski L, Bremer C, Petrovsky A, Weissleder R. Oligomerization of paramagnetic substrates result in signal amplification and can be used for MR imaging of molecular targets. Mol Imaging 2002;1:16–23.

[26] Aime S, Botta IM, Fedeli F, Gianolio E, Terreno E, Anelli P. High-relaxivity contrast agents for magnetic resonance imaging based on multisite interactions between a beta-cyclodextrin oligomer and suitably functionalized GdIII chelates. Chemistry 2001;7: 5261–9.

[27] De Leon-Rodriguez LM, Ortiz A, Weiner AL, Zhang S, Kovacs Z, Kodadek T, et al. Magnetic resonance

imaging detects a specific peptide-protein binding event. J Am Chem Soc 2002;124:3514–5.

[28] Nivorozhkin AL, Kolodziej AF, Caravan P, Greenfield MT, Lauffer RB, McMurry TJ. Enzyme-activated Gd^{3+} magnetic resonance imaging contrast agents with a prominent receptor-induced magnetization enhancement. Angew Chem Int Ed Engl 2001;40:2903–6.

[29] Moats RA, Fraser SE, Meade TJ. A smart magnetic resonance imaging agent that reports on specific enzyme activity. Angew Chem Int Ed Engl 1997;36:726–8.

[30] Louie AY, Huber MM, Ahrens ET, Rothbacher U, Moats R, Jacobs RE, et al. In vivo visualization of gene expression using magnetic resonance imaging. Nat Biotechnol 2000;18:321–5.

[31] Li WH, Parigi G, Fragai M, Luchinat C, Meade TJ. Mechanistic studies of a calcium-dependent MRI contrast agent. Inorg Chem 2002;41:4018–24.

[32] Zhang S, Wu K, Sherry AD. A novel pH-sensitive MRI contrast agent. Angew Chem Int Ed Engl 2001; 38:3192–4.

[33] Raghunand N, Howison C, Sherry AD, Zhang S, Gillies RJ. Renal and systemic pH imaging by contrast-enhanced MRI. Magn Reson Med 2003; 49:249–57.

[34] Lowe MP, Parker D, Reany O, Aime S, Botta M, Castellano G, et al. pH-Dependent modulation of relaxivity and luminescence in macrocyclic gadolinium and europium complexes based on reversible intramolecular sulfonamide ligation. J Am Chem Soc 2001; 123:7601–9.

[35] Meade TJ, Taylor AK, Bull SR. New magnetic resonance contrast agents as biochemical reporters. Curr Opin Neurobiol 2003;13:597–602.

[36] Rety F, Clement O, Siauve N, Cuenod CA, Carnot F, Sich M, et al. MR lymphography using iron oxide nanoparticles in rats: pharmacokinetics in the lymphatic system after intravenous injection. J Magn Reson Imaging 2000;12:734–9.

[37] Harisinghani MG, Barentsz J, Hahn PF, Deserno WM, Tabatabaei S, van de Kaa CH, et al. Noninvasive detection of clinically occult lymph-node metastases in prostate cancer. N Engl J Med 2003;348:2491–9.

[38] Hahn PF, Saini S. Liver-specific MR imaging contrast agents. Radiol Clin North Am 1998;36:287–97.

[39] Enochs WS, Harsh G, Hochberg F, Weissleder R. Improved delineation of human brain tumors on MR images using a long-circulating, superparamagnetic iron oxide agent. J Magn Reson Imaging 1999; 9:228–32.

[40] Dodd SJ, Williams M, Suhan JP, Williams DS, Koretsky AP, Ho C. Detection of single mammalian cells by high-resolution magnetic resonance imaging. Biophys J 1999;76(1 Pt 1):103–9.

[41] Dodd CH, Hsu HC, Chu WJ, Yang P, Zhang HG, Mountz Jr JD, et al. Normal T-cell response and in vivo magnetic resonance imaging of T cells loaded with HIV transactivator-peptide-derived superparamagnetic nanoparticles. J Immunol Methods 2001;256(1–2): 89–105.

[42] Bulte JW, Zhang S, van Gelderen P, Herynek V, Jordan EK, Duncan ID, et al. Neurotransplantation of magnetically labeled oligodendrocyte progenitors: magnetic resonance tracking of cell migration and myelination. Proc Natl Acad Sci U S A 1999;96:15256–61.

[43] Sipe JC, Filippi M, Martino G, Furlan R, Rocca MA, Rovaris M, et al. Method for intracellular magnetic labeling of human mononuclear cells using approved iron contrast agents. Magn Reson Imaging 1999;17: 1521–3.

[44] Arbab AS, Bashaw LA, Miller BR, Jordan EK, Bulte JW, Frank JA. Intracytoplasmic tagging of cells with ferumoxides and transfection agent for cellular magnetic resonance imaging after cell transplantation: methods and techniques. Transplantation 2003;76: 1123–30.

[45] Modo M, Cash D, Mellodew K, Williams SC, Fraser SE, Meade TJ, et al. Tracking transplanted stem cell migration using bifunctional, contrast agent-enhanced, magnetic resonance imaging. Neuroimage 2002;17: 803–11.

[46] Lewin M, Carlesso N, Tung CH, Tang XW, Cory D, Scadden DT, et al. Tat peptide-derivatized magnetic nanoparticles allow in vivo tracking and recovery of progenitor cells. Nat Biotechnol 2000;18:410–4.

[47] Weissleder R, Cheng HC, Bogdanova A, Bogdanov Jr A. Magnetically labeled cells can be detected by MR imaging. J Magn Reson Imaging 1997;7:258–63.

[48] Allport JR, Weissleder R. In vivo imaging of gene and cell therapies. Exp Hematol 2001;29:1237–46.

[49] Hoehn M, Kustermann E, Blunk J, Wiedermann D, Trapp T, Wecker S, et al. Monitoring of implanted stem cell migration in vivo: a highly resolved in vivo magnetic resonance imaging investigation of experimental stroke in rat. Proc Natl Acad Sci U S A 2002;99: 16267–72.

[50] Jendelova P, Herynek V, DeCroos J, Glogarova K, Andersson B, Hajek M, et al. Imaging the fate of implanted bone marrow stromal cells labeled with superparamagnetic nanoparticles. Magn Reson Med 2003;50:767–76.

[51] Zelivyanskaya ML, Nelson JA, Poluektova L, Uberti M, Mellon M, Gendelman HE, et al. Tracking superparamagnetic iron oxide labeled monocytes in brain by high-field magnetic resonance imaging. J Neurosci Res 2003;73:284–95.

[52] Moore A, Basilion JP, Chiocca EA, Weissleder R. Measuring transferrin receptor gene expression by NMR imaging. Biochim Biophys Acta 1998;1402: 239–49.

[53] Moore A, Josephson L, Bhorade RM, Basilion JP, Weissleder R. Human transferrin receptor gene as a marker gene for MR imaging. Radiology 2001;221: 244–50.

[54] Bhorade R, Weissleder R, Nakakoshi T, Moore A, Tung CH. Macrocyclic chelators with paramagnetic cations are internalized into mammalian cells via a HIV-tat derived membrane translocation peptide. Bioconjug Chem 2000;11:301–5.

[55] Bendszus M, Stoll G. Caught in the act: in vivo mapping of macrophage infiltration in nerve injury by magnetic resonance imaging. J Neurosci 2003;23: 10892–6.

[56] Bryant Jr LH, Brechbiel MW, Wu C, Bulte JW, Herynek V, Frank JA. Synthesis and relaxometry of high-generation (G = 5, 7, 9, and 10) PAMAM dendrimer-DOTA-gadolinium chelates. J Magn Reson Imaging 1999;9:348–52.

[57] Josephson L, Tung CH, Moore A, Weissleder R. High-efficiency intracellular magnetic labeling with novel superparamagnetic-Tat peptide conjugates. Bioconjug Chem 1999;10:186–91.

[58] Lacorazza HD, Flax JD, Snyder EY, Jendoubi M. Expression of human beta-hexosaminidase alpha-sub-unit gene (the gene defect of Tay-Sachs disease) in mouse brains upon engraftment of transduced progenitor cells. Nat Med 1996;2:424–9.

[59] Weissleder R, Moore A, Mahmood U, Bhorade R, Benveniste H, Chiocca EA, et al. In vivo magnetic resonance imaging of transgene expression. Nat Med 2000;6:351–5.

[60] Weissleder R, Simonova M, Bogdanova A, Bredow S, Enochs WS, Bogdanov Jr A. MR imaging and scintigraphy of gene expression through melanin induction. Radiology 1997;204:425–9.

[61] Enochs WS, Petherick P, Bogdanova A, Mohr U, Weissleder R. Paramagnetic metal scavenging by melanin: MR imaging. Radiology 1997;204:417–23.

[62] Artemov D, Mori N, Ravi R, Bhujwalla ZM. Magnetic resonance molecular imaging of the Her-2/neu receptor. Cancer Res 2003;63:2723–7.

[63] Artemov D, Mori N, Okollie B, Bhujwalla ZM. MR molecular imaging of the Her-2/neu receptor in breast cancer cells using targeted iron nanoparticles. Magn Reson Med 2003;49:403–8.

[64] Zhao M, Beauregard DA, Loizou L, Davletov B, Brindle KM. Non-invasive detection of apoptosis using magnetic resonance imaging and a targeted contrast agent. Nat Med 2001;7:1241–4.

[65] Schellenberger EA, Hogemann D, Josephson L, Weissleder R. Annexin V–CLIO: a nanoparticle for detecting apoptosis by MRI. Acad Radiol 2002; 9(Suppl 2):S310–1.

[66] Zhao M, Josephson L, Tang L, Weissleder R. Magnetic sensors for protease arrays. Angew Chem Int Ed Engl 2003;42:1375–8.

[67] Perez JM, Josephson L, O'Loughlin T, Hogemann D, Weissleder R. Magnetic relaxation switches capable of sensing molecular interactions. Nat Biotechnol 2002;20:816–20.

[68] Perez JM, Simeone FJ, Saeki Y, Josephson L, Weissleder R. Viral-induced self-assembly of magnetic nanoparticles allows the detection of viral particles in biological media. J Am Chem Soc 2003;125: 10192–3.

[69] Aboagye EO, Artemov D, Senter PD, Bhujwalla ZM. Intratumoral conversion of 5-fluorocytosine to 5-fluo-rouracil by monoclonal antibody-cytosine deaminase conjugates: noninvasive detection of prodrug activation by magnetic resonance spectroscopy and spectroscopic imaging. Cancer Res 1998;58:4075–8.

[70] Stegman LD, Rehemtulla A, Beattie B, Kievit E, Lawrence TS, Blasberg RG, et al. Noninvasive quantitation of cytosine deaminase transgene expression in human tumor xenografts with in vivo magnetic resonance spectroscopy. Proc Natl Acad Sci U S A 1999;96:9821–6.

[71] Dresselaers T, Theys J, Nuyts S, Wouters B, de Bruijn E, Anne J, et al. Non-invasive 19F MR spectroscopy of 5-fluorocytosine to 5-fluorouracil conversion by recombinant *Salmonella* in tumours. Br J Cancer 2003; 89:1796–801.

[72] Podo F. Tumour phospholipid metabolism. NMR Biomed 1999;12:413–39.

[73] Negendank W. Studies of human tumours by MRS: a review. NMR Biomed 1992;5:303–24.

[74] Koretsky AP, Brosnan MJ, Chen LH, Chen JD, vanDyke T. NMR detection of creatine kinase expressed in liver of transgenic mice: determination of free ADP levels. Proc Natl Acad Sci U S A 1990;87: 3112–6.

[75] Auricchio A, Zhou R, Wilson JM, Glickson JD. In vivo detection of gene expression in liver by 31P nuclear magnetic resonance spectroscopy employing creatine kinase as a marker gene. Proc Natl Acad Sci U S A 2001;98:5205–10.

[76] Askenasy N, Koretsky A. Transgenic livers expressing mitochondrial and cytosolic CK: mitochondrial CK modulates free ADP levels. Am J Physiol Cell Physiol 2002;282:C338–46.

[77] Walter G, Barton ER, Sweeney HL. Noninvasive measurement of gene expression in human muscle. Proc Natl Acad Sci U S A 2000;97:5151–5.

[78] Shulman RG, Rothman DL. 13C NMR of intermediary metabolism: implications for systemic physiology. Annu Rev Physiol 2001;63:15–48.

[79] Moreno A, Ross BD, Bluml S. Direct determination of the *N*-acetyl-L-aspartate synthesis rate in the human brain by (13)C MRS and [1-(13)C]glucose infusion. J Neurochem 2001;77:347–50.

[80] Jones JG, Carvalho RA, Franco B, Sherry AD, Malloy CR. Measurement of hepatic glucose output, Krebs cycle, and gluconeogenic fluxes by NMR analysis of a single plasma glucose sample. Anal Biochem 1998; 263:39–45.

[81] Artemov D, Solaiyappan M, Bhujwalla ZM. Magnetic resonance pharmacoangiography to detect and predict chemotherapy delivery to solid tumors. Cancer Res 2001;61:3039–44.

[82] Poptani H, Bansal N, Jenkins WT, Blessington D, Mancuso A, Nelson DS, et al. Cyclophospha-mide treatment modifies tumor oxygenation and glycolytic rates of RIF-1 tumors: 13C MRS, Eppendorf electrode and redox scanning. Cancer Res 2003;63: 8813–20.

[83] Golman K, Axelsson O, Johannesson H, Mansson S, Olofsson C, Petersson JS. Parahydrogen-induced polarization in imaging: subsecond 13C angiography. Magn Reson Med 2001;46:1–5.

[84] Ardenkjaer-Larsen JH, Fridlund B, Gram A, Hansson G, Hansson L, Lerche MH, et al. Increase in signal-to-noise ratio of > 10,000 times in liquid-state NMR. Proc Natl Acad Sci U S A 2003;100:10158–63.

[85] Golman K, Ardenkjaer-Larsen JH, Petersson JS, Mansson S, Leunbach I. Molecular imaging with endogenous substances. Proc Natl Acad Sci U S A 2003; 100:10435–9.

ELSEVIER
SAUNDERS

Radiol Clin N Am 43 (2005) 221–234

RADIOLOGIC
CLINICS
of North America

Non-PET functional imaging techniques: optical

Xavier Intes, PhD[a],*, Britton Chance, PhD, ScD[b]

[a]*Biomedical Optical Imaging, Advanced Research Technologies (ART), 2300 Alfred-Nobel Boulevard, Saint-Laurent, Quebec H4S 2A4, Canada*
[b]*Department of Biophysics, Physical Chemistry, and Radiologic Physics, University of Pennsylvania School of Medicine, 250 Anatomy–Chemistry Building, Philadelphia, PA 19104, USA*

Optical imaging techniques for medical applications have been receiving more and more attention in the last decade [1]. The promises of the techniques are manifold and many medical fields can potentially benefit from recent research developments in this area. Mainly, the goal of these optical approaches is to characterize optical properties of tissue using light from the ultraviolet to the infrared spectral region. The specific light-tissue interaction reveals fundamental properties of the biologic tissues, such as structure, physiology, and molecular function. In turn, these fundamental properties enable tracking non-invasively and with low-power sources specific biochemical events that are of interest to the medical community.

Light examination of tissue is already well established as a modality in medicine, especially optical surface imaging as commonly practiced in endoscopy or ophthalmology. These areas are still actively investigated as new approaches emerge, bringing more in-depth monitoring of epithelial tissue [2–5]. Moreover, some intrinsic compounds, such as NADH or flavins fluorescence, are re-emerging as new modalities [6], providing additional discrimination between healthy and diseased tissues [7–9].

Light propagation in biologic samples is highly dependent, however, on the wavelength selected. The most favorable spectral window in terms of depth penetration is situated in the near-infrared (NIR) range ($\lambda \in [600–1000]$ nm). NIR techniques are the optical techniques of choice to image large organs. In this spectral range, biologic tissues exhibit relatively weak absorption [10] allowing imaging through several centimeters of a sample. Outside this spectral window, the strong absorption of hemoglobin and water, respectively, for lower and higher wavelengths, restricts the optical examination to shallow interrogation. This article focuses on diffuse optical techniques based on NIR radiation.

Tissue optics

The interaction of light with tissue depends on local cellular and structural properties. Biologic tissues are composed of many different molecules that are bound into a vast variety of small and large molecules. Cells are composed of this large variety of molecules. The compositions of these molecules as their structural properties are the origin of light diffusion, light absorption, and fluorescence emission. In the NIR spectral window, scattering is the main process occurring during the propagation of light in the tissue [11]. Most photons emerging from the sample surface have followed a random path and probed deep volumes. Scattering is mainly caused by the refractive index variations both between and

This article is supported in part by NIH Grants CA87046, CA72895, CA110173, RR02305, NS36633, and HL44125.

* Corresponding author.

E-mail address: xintes@art.ca (X. Intes).

within a cell. Structural fibers, mitochondria, and nuclei in a background of cytoplasm and extracellular fluid are the origin for the main part of these index variations. NIR diffuse techniques are sensitive to local light-scattering signature. Because of the diffuse nature of the photon migration the structural information is blurred, and retrieving high-resolution structural information is hardly feasible. Nevertheless, the initial appeal of the technique resides in the main chromophores accountable for the absorption.

Light absorption in tissue originates from many different analytes. The main relevant chromophores are oxyhemoglobin and deoxyhemoglobin, melanin, water, lipids, porphyrins, NADH, flavins, and other structural components. In the NIR spectral range, however, the chromophores exhibiting significant extinction coefficients can be limited to four as shown in Fig. 1 (melanin is overlooked because of its confinement to the normal skin): (1) oxyhemoglobin, (2) deoxyhemoglobin, (3) water, and (4) lipids. NIR interrogation of tissue at multiple wavelengths correlated with appropriate photon propagation models provides the average or local quantitative concentrations of these compounds. Consequently, NIR optical techniques allow noninvasive monitoring of the metabolic activity of deep tissue through the hemoglobin concentration and oxygen saturation. This monitoring, combined with the inexpensive cost of instrumentation, opens many potential medical applications to NIR techniques.

Instrumentation

Three major experimental techniques exist in the field of NIR diffuse optical imaging. They are divided in three general categories that are defined by the time dependence of the source intensity impinging on the tissues. These three methods are referred to as continuous-wave (CW), frequency-domain photon migration, and time-domain photon migration.

The CW approach uses light source with constant amplitude or modulated to a few kilohertz [12–15]. The measured amplitude decay of the incident light is related to the macro-optical properties of the medium investigated. Because of the intrinsic limited information gathered with CW technique, however, scattering and absorption characteristics cannot easily be differentiated [16]. Only by selecting accordingly the spectral information collected and using appropriate preconditioning can one separate the scattering and absorption contribution [17,18]. Furthermore, intensity data are significantly sensitive to the surface interaction (the excitation fluence is exponentially attenuated from the tissue surface) and great care should be provided to have an efficient optode-tissue coupling. Nevertheless, CW techniques are popular because of their robustness, their relative inexpensive costs, their wide spectral range, and their fast acquisition speed (Fig. 2). They are well suited to follow dynamic events but rather inadequate when absolute estimates are required.

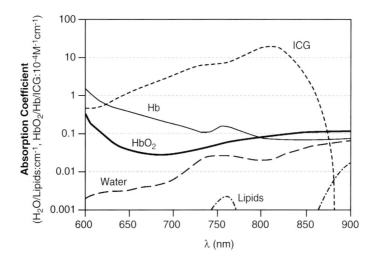

Fig. 1. Extinction coefficient spectra for hemoglobin and indocyanine green (ICG). These data are obtained from Scott Prahl's web page (available at: http://omlc.ogi.edu/spectra/). ICG's spectrum corresponds to 6.5μM dissolved in plasma. Hb, hemoglobin. (*Adapted from* Licha K. Contrast agents for optical imaging. Topics in Current Chemistry 2002;222:1–29; with permission.)

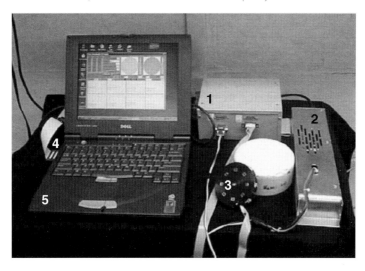

Fig. 2. LEDs imager: (1) control box, (2) power supply, (3) source-detector pad, (4) DAQ card, and (5) laptop. (*From* Lin Y, Lech G, Nioka S, Intes X, Chance B. Noninvasive, low-noise, fast imaging of blood volume and deoxygenation changes in muscles using LED continuous-wave imager. Rev Sci Instrum 2002;73:3065–74; with permission.)

The second instrumentation approach consists of modulating sinusoidally the laser source. Frequency-domain photon migration techniques record the amplitude modulation decay and phase shift with respect to the incident wave after propagation in the tissue [19–21]. Generally, the modulation frequency ranges from 10 MHz to 1 GHz, with many instruments in the range of 100 MHz. Single or sweeping frequency instruments are used. Conversely to CW technique, the frequency-domain photon migration technique provides a measurement set that enables independent retrieval of the absorption and scattering properties of the medium probed at a single wavelength. In addition, when probing tissue in the fluorescent mode, frequency-domain photon migration techniques recover spatial maps of the fluorophore concentration and lifetime. The systems need to be calibrated with well-characterized phantoms [22] or multidistance scheme, however, to provide absolute estimate of the absorption and scattering coefficients [23].

Time-domain photon migration uses subnanosecond laser pulses and relevant detection technology to monitor the biologic samples [24–27]. The photon times of flight are recorded to provide a histogram of the photon distribution as a function of time as they leave the tissue. The temporal point spread function recorded is then used to calculate the distribution of the photon paths in tissue. Accurate estimates of the absolute tissue absorption and scattering are subsequently achievable. It provides the wealthiest data set of all NIR instrumental techniques. It is comparable with multifrequency frequency-domain pho-

ton migration by Fourier transform and CW by integration of the photon counts. Time-domain photon migration allows selecting the desired data type to retrieve the appropriate information sought. Time-domain photon migration, however, is the most expensive and more technically challenging technique to deploy.

Combination of these different experimental techniques in the same instrument is feasible. Weaknesses of one approach then can be alleviated by providing complementary information gathered by another approach [15,28]. Such a system could allow acquisition of an instrument with a wide spectral range, dense detector array, and fast acquisition for absolute measurements.

Theory

The theoretical frame of laser light propagation is usually based on the Maxwell equations [29]. In the case of light propagation in tissues, however, the complexity of the numerous interaction light-cells forbids using such an approach. The importance of optical techniques for biomedical applications was underscored because of the lack of appropriate theoretical frame. This fact was the reason of the demise of such techniques as diaphanography [30,31].

A breakthrough was achieved when it was realized that light propagation in diffuse media was akin to other physics fields, such as neutron transport and heat transport [32–34]. Then, the light transport was cast based on the radiative transport equation [35]. With such models, it is possible to relate the NIR measurements to the macro-optical properties of the tissue that are the absorption, the scattering, and the mean cosine of the scattering phase function describing the anisotropic character of the light diffusion [36]. Moreover, in the case of predominant scattering, the diffusion equation that is an approximation (P1) of the radiative transport equation is preferred because of its simpler mathematical expression. The problem is then rescaled as an isotropic scattering problem depending on two parameters: the absorption and the reduced scattering (generally referred as scattering for simplicity later on in this article and in the field).

Its mathematical expression both in the frequency-domain and the time-domain can be solved analytically for planar geometries (the CW case corresponds to a null frequency) [37,38]. In the case of heterogeneous media, the diffusion equation also can be solved analytically by using perturbative approaches, such as the Born or the Rytov approximation [39]. For complex boundary conditions, however, numerical methods or more refined analytical algorithms [40] are necessary to model accurately the light propagation, leading to an increase in the computational burden.

Two different approaches are used to estimate the optical properties of the medium: near-infrared spectroscopy (NIRS) and diffuse optical tomography (DOT). NIRS was the first approach used to establish the potential of diffuse optical techniques [41]. NIRS estimates the optical properties of the tissue probed by one source-detector pair. NIRS is based on the assumption of a homogeneous tissue investigated. It retrieves the average optical properties of the volume probed by the light. Because of the scattering events, the photons are probing a large volume that has a banana shape. NIRS suffers from the partial volume effect (low sensitivity to focal changes in the optical parameters) when no a priori spatial information is available [42]. Moreover, because of the limited redundant information collected, NIRS is extremely sensitive to the quality of the coupling optode-tissue [43]. This approach, however, is well suited for fast estimation of the functional state of biologic tissue in the case of differential measurements and mathematically straightforward.

DOT is a more ambitious approach that relies on a data set collected with an increased number of source-detector pairs [44]. DOT uses measurements recorded from tissue using multiple optical source-detector pairs and retrieves (reconstructs) the targeted chromophore distribution by synthesizing the measurements through solution of an inverse problem [45]. Similar to other tomographic approaches, such as radiographic CT, PET, or single-photon emission CT, DOT first constructs the forward problem, which predicts the photon propagation for a known medium, and then inverts the problem. DOT falls in the class of nonlinear ill-posed inverse scattering problem, which presents many challenges. DOT has shown a steady growth in the last decade, however, because it provides a quantified estimate of the local concentration of absorption, scattering, blood volume, oxygenation, or contrast agent uptake noninvasively. It is still a very active research area with constant progress toward more accurate, more robust, and faster algorithms.

Applications

NIR optical imaging techniques are likely to be applied to numerous medical applications. To date, three major applications are investigated: (1) brain imaging for functional or stroke monitoring, (2) breast cancer detection-characterization, and (3) muscle imaging for physiology monitoring. For all these applications, optical imaging is likely to play an important role in clinical settings.

Brain imaging

Jobsis [41] was the first to report monitoring continuously cerebral oxygenation and hemodynamics noninvasively in human by means of NIRS. Since then, optical measurements of the brain have received increased and steady interest. These investigations of the potential application of NIRS to neuroimaging have contributed greatly to improvements in the apparatus and better understanding of the optical signal wealth [46].

To date, optical measurements of the brain aim to reveal information about the hemodynamics of the brain tissue and possibly about scattering changes related to neuron activity [47]. Then, the information provided by NIR techniques complement existing neuroimaging techniques, such as electroencephalography, PET, single-positron emission CT, magnetoencephalography, and functional MR imaging. Optical techniques are especially attractive because of their excellent temporal resolution, their low-cost, and their portability even though they posses a relatively poor resolution. Moreover, subjects can be examined under normal conditions without their motion being severely restricted and noninvasively

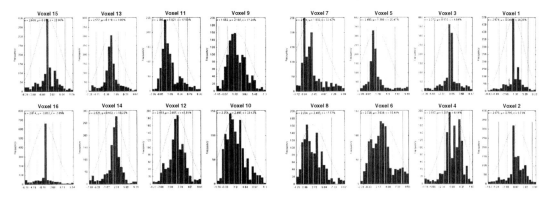

Fig. 3. Histograms of prefrontal activation data captured while subjects solved anagrams show number of tests as a function of postsolution oxygenation; histograms are listed by position on the probe. (*From* Chance B, Nioka S, Chen Y. Shining new light on brain function. OE Magazine 2003;3:16–9; with permission.)

during a long period of time. Functional mapping studies of recognized difficult populations, such as infants and small children, are feasible conversely to some existing modalities.

The main physiologic markers targeted by optical brain studies are the oxyhemoglobin and deoxyhemoglobin. More precisely, optical measurements track the spatial and temporal changes in these two markers relative to a functional activation. The amplitude, the dynamics, and the relative contributions of these chromophores are the parameters of interest. Numerous preliminary studies have been reported in various functional brain imaging applications, such as in the visual system [48], the auditory system [49], language stimuli [49,50], and problem solving (Fig. 3) [51].

Optical techniques have potentially an important role to play in the monitoring of ischemic and hemorrhagic stroke [52,53]. Optical techniques are well suited for early detection of hemorrhage and discrimination between ischemic and hemorrhagic stroke leading to a better management of the patient

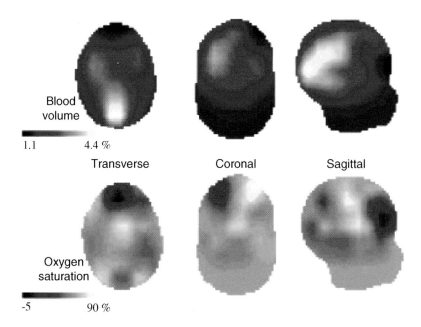

Fig. 4. Transverse, coronal, and sagittal slices across the three-dimensional images of estimated blood volume and fractional oxygen saturation. (*From* Hebden J, Gibson A, Yusof R, Everdell N, Hillman E, Delpy E, et al. Three dimensional optical tomography of the premature infant brain. Phys Med Biol 2002;47:4155–66; with permission.)

treatment. Furthermore, optical techniques offer the advantage to monitor in real-time over a long period the evolution of the stroke and the efficiency of the treatment.

Hemodynamics, however, is an indirect monitoring of neuron activity. Optical techniques are also sensitive to more direct neuronal activity markers. Neuronal activity induces changes in the index of refraction of the neuronal membranes (fast response) and cell swelling (slow response), which in turn produces contrast in the scattering properties [47]. Such changes in scattering signals have been reported during brain activation [54,55]. Such an approach is elusive, however, because of the weakness of the signal. Identically, metabolic markers, such as cytochrome oxidase, are proposed using diffuse optical techniques [56,57]. Indeed, cytochrome aa_3 has a variable NIR signal depending on its redox state and relates to the intracellular O_2 availability. Hence, information about intracellular metabolism is reachable through heavy HbO_2 interference (the NIR spectra are similar). Unfortunately, these measurements are the most difficult to achieve and interpret.

The lead difficulties in the case of brain imaging reside in the complex structures of the brain. Sharp changes in the optical properties exist and such complex boundaries between different kinds of tissues induce difficulties in modeling light propagation [58,59] Also, difficulties arise from the complexity of the responses to activation residing almost exclusively in the gray matter and in localized regions of the brain, which change depending on the source, nature, and duration intensity of activation and the size of the neural network. It has been difficult to perform DOT in highly localized regions of the brain; most studies are limited to NIRS or optical tomography with depth penetration appropriate to the cortical layer. Many efforts are put forward to produce more flexible apparatuses and more accurate three-dimensional imaging algorithm [60]. The most extensive studies have been performed in the CW mode and paradoxically the first detailed time-domain multisource, multidetector systematic study of the infant brain (Fig. 4) [61] containing a ventricular hemorrhage, has resulted in poorly understood underestimation of the ventricular hemorrhage as

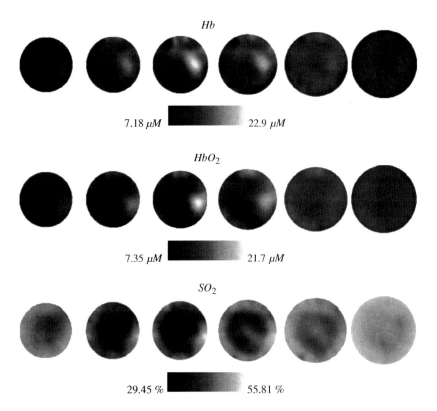

Fig. 5. Reconstructed images of Hb, HbO$_2$, and SO$_2$ of a patient with a 59-mm invasive carcinoma. (*From* Dehghani H, Pogue BW, Poplack SP, Paulsen KD. Multiwavelength three-dimensional near-infrared tomography of the breast: initial simulation, phantom, and clinical results. Appl Opt 2003;42:135–45; with permission.)

compared with many measurements made with simple CW apparatus on well-verified (CT scan) brain bleeds.

Breast imaging

Breast imaging is an excellent candidate for the application of optical techniques. The potential of light as a tool for breast cancer detection and characterization was already highlighted in the late 1920s by the work of Cutler [62]. Even with enhancement in the technology, transillumination was abandoned in the beginning of the 1990s because of poor sensitivity and a high number of false-positives [44]. Improvement in technologies, such as the modeling of light propagation, resurrected the interest in optical mammography in the mid-nineties.

NIR diffuse optical techniques are intrinsically sensitive to the principal components of the breast: blood, water, and adipose tissue. Numerous studies demonstrated the exquisite sensitivity of optical techniques to breast tissue structure and function

with healthy volunteers. Mainly, these optical parameters have been shown to be dependent on demographic factors. The major parameters impacting the tissue properties are the hormone levels during the menstrual cycle [63], menopausal status, age, body mass index, and hormone-replacement therapy [64–67]. Those studies are fundamental to obtain baseline values to assess the adequate sensitivity needed to discriminate healthy and diseased tissues.

Detection of lesions is based on the functional and structural contrast between normal and diseased tissue in the same patient. These contrasts are generated by the progression of the disease, which induces an increase in tumor cell density, nuclear volume fraction, tumor vasculature, and metabolic activity for both glucose and oxygen [68]. In turn, these modifications generate specific optical cancer signatures not attainable by other structural breast imaging modalities. The functional information revealed by the local quantification of oxyhemoglobin and deoxyhemoglobin gives insight into the angiogenesis [69] and the hypermetabolic state of

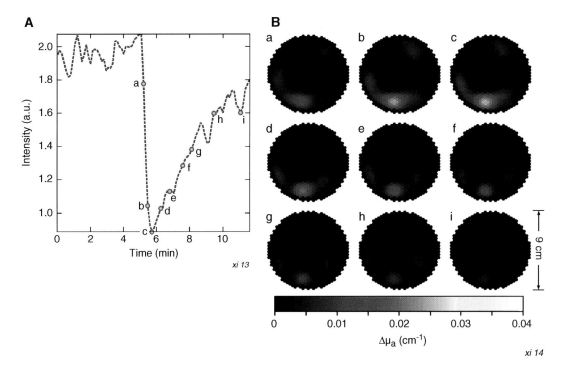

Fig. 6. (*A*) The dashed curve represent the optical intensity drop associated with the ICG-uptake for a source-detector pair (not capturing mass area) and from all time data; the dots represent the selected time used for display in Fig. 6B. (*B*) Differential absorption reconstructions for the time selected in Fig. 6A using data gathered form a fan beam configuration using 16 sources and 16 detectors at one wavelength. The frames are normalized to the same color bar. The reconstructions are arranged in row corresponding to the time course. The maximum uptake area was diagnosed as a fibroadenoma afterward by biopsy. (*From* Intes X, Ripoll J, Chen Y, Nioka S, Yodh A, Chance B. In vivo continuous-wave optical breast imaging enhanced with indocyanine. Green Med Phys 2003;30:1039–47; with permission.)

the tumor [70]. Targeting these specific correlates of tumor malignancy has been the goal of the actual studies. Preliminary clinical data have already reported breast cancer detection and characterization based on these two parameters (Fig. 5) [71–75]. Although statistical data indicate that there is only twofold to fourfold contrast between normal and tumorous structures for the blood volume, a tumor as small as 5 mm has been detected with current apparatus. Clinical trials are still ongoing to establish the specificity and sensitivity of optical technique, but preliminary results suggest that they could be around 90% accurate. Furthermore, contrast agents have been used successfully with this technique. To date, these studies are limited to a Food and Drug Administration approved blood pooling contrast agent, indocyanine green. This compound is an intravascular contrast agent that may extravasate through vessels of high permeability [76]. In vivo clinical validation with MR imaging coregistration [77] and enhanced diagnostic content with pharma-cokinetics have been demonstrated (Fig. 6) [78]. Finally, new avenues of optical detection and characterization of tumors are ongoing, such as the mapping of tissue refractive index variations, which is similar to phase-contrast radiographic CT [79].

Breast imaging forms quite a different kind of challenge to the NIR technology because a very simple technique collates angiogenesis and hypermetabolism in a two-dimensional monogram. This imaging has had reasonable success and has been operating for over 5 years (Figs. 2 and 7). The breast is significantly more heterogeneous than the brain, and also has the problem of not permitting active responses, as do the brain and muscle. Absolute technologies are needed for breast cancer detection that could detect objects even smaller than in the brain (ie, cancers as small as 3 mm with contrast ratios as small as 2:1).

Muscle imaging

Noninvasive monitoring of muscle with NIR light can be tracked back to the 1930s with Millikan's [80] work on cat muscle. Since then, the study of human peripheral muscle has been an active research area [81] that is mainly dedicated to monitoring muscle oxygenation [82,83] under different physiologic or pathologic stresses [84–88].

The ability of NIR system to acquire fast data that are sensitive to hemoglobin, myoglobin, blood flow, and oxygen consumption has drawn the interest of physiologists to make NIR techniques a method of choice in muscle dynamics monitoring (Figs. 2 and 8).

NIR techniques provide a unique noninvasive measurement of oxygenation in local muscle tissue, which was not available previously. Tissue oxygenation is defined by the rate of oxygen consumption by the muscles versus oxygen delivery to the muscle. NIR techniques measure the balance between the uptake and the delivery of oxygen to tissues [89].

Although NIR signals reflect the changes in hemoglobin and myoglobin oxygen saturation in the muscle, decoupling the relative contribution of hemoglobin and myoglobin is rather difficult to achieve. Some studies suggest that the NIR signal is primarily derived from hemoglobin [90], whereas others suggest that it is primarily derived from myoglobin [91], as proved in simultaneous studies with ^{1}H nuclear MR imaging measurements. Furthermore, other studies have shown that NIR mea-

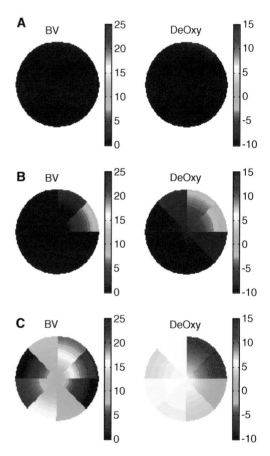

Fig. 7. Differential blood volume and deoxygenation of a tumor versus normal-model (*A*), tumor-model (*B*), and tumor-normal (*C*). The tumorous area exhibits higher total blood and higher deoxygenated blood content. The data were gathered using a simple hand-held probe as depicted in Fig. 2. BV, blood volume; DeOxy, deoxygenation.

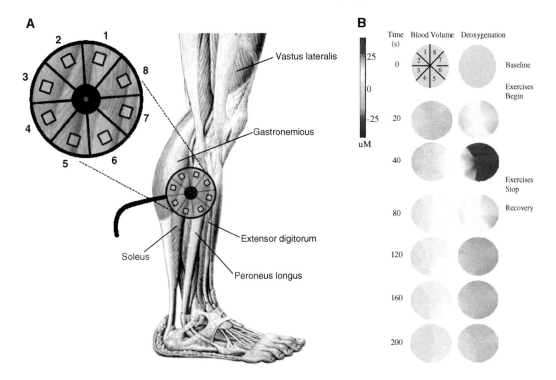

Fig. 8. (*A*) Source-detector probe position on extensor muscles (peroneus longus and extensor digitorum) and flexor muscles (gastrocnemius and soleus). (*B*) Functional imaging of anterior tibialis–lateral peroneus and gastrocnemius muscle. (*From* Lin Y, Lech G, Nioka S, Intes X, Chance B. Noninvasive, low-noise, fast imaging of blood volume and deoxygenation changes in muscles using LED continuous-wave imager. Rev Sci Instrum 2002;73:3065–74; with permission.)

surement of human muscle correlates with venous hemoglobin saturation [90,92]. At work rates above the lactic acid threshold, however, relative contribution of myoglobin affecting the NIR signal may be greater [93].

These facts suggest that both HbO_2 [94] and MbO_2 values have great potential to evaluate the effectiveness of training in developing the muscle capillary network for best extraction of oxygen and delivery to mitochondria for particular exercise

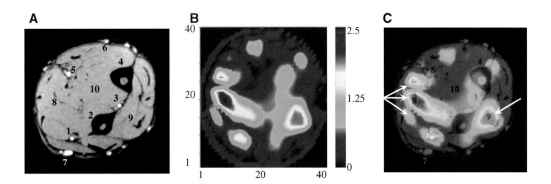

Fig. 9. (*A*) MR image of right forearm. Radial artery (*1*), radius (*2*), interosseous artery (*3*), ulna (*4*), ulnar artery (*5*), basilic vein (*6*), cephalic vein (*7*), flexor digitorum superficialis (*8*), extensor digitorum (*9*), and flexor digitorum profundus (*10*). (*B*) Amplitude of Fourier transform at finger flex frequency for absorption coefficient at 780 nm. (*C*) Overlay image. (*From* Graber HL, Zhong S, Pei Y, Schmitz CH, Arif I, Hira J. Dynamic imaging of muscle activity by optical tomography. Presented at the OSA Biomedical Topical Meetings. Miami Beach, Florida, April 2–5, 2000; with permission.)

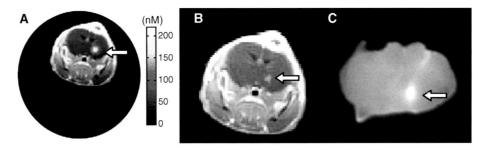

Fig. 10. NIR fluorescence imaging. Examples of fluorescence imaging using a cathepsin Bactivatable imaging probe. (*A, B*) Enzyme activity in a 9-L glioma model in a live mouse. The image in Fig. 10A is superimposed onto an MR image shown separately in Fig. 10B with gadolinium enhancement of the glioma. (*C*) In vitro fluorescence reflectance imaging (FRI) of the axial brain section corresponding to the MR and fluorescence molecular tomography (FMT) images. The tumor position is indicated by the arrow. (*From* Ntziachristos V, Tung CH, Bremer C, Weissleder R. Fluorescence molecular tomography resolves protease activity in vivo. Nat Med 2002;8:757–60; with permission.)

regimens [95]. Diffuse optical techniques are providing new insight in athletic training [96], geriatrics [97], and muscle disease diagnostics [98].

The NIRS has been applied as a main technology for muscle monitoring not only because of its fast response but also the simplicity of the apparatus. The optode-tissue coupling can be efficiently ensured with such apparatus and maintained during exercise. NIRS, however, provides bulk physiologic information that can be affected by structural parameters, such as a fat layer or melanin [99], or by physiologic events, such as spatiotemporal heterogeneous functional pattern of the muscle [100–102]. New technologic advances enable the gathering of data from multiple source-detectors in time settings relevant to the muscle physiology. Then, cross-sectional imaging of the muscle dynamics may be feasible and able to reveal the vascular responses to exercise (Fig. 9) [103].

Future outlook

As clinicians assist in the emergence of a new medical modality, new developments enhance the brightness of its future. The developments of new contrast agents that target specific molecular events [104–106] are particularly promising in revolutionizing the field of radiology. By specifically binding [107,108] or being activated in tumors (Fig. 10) [109], detection can be achieved in the early stages of molecular changes before structural modification [110]. These technologies are still confined to small animal models [111] and the translation to human imaging is foreseen as challenging but imminent.

Another exciting avenue of development of the technology is its ability to perform concurrent examination with other modalities. The potential of the technique to work simultaneously with currently well-established medical modalities, such as radiographic [112], ultrasound [113,114], and MR imaging [115–117], has been proved and is expected to allow new medical tools providing anatomic, functional, and eventually molecular maps of the probed organ. The gain is even more substantial when fusion-imaging algorithms are used. Hence, inherent weaknesses of diffuse optical technique can be alleviated, with the benefit of more accurate quantification [118,119].

Continuous development in instrumentation, algorithm, and molecular probes brings diffuse optical techniques closer to the clinical world. Initiatives, such as the Network for Translational Research in Optical Imaging funded by the National Cancer Institute, bring together multiple academic institutions and industrial partners, and facilitate the implementation of optical techniques into clinical practice.

Acknowledgments

The authors are grateful to J. Im for exciting insights on muscle physiology.

References

[1] Kincade K. Optical diagnostics continue migration from bench top to bedside. Laser Focus World 2004; 130–4.
[2] Farkas D, Becker D. Application of spectral imaging: detection and analysis of human melanoma and its precursor. Pigment Cell Res 2001;14:2–8.

[3] Zonios G, Bykowski J, Kollias N. Skin melanin, hemoglobin, and light scattering properties can be quantitatively assessed in vivo using diffuse reflectance spectroscopy. J Invest Dermatol 2001;117: 1452–7.

[4] Bono A, Tomatis S, Bartoli C, Tragni G, Tadaelli G, Maurichi A, et al. The ABCD system of melanoma detection: a spectrophotometric analysis of the *A*symmetry, *B*order, *C*olor, and *D*imension. Cancer 1999; 85:72–7.

[5] Popp A, Valentine M, Kaplan P, Weitz D. Microscopic origin of light scattering in tissue. Appl Opt 2003;42:2871–80.

[6] Wagnieres G, Star W, Wilson B. In vivo fluorescence spectroscopy and imaging for oncological applications. Photochem Photobiol 1998;68:603–32.

[7] Ramanujam N, Follen M, Mahadevan-Janson A, Thomsen S, Staerkel G, Malpica A, et al. Cervical cancer detection using a multivariate statistical algorithm based on laser-induced fluorescence spectra at multiple wavelength. Photochem Photobiol 1996; 64:720–35.

[8] Stepp H, Sroka R, Baumgartner R. Fluorescence endoscopy of gastrointestinal diseases: basic principles, techniques, and clinical experience. Endoscopy 1998;30:379–86.

[9] Moesta KT, Ebert B, Handke T, Nolte D, Nowak C, Haensch WE, et al. Protoporphyrin IX occurs naturally in colorectal cancers and their metastases. Cancer Res 2001;61:991–9.

[10] Cheong W, Prahl S, Welch A. A review of the optical properties of biological tissues. IEEE J Quantum Electron 1990;26:2166–85.

[11] Yodh AG, Chance B. Spectroscopy and imaging with diffusing light. Phys Today 1995;48:34–40.

[12] Lin Y, Lech G, Nioka S, Intes X, Chance B. Noninvasive, low-noise, fast imaging of blood volume and deoxygenation changes in muscles using LED continuous-wave imager. Rev Sci Instrum 2002;73: 3065–74.

[13] Schmitz C, Locker M, Lasker J, Hieslscher A, Barbour R. Instrumentation for fast optical tomography. Rev Sci Instrum 2002;73:429–39.

[14] Siegel A, Marota J, Boas DA. Design and evaluation of a continuous-wave diffuse optical tomography system. Opt Express 1999;4:287–98.

[15] Culver JP, Choe R, Holboke MJ, Zubkov L, Durduran T, Slemp A, et al. Three-dimensional diffuse optical tomography in the parallel plane transmission geometry: evaluation of a hybrid frequency domain continuous wave clinical system for breast imaging. Med Phys 2003;30:235–47.

[16] Arridge S, Lionheart W. Nonuniqueness in diffusion-based optical tomography. Opt Lett 1998;23:882–4.

[17] Corlu A, Durduran T, Choe R, Schweiger M, Hillman EM, Arridge SR, et al. Uniqueness and wavelength optimization in continuous-wave multispectral diffuse optical tomography. Opt Lett 2003;28:2339–41.

[18] Pei Y, Graber H, Barbour R. Normalized-constraint algorithm for minimizing inter-parameter crosstalk in DC optical tomography. Opt Express 2001;9:97–109.

[19] McBride TO, Pogue BW, Jiang S, Österberg UL, Paulsen K. A parallel-detection frequency-domain near-infrared tomography system for hemoglobin imaging of the breast in vivo. Rev Sci Instrum 2001;72:1817–24.

[20] Chance B, Cope M, Gratton E, Ramanujam N, Tromberg B. Phase measurement of light absorption and scatter in human tissue. Rev Sci Instrum 1998; 69:3457–81.

[21] Pham TH, Coquoz O, Fishkin JB, Anderson E, Tromberg BJ. Broad bandwidth frequency domain instrument for quantitative tissue optical spectroscopy. Rev Sci Instrum 2000;71:2500–13.

[22] McBride T, Pogue B, Osterberg U, Paulsen K. Strategies for absolute calibration of near infrared tomographic tissue imaging. Adv Exp Med Biol 2003;530:85–99.

[23] Fantini S, Franceschini MA, Gratton E. Semi-infinite geometry boundary problem for light migration in highly scattering media: a frequency-domain study in the diffusion approximation. J Opt Soc Am B 1994;11:2128–38.

[24] Eda H, Oda I, Ito Y, Wada Y, Oikawa Y, Tsunazawa Y, et al. Multichannel time-resolved optical tomographic imaging system. Rev Sci Instrum 1999;70: 3595–602.

[25] Ntziachristos V, Ma X, Yodh AG, Chance B. Multichannel photon counting instrument for spatially resolved near infrared spectroscopy. Rev Sci Instrum 1999;70:193–201.

[26] Schmidt F, Fry M, Hillman E, Hebden J, Delpy D. 32-channel time-resolved instrument for medical optical tomography. Rev Sci Instrum 2000;71:256–65.

[27] Intes X, Yu J, Yodh AG, Chance B. Development and evaluation of a multi-wavelength multi-channel time resolved optical instrument for NIR/MRI mammography co-registration. In: Proceedings of the IEEE 28th Annual Northeast Bioengineering Conference (IEEE Cat. No.02CH37342). Piscataway (NJ): IEEE; 2002. p. 91–2.

[28] Bevilacqua F, Berger A, Cerussi A, Jakubowski D, Tromberg B. Broadband absorption spectroscopy in turbid media by combining frequency-domain and steady-state methods. Appl Opt 2000;39:6498–507.

[29] Born M, Wolf E. Principles of optics. Cambridge (UK): Cambridge University Press; 1999.

[30] Carlsen E. Transillumination light scanning. Diagn Imaging 1982;4:28–34.

[31] Alveryd A, Andersson I, Aspegren K, Balldin G, Bjurstam N, Edstrom G, et al. Light scanning versus mammography for the detection of breast cancer in screening and clinical practice. Cancer 1990;65: 1671–7.

[32] Case KM, Zweifel PF. Linear transport theory. Reading: Addison-Wesley Publishing; 1967.

[33] Chandrasekhar S. Radiative transfer. New York: Dover; 1960.

[34] Morse PM, Feschbach H. Methods of theoretical physics. New York: McGraw-Hill; 1953.

[35] Ishimaru A. Wave propagation and scattering in random media. New York: Academic Press; 1978.

[36] Klose AD, Hielscher AH. Iterative reconstruction scheme for optical tomography based on the equation of radiative transfer. Med Phys 1999;26:1698–707.

[37] Patterson M, Chance B, Wilson BC. Time resolved reflectance and transmittance for the non-invasive measurement of tissue optical properties. Appl Opt 1989;28:2331–6.

[38] Haskell RC, Svaasand LO, Tsay T, Feng T, McAdams MS, Tromberg BJ. Boundary conditions for the diffusion equation in radiative transfer. J Opt Soc Am A Opt Image Sci Vis 1994;11:2727–41.

[39] O'Leary M. Imaging with diffuse photon density waves. Philadelphia: University of Pennsylvania; 1996.

[40] Ripoll J, Ntziachristos V. Iterative boundary method for diffuse optical tomography. J Opt Soc Am A Opt Image Sci Vis 2003;20:1103–10.

[41] Jobsis F. Noninvasive infrared monitoring of cerebral and myocardial sufficiency and circulatory parameters. Science 1977;198:1264–7.

[42] Boas D, Gaudette T, Strangman G, Cheng X, Marota J, Mandeville J. The accuracy of near infrared spectroscopy and imaging during focal changes in cerebral hemodynamics. Neuroimage 2001;13: 76–90.

[43] Boas D, Gaudette T, Arridge S. Simultaneous imaging and optode calibration with diffuse optical tomography. Opt Express 2001;8:263–70.

[44] Boas D, Brooks D, Miler E, DiMarzio C, Kilmer M, Gaudette R, et al. Imaging the body with diffuse optical tomography. IEEE Signal Process Mag 2001; 18:57–74.

[45] Arridge S. Optical tomography in medical imaging. Inverse Problems 1999;15:R41–93.

[46] Strangman G, Boas D, Sutton J. Non-invasive neuroimaging using Near-Infrared light. Biol Psychiatry 2002;52:679–93.

[47] Villringer A, Chance B. Non-invasive optical spectroscopy and imaging of human brain function. Trends Neurosci 1997;20:435–42.

[48] Wobst P, Wenzel R, Kohl M, Obrig H, Villringer A. Linear aspects of changes in deoxygenated hemoglobin concentration and cytochrome oxidase oxidation during brain activation. Neuroimage 2001;13: 520–30.

[49] Sato H, Takeuchi T, Satai K. Temporal cortex activation during speech recognition: an optical topography study. Cognition 1999;73:55–66.

[50] Watanabe E, Maki A, Kawaguchi F, Takashiro K, Yamashita Y, Koizumi H, et al. Non-invasive assessment of language dominance with near-infrared spectroscopic mapping. Neurosci Lett 1998;256: 49–52.

[51] Chance B, Nioka S, Chen Y. Shining new light on brain function. OE magazine 2003;3:16–9.

[52] Kirkpatrick P, Lam J, Al-Rawi P, Smielewski P, Czosnyka M. Defining thresholds for critical ischemia by using near-infrared spectroscopy in the adult brain. J Neurosurg 1998;89:389–94.

[53] Stankovic M, Maulik D, Rosenfeld W, Stubblefield P, Kofinas A, Gratton E, et al. Role of frequency domain optical spectroscopy in the detection of neonatal brain hemorrhage: a newborn piglet study. J Matern Fetal Med 2000;9:142–9.

[54] Steinbrink J, Kohl M, Obrig H, Curio G, Syre F, Thomas F, et al. Somatosensory evoked fast optical intensity changes detected non-invasively in the adult human head. Neurosci Lett 2000;291:105–8.

[55] Gratton G, Fabiani M. Shedding light on brain function: the event related optical signal. Trends Cogn Sci 2001;5:357–63.

[56] Quaresima V, Springett R, Cope M, Wyatt J, Delpy D, Ferrari M, et al. Oxidation and reduction of cytochrome oxidase in the neonatal brain observed by in vivo near-infrared spectroscopy. BBA-Bioenergetics 1998;1366:291–300.

[57] Heekeren H, Kohl M, Obrig H, Wenzel R, von Pannwitz W, Matcher S, et al. Noninvasive assessment of changes in cytochrome-c oxidase oxidation in human subjects during visual stimulation. J Cereb Blood Flow Metab 1999;19:592–603.

[58] Schweiger M, Arridge S. Optical tomographic reconstruction in a complex head model using a priori region boundary information. Phys Med Biol 1999; 44:2703–21.

[59] Fukui Y, Ajichi Y, Okada E. Monte Carlo prediction of near-infrared light propagation in realistic adult and neonatal head models. Appl Opt 2003;42: 2881–7.

[60] Bluestone A, Abdoulaev G, Schmitz C, Barbour R, Hielscher A. Three dimensional optical tomography of hemodynamics in the human head. Opt Express 2001;9:272–86.

[61] Hebden J, Gibson A, Yusof R, Everdell N, Hillman E, Delpy E, et al. Three dimensional optical tomography of the premature infant brain. Phys Med Biol 2002;47:4155–66.

[62] Cutler M. Transillumination as an aid in the diagnosis of breast lesions. Surg Gynecol Obstet 1929;48: 721–9.

[63] Cubeddu R, D'Andrea C, Pifferi A, Taroni P, Torricelli A, Valentini G. Effects of the menstrual cycle on the red and near-infrared optical properties of the human breast. Photochem Photobiol 2000; 72–73:383–91.

[64] Durduran T, Choe R, Culver J, Zubkov L, Holboke M, Giammarco J, et al. Bulk optical properties of healthy female breast tissue. Phys Med Biol 2002;47: 2847–61.

[65] Shah N, Cerussi A, Eker C, Espinoza J, Butler J, Fishkin J, et al. Noninvasive functional optical spectroscopy of human breast tissue. Proc Natl Acad Sci U S A 2001;98:4420–5.

[66] Cerussi A, Berger A, Bevilacqua F, Shah N, Jakubowski D, Butler J, et al. Sources of absorption

and scattering contrast for near-infrared optical mammography. Acad Radiol 2001;8:211–8.

[67] Srinivasan S, Pogue B, Jiang S, Dehghani H, Kogel S, Soho S, et al. Interpreting hemoglobin and water concentration, oxygen saturation, and scattering measured in vivo by near-infrared breast tomography. Proc Natl Acad Sci U S A 2003;100:12349–54.

[68] Tromberg B, Shah N, Lanning R, Cerussi A, Espinoza J, Pham T, et al. Non-invasive in vivo characterization of breast tumors using photon migration spectroscopy. Neoplasia 2000;2:26–40.

[69] Atiqur Rahman M, Toi M. Anti-angiogenic therapy in breast cancer. Biomed Pharmacother 2003;57: 463–70.

[70] Hockel M, Vaupel P. Biological consequences of tumor hypoxia. Semin Oncol 2001;28:36–41.

[71] McBride T, Pogue B, Jiang S, Osterberg U, Paulsen K. Initial studies of *in-vivo* absorbing and scattering heterogeneity in near-infrared tomographic breast imaging. Opt Lett 2001;26:822–4.

[72] Jiang H, Iftimia N, Eggert J, Fajardo L, Klove K. Near-infrared optical imaging of the breast with model-based reconstruction. Acad Radiol 2002;9: 186–94.

[73] Franceschini M, Moesta K, Fantini S, Gaida G, Gratton E, Jess H, et al. Frequency-domain techniques enhance optical mammography: initial clinical results. Proc Natl Acad Sci U S A 1997;94:6468–73.

[74] Colak S, van der Mark M, Hooft G, Hoogenraad J, van der Linden E, Kuijpers F. Clinical optical tomography and NIR spectroscopy for breast cancer detection. IEEE Journal of Selected Topics in Quantum Electronics 1999;5:1143–58.

[75] Holboke M, Tromberg B, Li X, Shah N, Fishkin J, Kidney D, et al. Three dimensional diffuse optical mammography with ultrasound localization in a human subject. J Biomed Opt 2000;5:237–47.

[76] Desmettre T, Devoiselle J, Mordon S. Fluorescent properties and metabolic features of indocyanine green (ICG) as related to angiography. Surv Ophthalmol 2000;45:15–27.

[77] Ntziachristos V, Yodh A, Schnall M, Chance B. Concurrent MRI and diffuse optical tomography of breast after indocyanine green enhancement. Proc Natl Acad Sci U S A 2000;97:2767–72.

[78] Intes X, Ripoll J, Chen Y, Nioka S, Yodh A, Chance B. In vivo continuous-wave optical breast imaging enhanced with indocyanine green. Med Phys 2003; 30:1039–47.

[79] Jiang H, Xu Y. Phase-contrast imaging of tissue using near-infrared diffusing light. Med Phys 2003;30: 1048–51.

[80] Millikan GA. Photometric methods of measuring the velocity of rapid reactions. III. A portable microapparatus applicable to an extended range of reactions. Proc R Soc A 1936;155:277–92.

[81] Quaresima V, Lepanto R, Ferrari M. The use of near infrared spectroscopy in sports medicine. J Sports Med Phys Fitness 2003;43:1–13.

[82] Kowalchuk J, Rossiter H, Ward S, Whipp B. The effect of resistive breathing on leg muscle oxygenation using near-infrared spectroscopy during exercise in men. Exp Physiol 2002;87:601–11.

[83] Miura H, Araki H, Matoba H, Kitagawa K. Relationship among oxygenation, myoelectric activity, and lactic acid accumulation in vastus lateralis muscle during exercise with constant work rate. Int J Sports Med 2000;21:180–4.

[84] McKinley B, Marvin R, Cocanour C, Moore F. Tissue hemoglobin O_2 saturation during resuscitation of traumatic shock monitored using near infrared spectrometry. J Trauma 2000;48:637–42.

[85] Garr J, Gentilello L, Cole P, Mock C, Matsen F. Monitoring for compartment syndrome using near-infrared spectroscopy: a noninvasive, continuous, transcutaneous monitoring technique. J Trauma 1999;46: 613–6.

[86] Chance B, Bank W. Genetic disease of mitochondrial function evaluated by NMR and NIR spectroscopy of skeletal tissue. Biochim Biophys Acta 1995;1271: 7–14.

[87] Matsui S, Tamura N, Hirakawa T, Kobayashi S, Takekoshi N, Murakami E. Assessment of working skeletal muscle oxygenation in patients with chronic heart failure. Am Heart J 1995;129:690–5.

[88] Wolf U, Wolf M, Choi J, Levi M, Choudhury D, Hull S, et al. Localized irregularities in hemoglobin flow and oxygenation in calf muscle in patients with peripheral vascular disease detected with near-infrared spectrophotometry. Vasc Surg 2003;37:1017–26.

[89] Hamaoka T, Iwane H, Shimomitsu T, Katsumura T, Murase N, Nishio S, et al. Noninvasive measurement of oxidative metabolism on working human muscles by near infrared spectroscopy. J Appl Physiol 1996; 81:1410–7.

[90] Mancini D, Bolinger L, Li H, Kendrick K, Chance B, Wilson J. Validation of near-infrared spectroscopy in man. J Appl Physiol 1994;77:2740–7.

[91] Tran TK, Sailasuta N, Kreutzer U, Hurd R, Chung Y, Mole P, et al. Comparative analysis of NMR and NIRS measurements of intracellular PO_2 in human skeletal muscle. Am J Physiol 1999;276:R1682–90.

[92] Wilson J, Mancini D, McKully K, Ferraro N, Lanoce V, Chance B. Noninvasive detection of skeletal muscle under perfusion with near-infrared spectroscopy in patients with heart failure. Circulation 1989; 80:1668–74.

[93] Belardinelli R, Barstow TJ, Porszasz J, Wasserman K. Skeletal muscle oxygenation during constant work rate exercise. Med Sci Sports Exerc 1995;27:512–9.

[94] McCully KK, Iotti S, Kendrick K, Wang Z, Posner JD, Leigh J, et al. Simultaneous in vivo measurements of HbO_2 saturation and PCr kinetics after exercise in normal humans. J Appl Physiol 1994;77:5–10.

[95] Rundell K, Nioka S, Chance B. Hemoglobin/myoglobin desaturation during speed skating. Med Sci Sports Exerc 1997;29:248–58.

[96] Ferrari M, Binzoni T, Quaresima V. Oxidative

metabolism in muscle. Philos Trans R Soc Lond B Biol Sci 1997;352:677–83.

[97] McCully KK, Halber C, Posner JD. Exercise-induced changes in oxygen saturation in the calf muscles of elderly subjects with peripheral vascular disease. J Gerontol 1994;49:128–34.

[98] Szmedra L, Im J, Nioka S, Chance B, Rundell KW. Hemoglobin/myoglobin oxygen desaturation during Alpine skiing. Med Sci Sports Exerc 2001;33:232–6.

[99] Niwayama M, Lin L, Shao J, Kudo N, Yamamoto K. Quantitative measurement of muscle hemoglobin oxygenation using near-infrared spectroscopy with correction for the influence of a subcutaneous fat layer. Rev Sci Instrum 2000;71:4571–5.

[100] Miura H, McCully K, Hong L, Nioka S, Chance B. Regional difference of muscle oxygen saturation and blood volume during exercise determined by near infrared imaging device. Jpn J Physiol 2001;51: 599–606.

[101] Miura H, McCully K, Nioka S, Chance B. Relationship between muscle architectural features and oxygenation status determined by near infrared device. Eur J Appl Physiol 2004;91:273–8.

[102] Quaresima V, Colier W, van der Sluijs M, Ferrari M. Nonuniform quadriceps O_2 consumption revealed by near infrared multipoint measurements. Biochem Biophys Res Commun 2001;285:1034–99.

[103] Graber HL, Zhong S, Pei Y, Schmitz CH, Arif I, Hira J. Dynamic imaging of muscle activity by optical tomography. Presented at the OSA Biomedical Topical Meetings. Miami Beach, Florida, April 2–5, 2000.

[104] Weissleder R, Ntziachritos V. Shedding light onto live molecular targets. Nat Med 2003;9:123–8.

[105] Frangioni JV. In vivo near-infrared fluorescence imaging. Curr Opin Chem Biol 2003;7:626–34.

[106] Licha K. Contrast agents for optical imaging. Top Curr Chem 2002;222:1–29.

[107] Achilefu S, Dorshow R, Bugaj J, Rajagopalan R. Novel receptor-targeted fluorescent contrast agents for in-vivo tumor imaging. Invest Radiol 2000;35: 479–85.

[108] Chen Y, Zheng G, Zhang Z, Blessington D, Zhang M, Li H, et al. Metabolism enhanced tumor localization by fluorescence imaging: in vivo animal studies. Opt Lett 2003;28:2070–2.

[109] Weissleder R, Tung CH, Mahmood U, Bogdanov A. In vivo imaging with protease-activated near-infrared fluorescent probes. Nat Biotech 1999;17:375–8.

[110] Weinberg R. How does cancer arise. Sci Am 1996; 275:62–71.

[111] Lewis J, Achilefu S, Garbow JR, Laforest R, Welch MJ. Small animal imaging: current technology and perspectives for oncological imaging. Eur J Cancer 2002;38:2173–88.

[112] Li A, Miller EL, Kilmer ME, Brukilacchio TJ, Chaves T, Stott J, et al. Tomographic optical breast imaging guided by three-dimensional mammography. Appl Opt 2003;42:5181–90.

[113] Zhu Q, Huang M, Chen N, Zarfos K, Jagjivan B, Kane M, et al. Ultrasound-guided optical tomographic imaging of malignant and benign breast lesions: initial clinical results of 19 cases. Neoplasia 2003;5: 379–88.

[114] Holboke M, Tromberg B, Li X, Shah N, Fishkin J, Kidney D, et al. Three-dimensional diffuse optical mammography with ultrasound localization in a human subject. J Biomed Opt 2000;5:237–47.

[115] Ntziachristos V, Yodh AG, Schnall MD, Chance B. MRI-guided diffuse optical spectroscopy of malignant and benign breast legions. Neoplasia 2002;4: 347–54.

[116] Chen Y, Tailor D, Intes X, Chance B. Quantitative correlation between near-infrared spectroscopy (NIRS) and magnetic resonance imaging (MRI) on rat brain oxygenation modulation. Phys Med Biol 2003;48:417–27.

[117] Merritt S, Bevilacqua F, Durkin AJ, Cuccia DJ, Lanning R, Tromberg BJ, et al. Coregistration of diffuse optical spectroscopy and magnetic resonance imaging in a rat tumor model. Appl Opt 2003;42: 2951–9.

[118] Brooksby B, Dehghani H, Pogue B, Paulsen K. Near-infrared (NIR) tomography breast reconstruction with a priori structural information from MRI: algorithm development reconstructing heterogeneities. IEEE Journal of Selected Topics in Quantum Electronics 2003;9:199–209.

[119] Intes X, Maloux C, Guven M, Yazici B, Chance B. Diffuse optical tomography with physiological and spatial a priori constraints. Phys Med Biol 2004; 49:N155–63.

ELSEVIER
SAUNDERS

Radiol Clin N Am 43 (2005) 235–246

RADIOLOGIC
CLINICS
of North America

Hyperpolarized helium-3 MR imaging of pulmonary function

Masaru Ishii, MD, PhD[a],*, Martin C. Fischer, PhD[b], Kiarash Emami, MS[b],
Abass Alavi, MD[c], Zebulon Z. Spector, BS[b], Jiangsheng Yu, MS[b],
James E. Baumgardner, MD, PhD[d], Maxim Itkin, MD[b],
Stephen J. Kadlecek, PhD[b], Jianliang Zhu, MD[e], Michael Bono, BS[f],
Warren B. Gefter, MD[b], David A. Lipson, MD[g], Joseph B. Shrager, MD[e],
Rahim R. Rizi, PhD[b]

[a]Department of Otolaryngology–Head and Neck Surgery, Johns Hopkins University, 4940 Eastern Avenue, A5W, 595A,
Baltimore, MD 21224, USA
[b]Department of Radiology, University of Pennsylvania Health System, 3400 Spruce Street, Philadelphia, PA 19104, USA
[c]Division of Nuclear Medicine, Department of Radiology, Hospital of the University of Pennsylvania, Philadelphia,
Pennsylvania, USA
[d]Department of Anesthesiology, University of Pennsylvania Health System, 3400 Spruce Street, Philadelphia, PA 19104, USA
[e]Section of General Thoracic Surgery, University of Pennsylvania Health System, 3400 Spruce Street, Philadelphia,
PA 19104, USA
[f]AMICI, 518 Vincent Street, Spring City, PA 19475, USA
[g]Department of Pulmonary Medicine, University of Pennsylvania Health System, 3400 Spruce Street, Philadelphia,
PA 19104, USA

The primary function of the respiratory system is to supply enough oxygen to the body to meet its metabolic needs and to remove carbon dioxide formed as a by-product of metabolism [1]. To accomplish this, sufficient quantities of blood and air must be brought in close proximity to allow for the adequate exchange of gases. Conditions that perturb the effective exchange of gases are seen in virtually all respiratory disease processes; measures of lung function play an important role in the diagnosis, management, and treatment of pulmonary disorders. Recent advances in hyperpolarized (HP) contrast agents have led to new MR imaging–based pulmonary function tests. These tests may lead to a new paradigm in the management, treatment, and study of lung disease.

This work was supported by a grant from Phillip Morris USA, and NIH Grant RO1-HL64741.

* Corresponding author.
E-mail address: mishii3@jhmi.edu (M. Ishii).

Anatomy

The lung is a multilobed organ whose primary purpose is to efficiently exchange gases across a liquid and gas interface. This exchange occurs in the alveolar capillary unit. Here, inspired gases are brought in close proximity to the circulating blood. The large surface area of the blood-gas interface makes the lungs efficient organs for gas exchange. Repetitive branching of the airways results in the enormous expansion of the cross-sectional area of the airways, from 2.5 cm^2 at the level of the trachea to a total cross-sectional area of 5.6×10^7 cm^2 at the level of the alveoli.

The lungs have a dual circulation: the bronchial and pulmonary circulations. The bronchial circulation supplies nutrients to all except the alveolar structures; it consumes approximately 1% of the heart's throughput. The pulmonary circulation is involved primarily in pulmonary gas exchange; it also supplies nutrients to the alveolar membranes. Nearly the entire cardiac output is diverted into the pulmonary circulation. Pulmonary perfusion, Q, is a measure of blood flow in the pulmonary circulation; it is usually normalized by the mass of tissue comprising the region of interest. This parameter is important when studying disease states that affect pulmonary circulation, such as sickle cell anemia, pulmonary embolism, and pulmonary hypertension.

Pulmonary mechanics

To oxygenate the blood and eliminate carbon dioxide from the body, a fresh supply of air must be brought repeatedly to the gas exchange units of the lung (ie, the alveoli) by the respiratory pump [2]. The respiratory pump consists of the chest wall and respiratory muscles. A pressure gradient is created between the lips and the alveoli when the inspiratory muscles contract. As a result air flows toward the alveoli. The pressure gradient must overcome the elastic recoil of the pulmonary system, the frictional resistance to airflow, and the inertial resistance of the system, which results in the following equation of motion for the lung:

$$\Delta P = \frac{1}{C} \Delta V + R \dot{V} + I \ddot{V}. \quad (1)$$

Here ΔP, C, ΔV, R, I, $\dot{V}$, and $\ddot{V}$ represent driving pressure, compliance, change in lung volume, resistance, inertance, airflow, and rate of change of airflow, respectively. Under most circumstances, the force required to accelerate the lung tissues and tracheobronchial air column is small and the inertance term can be neglected.

Compliance represents a measure of lung stiffness, and is an important parameter for understanding and categorizing many destructive disease processes, such as emphysema [3,4]. Airflow, $\dot{V}$, is a measure of ventilation, and is discussed in greater detail later. Eq. 1 predicts that large resistances limit airflow, whereas small compliances restrict changes in lung volume. Eq. 1 is analogous to the equation of state for a serial resistor-capacitor circuit, where compliance plays the role of capacitance, airflow the role of current, and volume the role of charge. Note that diseased lungs can be modeled by resistor-capacitor circuits placed in parallel, where each resistor-capacitor circuit represents one functional unit of the lung. Predictions on ventilation and changes in lung volume follow accordingly.

Oxygen, perfusion, and ventilation perfusion ratios

To understand HP MR imaging of perfusion and ventilation-perfusion ratios, it is helpful to consider a simple experiment where the right lower lobar branch of the pulmonary artery of an animal is occluded and then the lungs are serially imaged after the inhalation of HP helium-3 (^{3}He) (Fig. 1) [5]. Here, 600 mL of HP ^{3}He gas were insufflated into a pig's lungs after balloon occlusion of the right lower lobar pulmonary artery. Images were obtained, during breath hold conditions, every 4 seconds using a two-dimensional fast gradient echo pulse sequence. Note how in the early time limit, the ^{3}He gas is homogeneously distributed throughout the lung fields, suggesting uniform ventilation throughout the lungs. Note also how the signal decays in an inhomogeneous fashion as time progresses. That is, signal in the right lower lobe supplied by the occluded artery decays faster than the signal in regions of the lung where perfusion is normal. In the long time limit, regions with low or no perfusion have low signal intensity, whereas

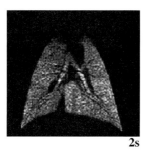 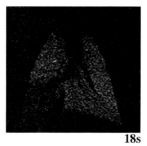 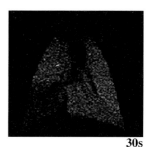

| 2s | 18s | 30s |

Fig. 1. HP ^{3}He MR images taken after 600 mL of HP ^{3}He with net activity 4.5 mmol was injected into the pig's lungs. The right inferior pulmonary artery was occluded with an 8-mm balloon catheter. TR of 7.3 ms; TE of 1.9 ms; matrix size 256 × 128; field of view 24 cm × 24 cm; slice thickness 2 cm; flip angle 5°.

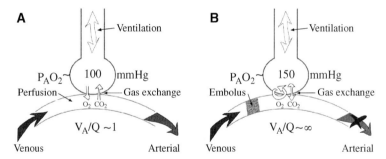

Fig. 2. Illustrations of alveolar capillary units. (*A*) Normal physiologic state. (*B*) Pulmonary embolism.

regions with high or normal perfusion have high signal intensity.

The reason for these signal discrepancies can be explained with the aid of the cartoon shown in Fig. 2. Consider a normal alveolar capillary unit. What looks like a Florence flask represents an alveolus, whereas the tube at the bottom of the illustration represents a capillary. Air in the lungs is exchanged with air in the atmosphere through the process of ventilation, supplying new oxygen to the alveoli. Deoxygenated blood enters the capillaries and absorbs oxygen from the alveoli before returning to the heart for circulation throughout the body. Note how the extraction of oxygen by hemoglobin keeps the alveolar partial pressure of oxygen (pO_2) roughly 50 mm Hg below the inspired pO_2. In the balloon occlusion case, or in pulmonary embolism, blood no longer flows through the pulmonary capillaries. As a result, oxygen is no longer extracted from the alveoli. If ventilation continues, then the alveolar pO_2 rises to a new steady state level. In this case, this level is 150 mm Hg.

During a breathhold experiment, one expects oxygen levels to remain constant in regions where perfusion is compromised, because new hemoglobin is not available to extract oxygen from the alveoli. Likewise, one expects oxygen levels to fall in regions where normal perfusion occurs. The consequence for HP ^{3}He MR imaging lies with the observation that the HP helium signal intensity decays or relaxes fastest in those regions with the highest oxygen tensions: the regions with vascular compromise [6]. The oxygen tension decreases in regions of the lung with normal perfusion, leaving less oxygen available to depolarize the helium, and resulting in relatively higher signal intensity.

These temporal changes in signal intensities can be used to detect pulmonary emboli greater than 4 mm in size (Fig. 3). When using this technique, early time images are obtained to rule out ventilation defects. Images acquired in the long time limit are used to localize perfusion defects. Because this is a gaseous contrast-based technique, no comments on perfusion in

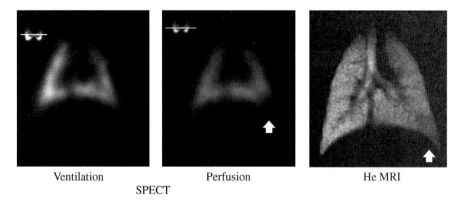

Fig. 3. Single-photon emission CT ventilation and perfusion images (*left*) and the corresponding long time limit HP ^{3}He image (*right*). A 3.8-mm glass bead was embolized into the left inferior pulmonary artery before the imaging experiment. A defect is seen in the lower right-hand corner of the single-photon emission CT perfusion and ^{3}He image, whereas ventilation appears homogeneous. TR of 6.4 ms; TE of 2.9 ms; matrix size 128 × 128; field of view 24 cm × 24 cm; slice thickness 2 cm; flip angle 5°. The MR image was taken 18 s after 600 mL of HP ^{3}He with net activity 4.5 mmol was injected into the pig's lungs.

regions of the lung with poor or absent ventilation can be made. This is an inherent limitation of this technique.

Regions of the lung with high oxygen tensions have correspondingly high ventilation-perfusion ratios because perfusion values tend to be small. Likewise, regions of the lung with restricted ventilation and normal perfusion (ie, small ventilation-perfusion ratios) have low oxygen tensions, because residual oxygen in these portions of the lung is absorbed by the circulating blood. This suggests a functional dependence of ventilation-perfusion ratios on local oxygen concentrations [7,8]. This observation is reviewed again in the section on ventilation-perfusion ratios. Before doing so, it is important to formalize the understanding of how oxygen affects HP [3]He signal intensities. These observations led to a method for determining local oxygen concentrations.

Oxygen measurements

The magnetization of polarized [3]He gas gradually decreases over time in the presence of oxygen [6].

This decrease is caused by dipole interactions between oxygen and helium molecules. The depolarization rate is strongly dependent on the pO_2 in the gas mixture because [3]He–oxygen interaction probabilities are a strong function of the relative concentrations of the two gas species. Measurements of the depolarization rate allows for the determination of the pO_2 [9–12]. The time-dependent evolution of pO_2, and consequently the oxygen depletion rate, can be obtained if the time-dependent behavior of the oxygen-induced depolarization rate is extracted from a time series of images. These measurements are complicated by the fact that HP [3]He gas is also partially depolarized by the radiofrequency pulses used for imaging [13–15]. This radiofrequency-induced depolarization is intrinsic to the MR imaging acquisition technique and needs to be distinguished from the oxygen-induced depolarization to allow for a precise pO_2 determination. Depolarization caused by boundary effects, inhomogeneous magnetic fields, and collisions with other gas species has been shown to be negligible over the time scale of an imaging experiment and is ignored [10,16–20].

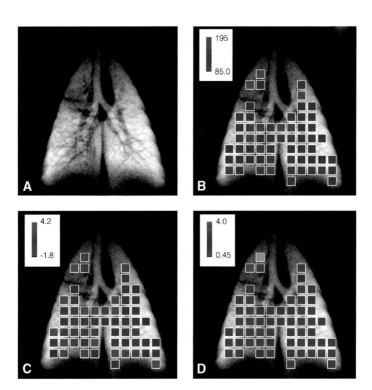

Fig. 4. Images are of a healthy porcine lung. (A) [3]He MR. (B) Oxygen. (C) Oxygen depletion rates. (D) Ventilation-perfusion ratios. Oxygen units are in mbar; oxygen depletion rates are in mbar/s.

Accounting for the dominant mechanisms of HP ^{3}He depolarization, the signal intensity of the i-th acquired image in a series can then be written as

$$A_i = A_0 \cos(\alpha)^{iN} \exp\left[- \int_0^{t_i} 1/_\xi pO_2(t')dt' \right], \quad (2)$$

where A_0 is a constant of proportionality, t_i denotes the acquisition start time of the i-th image, α represents the flip angle, N equals the number of phase encodes in an image, and $\xi = 2.6\ bar \cdot s$ at body temperature is an experimentally determined constant mapping of the pO_2 to the ^{3}He depolarization time constant. On the time scale of an imaging experiment the uptake of oxygen into the blood can be, to first order, assumed to be linear, for example

$$pO_2(t) = p_0 - Rt, \quad (3)$$

where p_0 and R represent the initial pO_2 and the oxygen depletion rate, respectively. Eq. 2 then simplifies to

$$A_i = A_0 \cos(\alpha)^{iN} \exp\left(-\frac{1}{\xi}\left[p_0 t_i - \frac{1}{2}Rt_i{}^2 \right] \right). \quad (4)$$

The desired parameters, p_0 and R, can be obtained using a fit procedure once an accurate estimate of the local flip angle, α, is obtained. A number of methods have been implemented to estimate α [21]. Perhaps the simplest method is to acquire two extra images with minimal interscan time during an imaging sequence. The effects of oxygen depolarization can be neglected if the interscan time for this extra set of images is kept at a minimum, and then an estimate for the local flip angle can be obtained from the change in intensity between the two images.

Fig. 4B shows local oxygen concentrations measured in a porcine lung using the double pulse acquisition method. Fig. 4A depicts a sample early time ^{3}He image used in the calculation. Fig. 5A plots a histogram of the pO_2 measured. Note how the values are centered on 140 mbar, values typically found in a healthy pig. Fig. 4C and Fig. 5B also show the oxygen degradation rate and the histogram of this value. The supraphysiologic and subphysiologic values are obtained in regions of the lung with low signal-to-noise and illustrate the inherent sensitivity of this technique to low signal-to-noise. Simulations indicate that signal-to-noise values greater than 20 are required to obtain meaningful data. Signal-to-noise values in the upper right lobe (see Fig. 4), from which many of the erroneous values originate, are in the range of 10 to 1. The effects of signal-to-noise on measurement accuracy are treated in greater detail elsewhere.

Perfusion

The effect of perfusion on ^{3}He signal intensities can be clarified with a second experiment. Consider a similar pig to the one discussed in the first experiment. Assume that the right lower lobar pulmonary artery is cannulated with an 8-mm balloon catheter. Three experiments are now performed where the local oxygen tensions in the lungs as a function of time are measured. During the first trial the balloon is deflated; during the second the balloon is inflated. The third experiment is performed after the pig is sacrificed. Sample images are depicted in Fig. 6. The pO_2 measured in the regions of interest depicted in Figs. 6 and 7 are plotted. Here the squares represent the dead pig, the crosses correspond to the balloon-

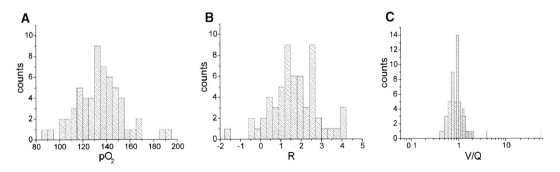

Fig. 5. Histograms of oxygen concentrations (*A*), oxygen depletion rates (*B*), and ventilation-perfusion ratios (*C*) illustrated in Fig. 4.

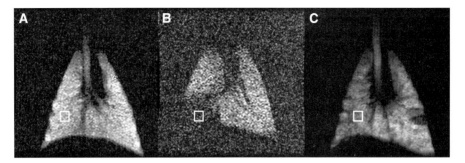

Fig. 6. ^{3}He MR images of a pig's lung. (*A*) Balloon deflated. (*B*) Balloon inflated. (*C*) Dead pig conditions. Note how images *A* and *C* appear homogenous, whereas the signal in the right lower lobe of *B*, supplied by the occluded artery, decays faster than elsewhere in the lung. TR of 7.3 ms; TE of 1.9 ms; matrix size 256 × 128; field of view 24 cm × 24 cm; slice thickness 2 cm; flip angle 5°. The MR images were taken 18 s after 600 mL of HP ^{3}He with net activity 4.5 mmol was injected into the pig's lungs.

occluded case, and the circles symbolize the deflated balloon experiment. Note how in the dead pig and the balloon-occluded experiment, the oxygen degradation rates are nearly zero, whereas in the deflated balloon case the slope is much greater, because oxygen is being extracted by the blood. Also note that the y intercepts for the deflated balloon example are lower than the balloon-occluded case and the dead pig case as expected. These images suggest that the slope of the temporal depletion line of oxygen is an important parameter when studying pulmonary perfusion. In essence, the slope of the temporal depletion lines gives a contrast mechanism for detecting perfusion abnormalities. It also serves as an index of pulmonary perfusion. The Fick principle needs to be examined in greater detail, however, to measure regional perfusion.

Consider the alveolar-capillary unit introduced in Fig. 2. Deoxygenated blood enters the capillaries and absorbs oxygen from the alveoli before returning to the heart for circulation throughout the body. Assume that the transit time of the blood through the capillaries is long enough so that the pO$_2$ in the blood approaches the pO$_2$ in the alveolus. This allows one to estimate the end-capillary oxygen concentration from alveolar oxygen tensions. This is a reasonable assumption under many physiologic conditions.

During breathhold conditions oxygen consumption in an alveolar capillary unit is governed by the Fick principle,

$$\frac{dO_2(t)}{dt} = Q \cdot (C_A O_2 - C_V O_2), \tag{5}$$

which relates oxygen consumption to the capillary perfusion rate and the oxygen concentration gradient between end-capillary and precapillary oxygen concentrations. Here $dO_2(t)/dt$, Q, $C_A O_2$, and $C_V O_2$ represent: oxygen consumption, local blood flow, arterial oxygen concentration, and venous oxygen concentration, respectively. Rearranging terms gives an expression for pulmonary perfusion in terms of alveolar oxygen depletion rates and capillary oxygen concentration gradients:

$$Q = \frac{dp_A O_2(t)}{dt} \frac{V}{P_B} \frac{1}{C_A O_2 - C_V O_2}, \tag{6}$$

where $dp_A O_2(t)/dt$, V, and P_B represent the rate of change of the alveolar pO$_2$, volume of the region of interest, and atmospheric pressure, respectively. It is assumed that the volume of the region of interest changes negligibly over the course of the experiment. Note that all of the terms on the right can be

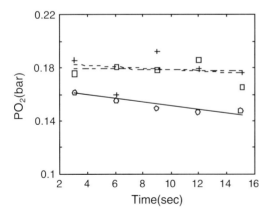

Fig. 7. Plots of the partial pressure of oxygen as a function of time for the regions of interest depicted in Fig. 6. Circles, crosses, and squares represent Figs. 6A, 6B, and 6C, respectively.

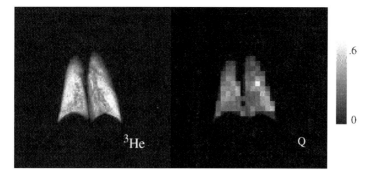

Fig. 8. HP ^{3}He image of a macaque monkey (*left*) and perfusion map (*right*). Units are in mL/min.

determined using ^{3}He MR imaging and venous blood gases. Eq. 6 illustrates why the oxygen degradation rate is an important parameter in lung function; essentially, it provides a measure of regional perfusion. This is the reason why the perfusion index (ie, the oxygen degradation rate, R) provides a contrast mechanism for localizing perfusion abnormalities.

Fig. 8 shows perfusion maps acquired in a macaque monkey. Blood parameters typical for humans were used to perform this calculation, because exact models for monkey blood are not available [22,23]. Note how the lung perfusion is relatively homogeneous throughout the lung fields.

Ventilation-perfusion ratios

Ventilation-perfusion ratios represent one of the most important parameters of lung function [7,8, 24–27]. To exchange gases most efficiently between blood and air, the lung needs to match ventilation and perfusion rates locally. The lung behaves most efficiently with respect to gas exchange in regions of the lung that are well ventilated and have high perfusion rates. Regions of the lung with high ventilation and low perfusion efficiently eliminate carbon dioxide and supply oxygen to the alveoli but are ineffective at oxygenating blood, because insufficient blood is supplied to respiratory exchange membrane. These regions of the lung waste ventilation and contribute to physiologic dead space. Similarly, portions of the lung with low ventilation and high perfusion rates supply high quantities of blood to the respiratory exchange membranes, but poorly oxygenate blood, because insufficient oxygen is supplied to the alveoli. These sections of the lung waste perfusion and contribute to physiologic shunt. The ventilation-perfusion ratio provides a measure of ventilation and perfusion matching. A ratio of one is ideal; high ratios are seen in pulmonary emboli, low ratios are

present in obstructive situations, such as the plugging of a bronchus with mucus [28–31].

Regional alveolar ventilation-perfusion ratios, V_A/Q, are related to local alveolar oxygen concentrations, p_AO_2, through a series of three balance equations and Dalton's law of partial pressures [32–34]. It is assumed that the pH, the partial pressure of carbon dioxide, p_VCO_2, and the partial pressure of oxygen, p_VO_2, of the mixed venous blood entering the lungs can be measured using blood gas analysis and that the fraction of oxygen in the inspired air, F_IO_2, remains constant during the time period of interest. It is further assumed that the F_IO_2 can be determined experimentally.

Begin by considering the steady-state balance equation for oxygen:

$$(V_I/Q)p_IO_2 - (V_A/Q)p_AO_2$$
$$= k(C_aO_2 - C_vO_2). \qquad (7)$$

Here C_aO_2, C_vO_2, V_I, and k represent end-capillary oxygen concentration, mixed venous oxygen concentration, total ventilation, and a constant of proportionality converting gas volumes between body temperature and pressure, saturated and standard temperature and pressure, dry, respectively. Note that C_vO_2 follows directly from the oxygen and carbon dioxide dissociation curves once venous pH, p_VCO_2, and p_VO_2 are known, whereas C_aO_2 remains an implicit function of the blood pH, the alveolar partial pressure of carbon dioxide, P_ACO_2 and the p_AO_2.

The steady-state balance equation for carbon dioxide, CO_2, gives,

$$(V_A/Q)P_ACO_2 = k(C_aCO_2 - C_vCO_2), \qquad (8)$$

where C_aO_2 and C_vCO_2 denote end-capillary carbon dioxide concentration and mixed venous carbon dioxide concentration, respectively. As with Eq. 7, C_aO2 remains an implicit function of P_ACO_2, while C_VCO_2 can be calculated from the oxygen and carbon dioxide dissociation curves.

For nitrogen, N_2, mass balance leads to

$$(V_I/Q)P_IN_2 - (V_A/Q)P_AN_2$$
$$= \lambda_{N2}(P_AN_2 - P_{vN2}), \tag{9}$$

where P_IN_2 and P_AN_2 are the inspired and alveolar nitrogen partial pressures, respectively, whereas λ_{N_2} represents the blood gas partition coefficient for nitrogen. P_{vN_2} is the mixed venous nitrogen partial pressure (calculated from a balance on mixed venous blood gas data).

Eqs. 7–9 represent three equations with four unknowns. A fourth equation follows from Dalton's law of partial pressures, which requires the partial pressures of all gases in the lung to sum to the barometric pressure:

$$P_AO_2 + P_ACO_2 + P_AN_2 = P_B - P_{H_2O}. \tag{10}$$

Here P_B is barometric pressure and P_{H_2O} is the water vapor pressure.

Eqs. 7–10 represent four equations with four unknowns, which can be solved simultaneously for the desired V_A/Q ratios. These equations are inherently nonlinear and an iterative procedure is required.

Fig. 4D illustrates the V_A/Q ratios calculated from the oxygen data presented in Fig. 4B. A histogram of the V_A/Q data is show in Fig. 5C. As expected, the V_A/Q ratios cluster in the neighborhood of one. The spurious high values are a consequence of the supraphysiologic oxygen values calculated in regions of the lung with low signal-to-noise and are not physiologic.

Ventilation

Many pulmonary disorders, such as emphysema and asthma, affect lung compliance and resistance, and affect pulmonary ventilation [35–37]. Emphysema, for example, is characterized by the enlargement of airspaces distal to the respiratory bronchioles brought about by destruction of elastin in the walls of the distal airways. This local destruction leads to increased compliance and a dynamic increase in expiratory airway resistance in emphysema. As a result regional ventilation is affected. Similarly, asthma is characterized by an increased responsiveness of the

airways to various stimuli. This increased responsiveness manifests itself as a narrowing of the airways that varies in severity and causes global and regional changes in airway resistance. Measures of these changes may play an important role in the diagnosis and management of such disease processes.

Fractional ventilation, r, is defined as the fraction of lung volume that is replaced during one inspiratory cycle:

$$r = \frac{V_{new}}{V_{new} + V_{old}}. \tag{11}$$

It represents the measure of ventilation most typically measured using HP MR imaging. Here, V_{old} denotes the gas volume that remains in the lung, whereas V_{new} is the volume that is replaced. The parameter $q = 1 - r$ describes the nonreplaced fraction. A method for determining q and r was originally proposed by Deninger et al [38]. In this method, local fractional ventilation was determined by imaging the buildup of HP ^{3}He gas in a region of the lung after successive HP ^{3}He breaths. A recursion relationship was developed to model the buildup of HP gases in the lung mathematically; a nonlinear fit of experimental data to this model allowed for the extraction of the desired fractional ventilation. Fractional ventilation varies with the inspiratory volume, and must be standardized if values are to be compared among subjects. The authors typically standardize to a subject's tidal volume.

To understand how fractional ventilation is determined, note that HP gas accumulates in the lungs following sequential inhalation of HP gas. The net magnetization, $M(j)$, in a volume element of interest after the j-th inhalation of HP gas, with initial magnetization M_{new}, is given by the following recursion relation:

$$M(j) = M_{new}(1 - q)\exp\left(\frac{-[j-1]\tau}{T_{1,ext}}\right)$$
$$+ M(j-1)q \exp\left(\frac{-\tau}{T_{1,O_2}}\right). \tag{12}$$

In this equation, τ is the time interval of respiration. $T_{1,ext}$ denotes the spin relaxation time of the external reservoir housing the HP gas during an imaging experiment, and T_{1,O_2} is the oxygen-induced relaxation time constant. The initial condition for this recursion relation requires that the net magnetization equals zero before the first helium breath. The first term in eq. 12 accounts for magnetization added to

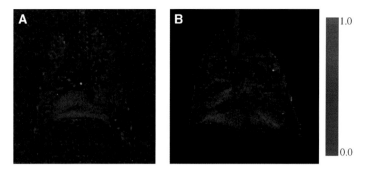

Fig. 9. (*A*) Fractional ventilation image in a normal lung. (*B*) Fractional ventilation image in an emphysematous lung. The color scale is proportional to the fractional ventilation. Note how the emphysematous lung is larger and less efficient at ventilation than the normal lung.

the region of interest following a new breath. The exponential component of this term accounts for spin relaxation that occurs in the inhalation reservoir. The second term accounts for the magnetization remaining from the previous breaths. The exponential term here accounts for magnetization lost because of dipole interactions with residual oxygen in the lungs. As expected T_{1,O_2} is a function of q.

Note that signal intensity measured after the j-th breath is proportional to the magnetization predicted by the recursive eq. 12. In this equation, one assumes an initial oxygen concentration before the inhalation of HP gas. $T_{1,ext}$ is measured experimentally and τ is

controlled during each experiment. The remaining parameters M_{new} and q are determined using a nonlinear fit procedure. The fractional ventilation follows from the relation, $r = 1 - q$.

It is informative to compare fractional ventilation maps of emphysematous and normal rats (Fig. 9). Note how the distribution of ventilations differs greatly between the normal and emphysematous rat. This difference is depicted more clearly by histograms of the distribution of fractional ventilations (Fig. 10). These histograms indicated that emphysematous rats are markedly less efficient than normal rats at ventilating their lungs. These types of

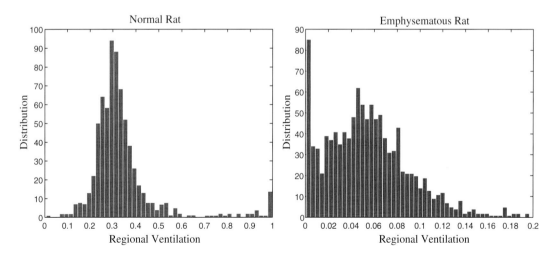

Fig. 10. Histograms of the distribution of regional ventilation in a normal (*left*) and emphysematous (*right*) rat. Range for normal and emphysematous ventilations are 0–1 and 0–0.2, respectively. Note how the emphysematous rat is far less efficient at ventilating its lungs than a normal rat.

measurements may play a role in monitoring the progression and treatment of chronic obstructive pulmonary disorders [39].

Diffusion

During a breathhold the pleural pressures rapidly equilibrate and the diffusion process drives mass transport of gases throughout the lungs. A gas molecule's current density, J, is proportional to the gradient of its concentration, ϕ:

$$J = -D\nabla\phi. \tag{13}$$

The constant of proportionality, D, is known as the *diffusion coefficient*. It gives a measure of the length scale of the diffusion process, and is itself related to the transport mean free path, l, by the following expression:

$$D = \frac{1}{3}cl. \tag{14}$$

Here c is the average speed of a gas molecule, and l represents the average distance a gas molecule travels before its direction is randomized. The gradient term in eq. 13 implies that gas molecules move from regions of high concentration to regions of low concentration. In the alveoli, pressure gradients are small, and diffusion plays a major role in determining the distribution of gases.

Diffusion coefficients for HP gases [40–42] and hydrogen-1 (^{1}H) are measured using similar techniques: bipolar gradients are applied before signal acquisition to dephase and rephase spins. Nuclear spins suffer a net phase shift proportional to their displacements before the rephrasing pulse. As a result the measured signal intensity is attenuated in the presence of diffusing spins. In the case of free diffusion, the MR signal intensity, S, is related to the free diffusion coefficient, D_0, by a simple exponential expression:

$$S = S_0 \exp(-bD_0). \tag{15}$$

Here, S_0 represents the signal intensity measured in the absence of diffusion-sensitizing gradients. The b value is a function related to the strength, duration, and shape of the bipolar gradients. The free diffusion coefficient for ^{3}He diffusing in air is 0.86 cm^2/s.

Interestingly, the average diffusion coefficient measured in a healthy lung is considerably lower, averaging about 0.20 cm^2/s. Because the diffusivity of a gas is characterized by the transport mean free path, one expects the diffusion coefficient for a gas to be identical within the lung and in free space. The interpretation of the results suggests MR imaging measures of diffusion are made over length scales larger than the diffusion length, and that the movement of the gas within the lung must be constrained by the boundaries of the airways. The apparent diffusion coefficient obtained represents a measure of the restrictions imposed on the movement of gases by the lung parenchyma. Measurements of the apparent diffusion coefficient in patients with emphysema, a destructive disease characterized by enlarged distal airways, average in the 0.55 cm^2/s range [43].

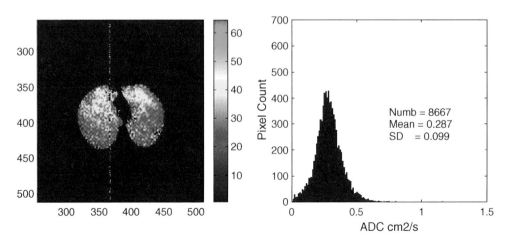

Fig. 11. Apparent diffusion coefficient measured in a coronal section of a normal human lung (*left*) and a histogram of values (*right*).

This value is much larger than those seen in the normal lung, suggesting that measures of the apparent diffusion coefficient may serve as a sensitive marker for destructive airway diseases, such as emphysema.

Sample apparent diffusion coefficient maps are depicted in Fig. 11 for a healthy human subject. As expected, the apparent diffusion coefficients are small, clustering around 0.3 cm^2/s.

Mathematical representations for MR imaging signal intensities after the application of a diffusion sensitizing pulse for simplified lung geometries follow from diffusion theory. These models have been used to determine estimate measures of airway size [44].

Summary

Recent advances in HP MR imaging contrast agents have led to novel tests of pulmonary function. Many of these tests show promise in the clinical arena.

References

[1] Kety SS. The theory and applications of the exchange of inert gas at the lungs and tissues. Pharmacol Rev 1951;3:1–41.

[2] Macklem PT. Respiratory mechanics. Annu Rev Physiol 1978;40:157–84.

[3] Gibson GJ. Lung volumes and elasticity. Clin Chest Med 2001;22:623–35.

[4] Shapiro MB, Bartlett RH. Pulmonary compliance and mechanical ventilation. Arch Surg 1992;127:485–6.

[5] Jalali A, Ishii M, Edvinsson JM, et al. Detection of simulated pulmonary embolism in a porcine model using hyperpolarized ^{3}He MRI. Magn Reson Med 2004;51:291–8.

[6] Saam B, Happer W, Middleton H. Nuclear relaxation of ^{3}He in the presence of O$_2$. Phys Rev A 1995;52: 862–5.

[7] West JB. Ventilation-perfusion relationships. Am Rev Respir Dis 1977;116:919–43.

[8] West JB, Wagner PD. Ventilation-perfusion relationships. In: Crystal RG, West JB, Weibel ER, et al, editors. 2nd edition. The lung, scientific foundations, vol. 2. Philadelphia: Lippincott-Raven; 1997. p. 1693–709.

[9] Deninger AJ, Eberle B, Bermuth J, et al. Assessment of a single-acquisition imaging sequence for oxygen-sensitive ^{3}He-MRI. Magn Reson Med 2002;47:105–14.

[10] Deninger AJ, Eberle B, Ebert M, et al. Quantification of regional intrapulmonary oxygen partial pressure evolution during apnea by ^{3}He MRI. J Magn Reson 1999;141:207–16.

[11] Fischer MC, Spector ZZ, Yu J, et al. Single-acquisition sequence for the measurement of oxygen partial pressure by hyperpolarized gas MRI. Magn Res Med 2004;52(4):766–73.

[12] Deninger AJ, Eberle B, Ebert M, et al. ^{3}He-MRI-based measurements of intrapulmonary PO$_2$ and its time course during apnea in healthy volunteers: first results, reproducibility, and technical limitations. NMR Biomed 2000;13:194–201.

[13] Johnson GA, Cates GD, Chen XJ, et al. Dynamics of magnetization in hyperpolarized gas MRI of the lung. Magn Reson Med 1997;38:66–71.

[14] MacFall JR, Charles HC, Black RD, et al. Human lung air spaces: potential for MR imaging with hyperpolarized He-3. Radiology 1996;200:553–8.

[15] Middleton H, Black RD, Saam B, et al. MR imaging with hyperpolarized 3He gas. Magn Reson Med 1995; 33:271–5.

[16] Cates GD, Schaefer SR, Happer W. Relaxation of spins due to field inhomogeneities in gaseous samples at low magnetic fields and low pressures. Phys Rev A 1988; 37:2877–85.

[17] Cates GD, White DJ, Chien TR, et al. Spin relaxation in gases due to inhomogeneous static and oscillating magnetic fields. Phys Rev A 1998;38:5092–106.

[18] Wu Z, Schaefer SR, Cates GD, et al. Coherent interactions of the polarized nuclear spins of gaseous atoms with the container walls. Phys Rev A 1988; 37:1161–75.

[19] Newbury NR, Barton AS, Cates GD, et al. Gaseous 3He-3He magnetic dipolar spin relaxation. Phys Rev A 1993;48:4411–20.

[20] Schearer LD, Walters GK. Nuclear spin-lattice relaxation in the presence of magnetic field gradients. Phys Rev 1965;139:1398–402.

[21] Markstaller K, Eberle B, Schreiber WG, et al. Flip angle considerations in ^{3}helium-MRI. NMR Biomed 2000;13:190–3.

[22] Severinghaus JW. Blood gas calculator. J Appl Phys 1966;21:1108–16.

[23] Severinghaus JW. Simple, accurate equations for human blood O2 dissociation computations. J Appl Phys 1979;46:599–602.

[24] Wagner PD, Laravuso RB, Uhl RR, et al. Continuous distributions of ventilation-perfusion ratios in normal subjects breathing air and 100% O$_2$. J Clin Invest 1974;54:54–68.

[25] Wagner PD, Saltzman HA, West JB. Measurements of continuous distributions of ventilation-perfusion ratios: theory. J Appl Phys 1974;36:588–99.

[26] West JB. Ventilation/perfusion inequality and overall gas exchange in computer models of the lung. Respir Physiol 1969;7:88–110.

[27] Rhodes CG, Valind SO, Brudin LH, et al. Quantification of regional V/Q ratios in humans by use of PET. I. Theory. J Appl Phys 1989;66:1896–904.

[28] Dantzker DR. Pulmonary embolism. In: Crystal RG, West JB, editors. The lung: scientific foundations. Philadelphia: Lippincott-Raven; 1997. p. 1601–6.

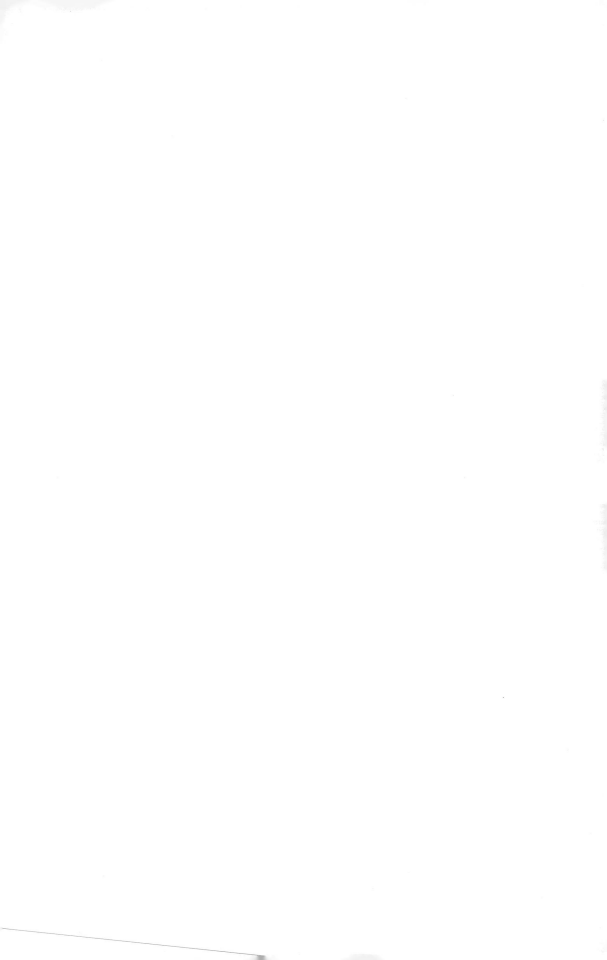

Changing Your Address?

Make sure your subscription changes too! When you notify us of your new address, you can help make our job easier by including an exact copy of your Clinics label number with your old address (see illustration below.) This number identifies you to our computer system and will speed the processing of your address change. Please be sure this label number accompanies your old address and your corrected address—you can send an old Clinics label with your number on it or just copy it exactly and send it to the address listed below.

We appreciate your help in our attempt to give you continuous coverage. Thank you.

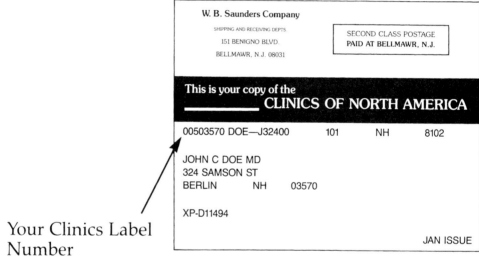

Your Clinics Label Number
Copy it exactly or send your label
along with your address to:
W.B. Saunders Company, Customer Service
Orlando, FL 32887-4800
Call Toll Free 1-800-654-2452

Please allow four to six weeks for delivery of new subscriptions and for processing address changes.